VOLUME ONE HUNDRED AND SIX

ADVANCES IN PARASITOLOGY

Giardia and Giardiasis, Part A

VOLUME ONE HUNDRED AND SIX

ADVANCES IN PARASITOLOGY

Giardia and Giardiasis, Part A

Edited by

M. GUADALUPE ORTEGA-PIERRES

*Departamento de Genética y Biología Molecular,
Centro de Investigación y de Estudios Avanzados del
Instituto Politécnico Nacional, Ciudad de México, México*

ELSEVIER

ACADEMIC PRESS
An imprint of Elsevier

Academic Press is an imprint of Elsevier
125 London Wall, London EC2Y 5AS, United Kingdom
The Boulevard, Langford Lane, Kidlington, Oxford OX5 1GB, United Kingdom
50 Hampshire Street, 5th Floor, Cambridge, MA 02139, United States
525 B Street, Suite 1650, San Diego, CA 92101, United States

First edition 2019

ISBN: 978-0-12-817720-4
ISSN: 0065-308X

For information on all Academic Press publications
visit our website at https://www.elsevier.com/books-and-journals

Publisher: Zoe Kruze
Acquisition Editor: Ashlie M. Jackman
Editorial Project Manager: Ana Claudia Garcia
Production Project Manager: Abdulla Sait
Cover Designer: Mark Rogers

Typeset by SPi Global, India

Contents

Contributors

Vanessa V. Angelova
Department of Biology, Georgetown University, Washington, DC, United States

Raúl Argüello-García
Departamento de Genética y Biología Molecular, Centro de Investigación y de Estudios Avanzados del Instituto Politécnico Nacional, Ciudad de México, México

Carmen Faso
Laboratory of Molecular Parasitology, Institute of Parasitology, University of Zurich (ZH), Zürich, Switzerland

Constanza Feliziani
Instituto de Investigación Médica Mercedes y Martín Ferreyra, INIMEC–CONICET–Universidad Nacional de Córdoba, Córdoba, Argentina

Marc Y. Fink
Department of Biology, Georgetown University, Washington, DC, United States

Annarita Fiorillo
Department of Biochemical Sciences "A. Rossi Fanelli", Sapienza University of Rome, Rome, Italy

Adrian B. Hehl
Laboratory of Molecular Parasitology, Institute of Parasitology, University of Zurich (ZH), Zürich, Switzerland

Marco Lalle
Department of Infectious Diseases, European Union Reference Laboratory for Parasites, Istituto Superiore di Sanità, Rome, Italy

M. Guadalupe Ortega-Pierres
Departamento de Genética y Biología Molecular, Centro de Investigación y de Estudios Avanzados del Instituto Politécnico Nacional, Ciudad de México, México

Andrea S. Rópolo
Instituto de Investigación Médica Mercedes y Martín Ferreyra, INIMEC–CONICET–Universidad Nacional de Córdoba, Córdoba, Argentina

Una Ryan
College of Science, Health, Education and Engineering, Murdoch University, Perth, WA, Australia

Steven M. Singer
Department of Biology, Georgetown University, Washington, DC, United States

María C. Touz
Instituto de Investigación Médica Mercedes y Martín Ferreyra, INIMEC–CONICET–Universidad Nacional de Córdoba, Córdoba, Argentina

Alireza Zahedi
College of Science, Health, Education and Engineering, Murdoch University, Perth, WA, Australia

Preface

Giardiasis is an intestinal disease of major socioeconomic importance worldwide. This disease is caused by members of the genus *Giardia* (Protista; order Diplomonadida), and affects ~30% of people in underprivileged communities, mostly in subtropical and tropical climes. Given its impact in these communities, the World Health Organization (WHO) has recently recognised giardiasis as a neglected tropical disease (NTD).

Of the eight recognised species of *Giardia*, only *G. duodenalis* infects humans. This species has eight (genetic) assemblages (A–H), of which predominantly assemblages A and B and respective subtypes are 'zoonotic', and cause human disease. Other assemblages infect animals including cattle, beavers, sheep, goats, domestic dogs and cats. The other species, including *Giardia agilis*, *G. ardeae*, *G. psittaci*, *G. muris*, *G. microti*, *G. peramelis* and *G. cricetidarum*, infect animals such as amphibians, birds, rodents and marsupials.

In humans, giardiasis is transmitted directly via the faecal-oral route through *Giardia* cyst-contaminated water or food. Clinical symptoms can be acute or chronic and include diarrhoea, steatorrhoea, nausea, abdominal pain, headache, vomiting, weight loss and/or malabsorption, which can lead to anaemia, stunting and cognitive delay as well as complications such as irritable bowel syndrome, chronic fatigue syndrome, food allergies or even reactive arthritis.

Given the major public health impacts of giardiasis, there has been extensive research of many facets of this disease and its causative agent(s) over the last decades. Given the significant technological advances in recent years, it seemed both timely and appropriate to focus on bringing together the latest published information on aspects of *Giardia* and giardiasis by some of the experts in the field. For this reason, I initiated discussions with the editors of *Advances in Parasitology* and proposed that we assemble a Thematic Issue on the topic.

The purpose of this issue (Volumes 1 and 2) was to target some exciting areas of molecular research on *Giardia*/giardiasis, not previously covered in great depth. Here, in Volume 1, the topics include: (a) the molecular and cellular biology of *Giardia* and the roles of particular proteins in essential functions and/or trafficking in the parasite; (b) the role of virulence factors secreted by *Giardia*; (c) innate and acquired immunity to *Giardia*; and (d) the molecular epidemiology of *Giardia*/giardiasis.

The first part of this volume is dedicated to aspects of molecular and cellular biology of *Giardia* and the role of particular molecules or molecular groups in essential functions and/or trafficking in the parasite. To explore how this parasite adapts to an ever-changing environment both within and outside of the host animal, Andrea S. Rópolo and co-authors (Chapter 1) provide an overview of unusual proteins in *Giardia* that are believed to have multifunctional properties, depending on their location in and/or requirement by the parasite. Importantly, they discuss the possible role of 'moonlighting proteins' in *Giardia* and explain why they believe this parasite might be a useful model for understanding the roles and functions of such proteins. Extending to another group of molecules, Marco Lalle and Annarita Fiorillo (Chapter 2) review the structures of members of the 14-3-3 protein family, and their functions in target recognition and regulatory mechanisms, and then focus on current knowledge of the biochemistry and biology of 14-3-3 protein in *Giardia* and propose that this protein may represent a drug target candidate. The authors emphasise the importance of this protein family as a distinctive example of phosphoserine/phosphothreonine-binding proteins which are 'at the crossroads' of multiple signalling pathways that regulate physiological and pathological cellular processes in *Giardia*. Then, the 'cytonauts', Carmen Faso and Adrian B. Hehl (Chapter 3), delve deep into the fascinating area of trafficking pathways in *Giardia*, and discuss *endo*- and *exo*-cytosis, organellar import and function. They provide innovative perspectives on open questions regarding organellar replication and inheritance, and discuss methods and approaches for the genetic manipulation of *Giardia*. These authors indicate how a better understanding of the subcellular organisation might provide a foundation for designing new strategies to interfere with parasite transmission and/or pathogenesis.

Subsequently, M. Guadalupe Ortega-Pierres and Raúl Argüello-García (Chapter 4) provide a comprehensive description of virulence factors secreted by *Giardia*, review their cytotoxic mechanisms and roles in the pathophysiology of giardiasis, and then assesses the potential of these secreted molecules as targets for drugs. In the context of the immunopathogenesis of giardiasis, Steven M. Singer and co-workers (Chapter 5) focus on reviewing data and information on innate and adaptive immunity to *Giardia*, published in the last decade, and discuss how improved knowledge of immunity is advancing our understanding of the pathogenesis and clinical outcomes of giardiasis. The authors comment how understanding immune responses against *Giardia* could identify mechanisms that lead to the diverse clinical outcomes, and might identify protective mechanisms and targets for vaccine development in the near future. In the final part of this volume, Una Ryan and Alireza Zahedi (Chapter 6) review the molecular epidemiology of giardiasis in a veterinary context. They discuss the current status of the species and assemblages of *Giardia*, and issues surrounding the assignment of host specificity and the zoonotic potential using current molecular markers and tools. These authors conclude that the transmission dynamics of *Giardia* is still poorly understood and that there is a need for the development of genetic tools, such as whole genome sequencing (WGS), that should have improved discriminatory power for *Giardia* isolates compared with those presently used.

Overall, this compilation of chapters provides new and exciting insights into aspects of the molecular and cellular biology of *Giardia*, host–parasite relationships (linked to immunity and immunopathogenesis) and the epidemiology of giardiasis. This volume sets the scene for Volume 2, which expands to a number of fundamental and applied areas of molecular research of *Giardia*/giardiasis.

To conclude, I sincerely thank all of the authors for their contributions to Volume 1 (see Contents), and Professors David Rollinson, Russell Stothard (Editors of *Advances in Parasitology*), Ms. Ana Garcia (Elsevier) and Professor Robin B. Gasser (The University of Melbourne) for their enthusiasm, discussions and support.

M. Guadalupe Ortega-Pierres
Department of Genetics and Molecular Biology Center for Research and Advanced Studies Mexico

CHAPTER ONE

Unusual proteins in *Giardia duodenalis* and their role in survival

Andrea S. Rópolo, Constanza Feliziani, María C. Touz*
Instituto de Investigación Médica Mercedes y Martín Ferreyra, INIMEC–CONICET–Universidad Nacional de Córdoba, Córdoba, Argentina
*Corresponding author: e-mail address: ctouz@immf.uncor.edu

Contents

Abstract

The capacity of the parasite *Giardia duodenalis* to perform complex functions with minimal amounts of proteins and organelles has attracted increasing numbers of scientists worldwide, trying to explain how this parasite adapts to internal and external changes to survive. One explanation could be that *G. duodenalis* evolved from a structurally complex ancestor by reductive evolution, resulting in adaptation to its parasitic lifestyle. Reductive evolution involves the loss of genes, organelles, and functions that commonly occur in many parasites, by which the host renders some structures and functions redundant. However, there is increasing data that *Giardia* possesses proteins able to perform more than one function. During recent decades, the concept of moonlighting was described for multitasking proteins, which involves only proteins with an extra independent function(s). In this chapter, we provide an overview of unusual proteins in *Giardia* that present multifunctional properties depending on the location

Advances in Parasitology, Volume 106
ISSN 0065-308X
https://doi.org/10.1016/bs.apar.2019.07.001

and/or parasite requirement. We also discuss experimental evidence that may allow some giardial proteins to be classified as moonlighting proteins by examining the properties of moonlighting proteins in general. Up to date, *Giardia* does not seem to require the numerous redundant proteins present in other organisms to accomplish its normal functions, and thus this parasite may be an appropriate model for understanding different aspects of moonlighting proteins, which may be helpful in the design of drug targets.

1. Introduction

For a few years now, the multidisciplinary approach to science has not only added new knowledge to the subject under study but has discovered phenomena that occur at the scale of molecules, macromolecules, organs, and organisms. In this collaborative work, scientists devoted to study various aspects in evolution, biology, medicine and informatics, among others, have contributed to understand how nature works. The most intriguing questions emerged after completion of the genome sequences of many different species, and the data obtained showed that genomes are very similar and that only few genes are required for life. Thus, new explanations were necessary to understand these new findings, and the discovery of multitasking or moonlighting proteins opened a new view on how genes have evolved and how these can have new functions.

Moonlighting proteins are proteins that perform multiple functions and have been described in mammals, yeast, parasites, plants, viruses, bacteria, and other organisms (Jeffery, 2015). One of the most frequently asked questions is how is it possible for a protein to generate a new function? The word "exaptation" has emerged for this exciting property of proteins, referring to the capacity of one protein to perform another, unpredicted, function. It is rarely found in nature that the same protein can correctly perform more than one function, but it has been suggested that multiple functions of a gene can be performed through gene duplication. However, how gene duplication results in an evolutionary moonlighting function for a protein is still an open question and will require more studies in different organisms (Espinosa-Cantu et al., 2015).

In *Giardia duodenalis*, the small number of genes discovered and the reduced set of intraorganelles present in this parasite suggested that it contains moonlighting proteins. Many protozoa parasites have the capacity for a quick adaptation since they had evolved to resist chemical treatments or to invade a new host. Understanding how new evolutionary traits originate, or others are lost, is important since this will provide answers that may have an immediate and practical impact on human health. In this chapter, we review proteins that play more than one function in *G. duodenalis* depending on the location and/or parasite requirement. We also discuss experimental evidence that may allow classifying some giardial proteins as moonlighting proteins in the context of the evolution of moonlighting proteins in eukaryotic cells.

2. Multifunctional giardial proteins

2.1 The giardial enzyme arginine deiminase

The studies performed in *Giardia duodenalis* on the enzyme arginine deiminase (gADI) were surprising right from the beginning of its study. Initial studies revealed that this enzyme, which is highly similar in sequence to the ADI of prokaryotic cells, was involved in the synthesis of ATP from L-Arg, later reports showed that it plays a dual function: as an arginine deiminase, acting on cytoplasmic free-arginine (L-Arg), and as a peptidyl-arginine deiminase (PAD), modifying protein-bonded arginine to citrulline in the cytoplasmic tail of variant-specific surface proteins (VSPs) (Touz et al., 2008). Interestingly, further studies showed that during encystation, this enzyme translocates to the nuclei during the last stage of differentiation into cyst, and is involved in the downregulation of this process. Moreover, its functions are not limited to the intracellular space, since this protein is secreted into the culture media (Ma'ayeh et al., 2017). This gADI consumes L-Arg, indirectly affecting nitric oxide (NO) production from the intestinal epithelial cells (IEC) (Banik et al., 2013). It also influences the proliferation of and cytokine secretion by dendritic and mast cells, thus manipulating the innate and adaptive host immune response (Banik et al., 2013). In the first part of this chapter, we discuss the multiple functions exerted by gADI, a protein that possibly acquires new functions during the life cycle of the parasite as a result of adaptation.

2.1.1 L-ARG Starvation

The arginine dihydrolase (ADH) pathway was first described in bacteria as a major source of energy and nitrogen (Cunin et al., 1986). In this pathway, arginine is catalysed to ornithine, ammonium and carbon dioxide, to generate ATP from ADP and phosphate. Initially, L-Arg is deiminated by the enzyme ADI to yield citrulline and NH4+. Then, the enzyme ornithine transcarbamylase (OTC) catalyses the conversion of citrulline into carbamoyl-phosphate and ornithine. Finally, the enzyme carbamate kinase (CK) uses carbamoyl phosphate to phosphorylate ADP to produce one ATP molecule. This pathway has been also described in Archaea and in some species of anaerobic eukaryotes, such as *Trichomonas vaginalis, Tritrichomonas foetus, Chlamydomonas reinhardtii, Hexamita inflate, Spironucleus salminicida* and in *Giardia duodenalis* (Andersson et al., 2007; Biagini et al., 2003; Edwards et al., 1992; Schofield et al., 1992; Yarlett et al., 1994; Zuniga et al., 2002). All these organisms are amitochondriate parasitic protists, belonging to the Parabasalia and Diplomonadida, both members of the Metamonada, a subgroup of Excavata. Recently, using genomic and transcriptomic sequences, an up-to-date survey and phylogenetic analysis of the enzymes of the ADH pathway were performed. This study showed the presence of all three enzymes in 10 other members of Metamonada and in non-metamonads (*Harpagon schusteri, Mastigamoeba balamuthi, Pygsuia biforma*), and the algae *Chlorella variabilis* and *Coccomyxa subelipsoidea* (Novak et al., 2016). However, further studies are needed to demonstrate whether these enzymes are functional in the ADH pathway in these organisms.

In *G. duodenalis*, the ADH pathway is the most important source of energy, producing seven- to eightfold more ATP by L-Arg consumption than from glycolysis (Schofield et al., 1992). *G. duodenalis* obtains L-Arg from the media, where L-Arg is transported by an antiport in exchange for ornithine. The intracellular amino acid pool of *G. duodenalis* is led by alanine, an amino acid that is three-fold greater than the second one which is glutamate. Both of these amino acids constitute 50% of the total amino acid pool. As for the amino acids of the ADH pathway, no arginine is detected, but there is a significant level of citrulline and ornithine. Considering that the ADH pathway is very active in *G. duodenalis*, the external L-Arg is rapidly degraded to ornithine and ammonia, and the presence of ornithine means that the limited step of the reaction is produced by OTC (Knodler et al., 1994). Moreover, both L-Arg and ornithine pass through the cell membrane in down concentration gradients (Brown et al., 1998). Thus, L-Arg metabolism regulates its own uptake via the synthesis and export of ornithine.

Nutrient depletion is a strategy used by many microorganisms to enable their own proliferation, competing with the host cell for the same biological niche. In mammals, L-Arg can be catabolized by nitric oxide synthetase (NOS), arginase (ARG), L-Arg glycine amidinotransferase, or L-Arg decarboxylase. Of these, the two main catabolic enzymes are NOS and ARG.

ARG hydrolyses L-Arg to L-ornithine, a precursor for the synthesis of polyamines and of L-proline. Polyamines are involved in cell growth and differentiation, while L-proline affects the production of collagen (Bronte and Zanovello, 2005). NOS has three isoforms that have been described in mammals (Alderton et al., 2001; Bogdan, 2001; Wu and Morris, 1998): two are constitutive (endothelial and neuronal) and one induced (iNOS), expressed mainly by IEC (Salzman et al., 1996). During the enzymatic reaction, L-Arg is metabolized by NOS to produce L-citrulline and NO, a highly reactive free radical essential for endothelial function, antitumor, and innate immune response (Daubener et al., 2009; Moncada et al., 1991; Peranzoni et al., 2007). NO is also an antimicrobial for a wide range of pathogenic bacteria and parasites (Clark and Rockett, 1996; James, 1995), and has multiple functions including a role in neurotransmission, in regulating the integrity of the mucosal barrier and of intestine muscle tone (Alican and Kubes, 1996). Epithelial cells depend on the availability of L-Arg present in the intestinal lumen for the production of NO; however, the arginine transport system in *G. duodenalis* has a transport capacity 10 or 20 times higher than that of the epithelial cells (Cendan et al., 1995; Knodler et al., 1995; Mailliard et al., 1995; Pan and Stevens, 1995). Therefore, *Giardia* trophozoites can indirectly reduce the production of NO produced by IEC, decreasing the innate immune response and facilitating its permanence in the small intestine (Eckmann et al., 2000).

2.1.2 Release of gADI to the extracellular medium

Svärd et al. (2017) have shown that gADI is released into the extracellular environment in vitro when the trophozoites interact with the epithelial cells. Thus, L-Arg consumption from the extracellular medium may be due, in part, to the incorporation of this amino acid by the parasite and also to the conversion of L-Arg to citrulline by the gADI enzyme present in the extracellular medium (Ringqvist et al., 2008). The lower availability of L-Arg impacts NO production by IEC and upon arginine withdrawal, there is a reduced expression of cell proliferation proteins and growth arrest in these cells. One possible explanation of this process is that polyamine synthesis is affected by L-Arg starvation, since a significant reduction of spermine levels was observed in parasite-host interaction (Stadelmann et al., 2012). Also, L-Arg depletion may produce, in the longer term, morphological changes in the villus, increased intestinal permeability, and diarrhoea (Scott et al., 2000).

Studies of the adaptive immune response, have shown that L-Arg consumption by ADI influences the expression of co-stimulatory molecules (CD83 and CD86) and the profile of pro- and anti-inflammatory cytokine secretion of human dendritic cells, which are key cells involved at the beginning of any immune response since these cells orchestrate the type of response that will be activated against the microorganism (Banik et al., 2013; Eckmann et al., 2000; Palm et al., 2003). Thus, by impairing the immune response, the parasite may colonize and remain in the small intestine. On the other hand, it was demonstrated that gADI is involved in mast cell activation, the population of cells that acts as a first line of defence against *G. duodenalis*. This metabolic enzyme was able to stimulate IL-6 and TNF-α secretion and, interestingly, may induce TNF-α secretion even in absence of arginine, supporting a direct role of gADI in mast cell activation (Yepez-Mulia et al., 2009). A direct role of gADI in immune cells was recently suggested in a study in which it was shown that *G. duodenalis* may release microvesicles (MVs) in response to different pH levels and calcium (Evans-Osses et al., 2017). Also, gADI was identified as one of the metabolic enzymes present in these MVs, and results from in vitro experiments with dendritic cells and isolated MVs showed that dendritic cells internalized *Giardia* MVs by endocytosis. As a result, upregulation of the activation marker CD25 was observed, suggesting that gADI induces a mild activation of dendritic cells. However, it is not clear how this enzyme induces this response (Evans-Osses et al., 2017).

2.1.3 gADI as a peptidyl arginine deiminase during growth

In eukaryotic cells, protein deimination is a process catalysed by enzymes named Peptidyl-Arginine Deiminases (PADs) that transform peptidyl-arginine into peptidyl-citrulline, in the presence of Ca^{2+} ions. Citrulline is not a classic amino acid and its name was given because it was first isolated from *Citrullus vulgaris* in 1914 (Anzilotti et al., 2010). The absence of tRNAs for this amino acid explains the presence of citrulline residues in a protein as a product of post-translational modification, which results in an increase in the molecular mass of the protein (0.984 Da), the loss of a positive charge for each modified arginine, a change in the isoelectric point (Orgovan and Noszal, 2011), and the ability to form hydrogen bonds and interaction with other proteins (Anzilotti et al., 2010; Vossenaar et al., 2003a). The replacement of a positively charged amino acid (arginine) by a neutral one (citrulline) through the action of PADs, induces conformational changes in the protein that lead, in many cases, to changes in its specific function

(Vossenaar et al., 2003a; Vossenaar et al., 2004). Although the chemical reaction catalysed by PADs is officially called deimination, the term citrullination is usually used, due to the formation of peptidyl-citrulline as a product of the reaction, and this term will be used in the this chapter.

Citrullination has been described in many physiological processes such as apoptosis (Liu et al., 2006), differentiation of keratinocytes (Ying et al., 2009), histone modification (Esposito et al., 2007; Vossenaar et al., 2003b), and also in pathologies such as cancer (Chang and Fang, 2010), Alzheimer (Ishigami et al., 2005), glaucoma (Bhattacharya et al., 2006), and in autoimmune diseases such as rheumatoid arthritis (Vossenaar et al., 2004) and multiple sclerosis (Moscarello et al., 2007). At the molecular level, it has been shown that citrullination influences the protein-protein interaction and cellular signalling, and to interfere with susceptibility to proteolytic degradation (Tutturen et al., 2010). Although the physiological role of PADs was evident by the use of enzyme inhibitors and from analysis of its the biological activity, the mechanisms that regulate the activity of PADs are less understood, though it is known that they are Ca^{2+} dependent (Vossenaar et al., 2003b). Further studies proposed that additional factors, such as other post-translational modifications, regulate the activity of PADs in vivo. This option is particularly plausible considering that numerous cellular signalling proteins undergo multiple post-translational modifications such as phosphorylation, acetylation and methylation, which regulate protein-protein interactions, enzymatic activity, and cellular localization (Slack et al., 2011).

Genome databases reveal the existence of five isoforms of PADs (PAD1-6) in mammals; the main difference between these proteins lies in their differential expression in certain tissues (Vossenaar et al., 2003b). However, in prokaryotes, only one enzyme capable of modifying both L-Arg and peptide-linked arginine was described in *Porphyromonas gingivalis*, a bacterium associated with the initiation and progression of periodontitis in adults (McGraw et al., 1999). Although it has not been evolutionarily related to other vertebrate PADs, ADI from *P. gingivalis* acted independently of Ca^{2+} and showed sequence homology with several arginine deiminases (Shirai et al., 2001). Even though the protein sequence of gADI shows a rather low homology with the sequence of prokaryotic ADI, it was clearly demonstrated that gADI participates in the ADH pathway, producing energy from L-Arg, as occurs in bacteria (Cunin et al., 1986). In the strain WB, gADI is encoded by the gene GL50803_112103, and the protein has a molecular mass of 64.13 kDa. Despite presenting two amino acid insertions at its C-terminal end, this enzyme has a highly conserved active site

(Trejo-Soto et al., 2016). This site is composed of residues Cys424, His280, and Glu226, and it has been postulated that these residues stabilize the interaction with the substrate. On the other hand, the amino acids that compose the catalytic pocket, such as Phe172 and the pairs Asp175/Asp182 and Arg194/Arg285, seem to be involved in the nucleophilic attack of water and in the stabilization of the transition state (Trejo-Soto et al., 2016).

The architecture of the active site and the disposition of the residues in gADI seem to be similar to those of other described PADs, so it was proposed that this enzyme may also act on peptidyl-arginines (Touz et al., 2008). Therefore, this possibility was addressed by testing the PAD activity of gADI during *Giardia* growth and encystation (Touz et al., 2008; Vranych et al., 2014). During trophozoite's growth, it was found that gADI interacts with the cytosolic tail of VSPs, a since this enzyme co-localizes with VSPs near the plasma membrane and directly interacts with the arginine present in the conserved cytoplasmic tail (CRGKA) of VSPs (Touz et al., 2008). The first evidence of VSPs citrullination was provided by using an antibody that recognizes only modified peptidyl-citrulline, and the PAD activity of gADI in VSPs was shown by testing direct citrullination of purified gADI-HA in the CRGKA peptide. The importance of such post-translational modification of VSPs is uncertain, but the functional significance of the citrullination of the cytoplasmic tail of VSP is directly related with the antigenic variation process (Touz et al., 2008). Antigenic variation in *Giardia*, as in other microorganisms, is a mechanism by which the parasite continuously switches its major VSPs at the plasma membrane. This process has been related to immunological evasion, but it also occurs spontaneously in culture, suggesting that this process is a survival mechanism (reviewed in (Nash, 2002). Further it was observed that the presence of high levels of specific monoclonal antibodies against VSPs induces cytotoxicity and the appearance of a population of trophozoites expressing a different VSP (Aggarwal and Nash, 1988; Nash and Aggarwal, 1986). When the arginine located in the cytosolic tail of VSPs is mutated, VSP switching does not occur, and overexpression of the gADI enzyme induces deregulation of the antigenic variation process (Touz et al., 2008). Therefore, this new function of gADI as a PAD directly involved in VSP switching provides more evidence in favour of considering this enzyme as a multitasking protein.

2.1.4 Role of gADI during encystation

During the encystation process, trophozoites undergo complex molecular and morphological changes in response to cholesterol deprivation in the final regions of the small intestine (Lujan et al., 1996). Svärd et al. observed that, during the last stages of encystation, there was a decrease in surface expression of the original VSP, now located in lysosome-like vacuoles (Svard et al., 1998). They relate these findings to an intense VSP recycling process. Biologically, this would favour greater infectivity of the cysts and the possibility of re-infections and chronic infections. Based on these observations it was analysed if there was a greater citrullination of the VSPs during the encysting process, which is directly related to the process of antigenic variation. No changes were observed in the citrullination pattern (Touz et al., 2008), but the location of gADI changed to the nuclei during the last stages of the encystation process. This suggests that gADI may be performing another function during differentiation, probably not related to the process of antigenic variation.

The mechanism of gADI translocation inside the nuclei has been partially described (Vranych et al., 2014). During encystation, a change was observed in the molecular mass of the enzyme from 65 to ~85 kDa, due to the addition of the protein SUMO to gADI (Touz et al., 2008). It is known that SUMOylation regulates nuclear transport, though the mechanisms of this important biological process have not been clearly defined (Melchior, 2000). gADI is SUMOylated in the lysine of position 101, located within a consensus motif of SUMOylation, and it is exposed according to the secondary structure predicted for the protein. The SUMOylation of gADI seems to be involved in the stabilization of the protein, considering that enriched low molecular weight bands were described in mutant cells (ADIK101A-HA), corresponding to probable degradation products of the enzyme in the absence of SUMOylation. Moreover, it was suggested that, although conjugation to gSUMO is not required for the protein to enter the nuclei, it may support the increase on the efficiency of the translocation (Vranych et al., 2014). Most SUMO substrates that localize in the core, including Sp100, HDAC4, Mdm2 and Smad4, require nuclear localization signals (NLS) for SUMOylation and, though the ψKXE motif is sufficient for in vitro SUMOylation, an NLS is often required for in vivo SUMOylation (Seeler and Dejean, 2003).

The NLSs represent, in eukaryotes, the classical and best understood path for transporting proteins to the nucleus, in the case of those that exceed 50 kDa. These signals are sequences of basic amino acids, recognized by a family of proteins named importins or karyopherins, which transport proteins through the nuclear envelope (Hodel et al., 2001). gADI shows two conserved NLSs in its sequence: one monopartite (PQRRREQ) and the other bipartite (RRGIVMGQFQAPQRRRE). Mutation on both motifs alters the translocation of the enzyme to the nucleus (Vranych et al., 2014).

SUMOylation alters the surface of the protein, affecting its interaction with other macromolecules, thus being able to interfere with or promote protein-protein interactions, masking binding sites, adding others that are present in SUMO or promoting conformational changes that reveal new surfaces on the target protein (reviewed in (Geiss-Friedlander and Melchior, 2007). Therefore, it was suggested that SUMOylation of gADI may expose the NLS for interaction with importins, favouring the shuttle of gADI from the cytoplasm to the nuclei during encystation (Vranych et al., 2014). However, the molecules involved in the development of the encystation process are unknown. Cholesterol deprivation seems to be the initial step, but the receptors involved and the molecular mediators that finally induce the process are still not known. Even less known are the signals involved in the induction of SUMOylation of gADI, and whether they are triggered at the beginning of encystation or during the last stages.

The functional effect of gADI localisation in the nuclei during encystation was evaluated, and these studies revealed that the translocation of ADI-HA to the nuclei reduces the production of cysts and silenced genes of the cyst wall proteins (CWPs) family, required for complete encystation, as well as for regulating the expression of transcription factors such as Myb-2 (Touz et al., 2008; Vranych et al., 2014). This effect occurs in the last stages of encystation in wild-type cells and early in transgenic cells that over-express ADI-HA, enhancing nuclear translocation and reducing the expression of CWPs and cyst formation. The question that arises is how this enzyme may regulate cyst gene expression. In eukaryotic cells, the PAD4 enzyme has been identified as a specific PAD for histone H3, regulating the methylation of arginine by the conversion of methyl-arginine to citrulline (Cuthbert et al., 2004), a process generally associated with gene silencing. In *Giardia*, inhibition of histone deacetylase has been shown to increase histone acetylation and induce transcriptional changes (Sonda et al., 2010) and, although methylation of histones H3 has also been suggested (Salusso et al., 2017), the methylation of arginines has not yet been studied. It would be interesting to analyse if methylation of arginines from histones occurs in *Giardia* during growth and encystation, and whether citrullination antagonizes the effect of arginine methylation, as has been observed in other eukaryotic cells (Wang et al., 2004). Since the modification of histones by acetylation was demonstrated in other cell types, it was proposed that gADI modifies histones by citrullination, which is closely related to the negative regulation of the encystation process (Vranych et al., 2014). In relation to this hypothesis, the only evidence of citrullination during encystation was found using anti-citrulline antibodies in wild-type cells, showing nuclear localisation in encysting cells. This suggests that histones are probably modified by the enzyme (Vranych et al., 2014). In this context, it would be interesting to show citrullination using other specific assays, ideally mass spectrometry, to determine the presence of citrulline instead of arginine in histones from encysting trophozoites.

The model proposed described a cascade of events that start with the SUMOylation of gADI, a signal that induces the enzyme to translocate to the nuclei. Once in the nuclei, gADI probably acts as PAD, and the deimination of histones results in a relaxation in the transcription of genes that eventually leads to a lower expression of the specific genes of encystation. Thus, downregulation of cyst protein expression would allow the completion of encystation process allowing the parasite to enter into its latency state.

gADI is a pivotal enzyme, which can modify both L-Arg and peptidyl-arginine (Fig. 1). It acts during the vegetative life of the parasite, producing

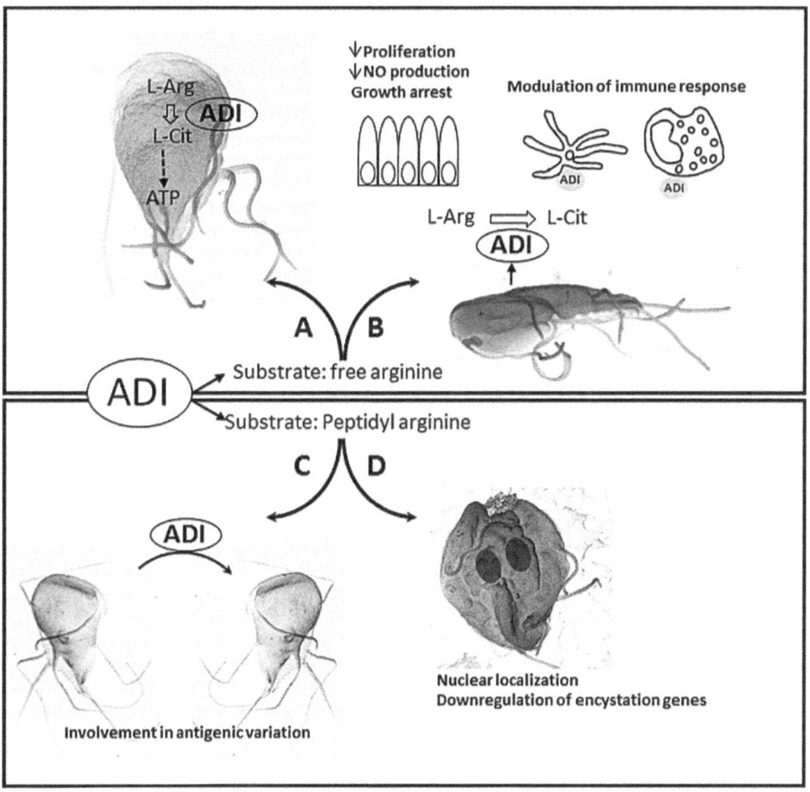

Fig. 1 Multiple roles played by gADI during *Giardia duodenalis* life cycle. (A) as a metabolic enzyme involved in ATP production; (B) with an immunomodulatory activity influencing IEC, dendritic cells and mast cells function; (C) regulating the antigenic variation process; (D) turning off the encystation specific genes during the last stage of differentiation.

energy, as well as regulating the antigenic variation process. It also has a role in the negative regulation of the encystation process. Moreover, this enzyme is released and acts both by sequestering L-Arg, decreasing the availability of this amino acid to the host cells, and also directly on the cells of the immune system, by a mechanism still unknown. Because gADI is not present in other eukaryotic organisms and is essential for the survival and differentiation of *Giardia*, it could be a possible therapeutic target or useful in the development of synthetic competitors to combat giardiasis.

2.2 The ENTH/ANTH/VHS monomeric adaptor superfamily

Budding from plasma membrane (PM) and mediated by clathrin, endocytic vesicles are formed f, and these internalize nutrients, receptors, and other cell surface proteins (Conner and Schmid, 2003b; McPherson et al., 2001). Clathrin also participates in protein trafficking from the trans region of the Golgi apparatus (*trans*-Golgi network or TGN) to the endosomal-lysosomal system (Brodsky et al., 2001; Hinners and Tooze, 2003). Although several studies have revealed the presence of complex molecular machinery underlying the formation and function of clathrin cages (CCs) and clathrin-coated vesicles (CCVs) at the PM (Slepnev and De Camilli, 2000; Takei and Haucke, 2001), little is known about the mechanisms by which these events occur in the TGN.

In recent decades, two new highly related protein modules have been identified, called the ENTH domain (Epsin N-Terminal Homology) and the ANTH domain (AP180 N-Terminal Homology), present in proteins involved in clathrin-mediated trafficking (Legendre-Guillemin et al., 2004) (Fig. 2).

2.2.1 ENTH domain identification

One of the best characterized members of the ENTH family is the protein epsin1, which was discovered in 1998 by virtue of its binding to another auxiliary factor, Eps15, thus it was called "the protein that interacts with Eps15" or, in abbreviated form, "epsin" (from Eps15 Interacting) (Chen et al., 1998). Subsequently, it was shown that epsin and its isoforms (epsin2a, epsin2b, epsin3), which are known now as classic epsin proteins, are expressed in all vertebrates, and are found in many cells and tissues, especially in active secretory cells. Another protein related to epsin, called epsinR (Epsin Related) (Mills et al., 2003), or enthprotin (Wasiak et al., 2002), or Clint (Kalthoff et al., 2002b), was also identified. Thus, the ENTH family in mammals includes classical epsin proteins (epsin1/2/3) and epsinR, and all have in common the presence of the ENTH highly conserved N-terminal domain (Fig. 2).

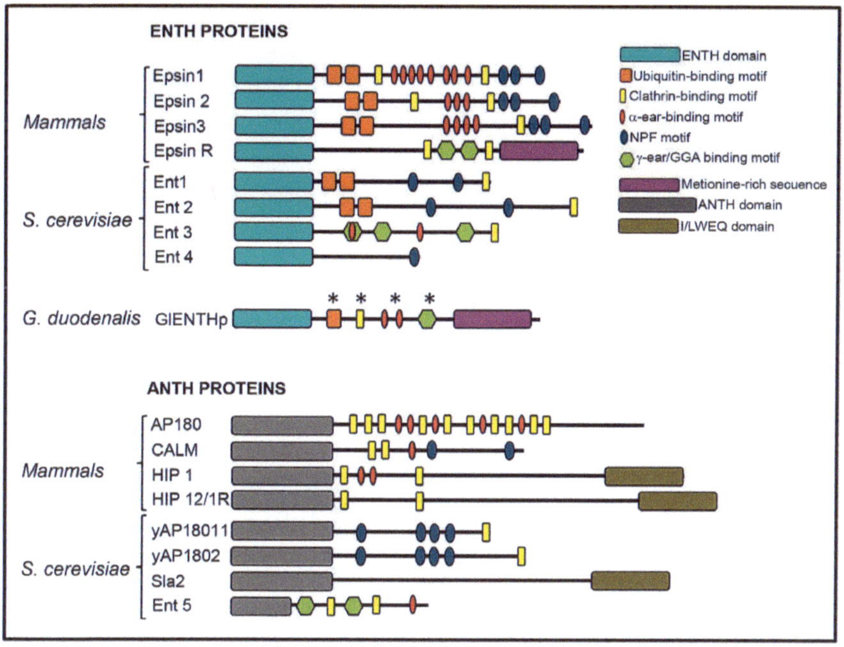

Fig. 2 Schematic representation of E/ANTH proteins of mammals, ***S. cerevisiae***, and *G. duodenalis*. The ENTH or ANTH domain is depicted in the N-terminus. Specific motifs within their C-terminal region are also represented. In the C-terminal region, they contain short peptide motifs and domains that mediate interactions with other proteins. I/LWEQ, allows the binding with actin. The motif for ubiquitin interaction (UIM) is a consensus site (EDExLxxAxxxSxxE/D) that mediates the interaction with ubiquitinated proteins. NPF motifs bind to Eps15 homology (EH) domain-containing proteins. EpsinR possess a methionine-rich domain (MRD), at the C-terminal region, whose function is unknown. The binding site to the γ/GAE appendix has a consensus sequence [D/E][G/A](0–1) F[G/A][D/E]⊠, where ⊠ is any hydrophobic amino acid. The clathrin interaction motifs encompass multiple sequences that bind to the clathrin heavy chain terminal domain, including DLL motifs and clathrin boxes of type I and II. The appendage-binding segment of AP-2 includes the DPW, DPF, and FxDxF motifs. Asterisks denote undefined presence or localization of the motifs.

2.2.2 The ENTH domain binds phosphatidylinositol phosphate

An important advance in understanding the function of the ENTH domain started with the observation that it binds phosphatidylinositol phosphate (PIP). Nuclear magnetic resonance and X-ray crystallography showed that phosphatidylinositol 4,5-bisphosphate ($PI4,5P_2$) binds to the ENTH domain of classical epsin-like proteins through basic residues. In contrast, the conserved ENTH domain of epsinR revealed that it possesses a different specificity to PIP binding, demonstrating preference for PI4P rather than $PI4,5P_2$ (Hirst et al., 2003).

2.2.3 The ENTH domain function

The generation of membrane curvature has been considered the most important function of the ENTH domain (Ford et al., 2002; Ritter and McPherson, 2006). This module has a compact α-helical structure that allows it to bind specifically to the PIPs that are found in certain regions of the membranes. Thus, the classical epsin proteins bind to $PI4,5P_2$, which is enriched in certain patches of the PM, while epsinR interacts with PI4P, present in the membrane of the TGN. Previously, it has been reported that the binding of PIPs to the ENTH domain induces the formation of an amphipathic helix (helix α_0), present at the NH_2-terminal end, which is inserted into the inner layer of the lipid bilayer and induces membrane curvature. Members of the ENTH family stimulate the assembly of soluble clathrin triskelion in clathrin cages, probably by or through the regions involved in protein assembly located outside this domain (Ahle and Ungewickell, 1986; Kalthoff et al., 2002a; Morgan et al., 2000). An attractive model is the one in which the proteins that contain ENTH modules are anchored to the membrane through their interaction with PIPs, leaving their C-terminal regions extended and available to recruit the other components, catalyse the assembly of clathrin, and classify the proteins to be transported (Kalthoff et al., 2002a; Wasiak et al., 2002; Wendland, 2002).

2.2.4 Epsin and endocytosis

The classical epsin proteins in mammals (epsin1/2/3) and in yeasts (Ent1/2), immediately after the ENTH domain and towards the C-terminal, possess two or three copies of ubiquitin-binding motifs (UIMs), which are involved in ubiquitinated membrane protein binding, concentrating these in the CCVs (Aguilar et al., 2003; Polo et al., 2002) (Fig. 2). Ubiquitination is a key regulator of the endocytosis signal of proteins present on the cell surface (Hicke and Riezman, 1996) and AP-2 is necessary for the recruitment of only a certain class of cargos to CCVs (Traub, 2003). It is possible, then, that the ENTH proteins are responsible for concentrating proteins to be transported independently of AP-2. Another possibility is that the two classes of adapters work cooperatively to recruit cargo molecules to the CCVs, since several E/ANTH proteins bind to AP-2 (Conner and Schmid, 2003a; Motley et al., 2006).

2.2.5 EpsinR and forward vesicular trafficking

The ENTH domain binding to PI4P and the C-terminal region interaction with other adapter proteins seem to be essential to recruit epsinR to the TGN (Hirst et al., 2003). Thus, through interactions with AP-1, GGA2, and clathrin, epsinR may stimulate the formation of CCVs in the vicinity of GGAs and AP-1, which will bind to the cytoplasmic domains of the receptors, thus allowing the concentration of these transmembrane proteins in the nascent CCVs (Wang et al., 2003).

2.2.6 Giardial ENTH protein

Vesicle trafficking is a key mechanism to establish and maintain subcellular compartmentalisation. Vesicles are assembled on the cytosolic side of a membranous donor compartment to then deliver specific cargo molecules to an appropriate acceptor compartment. CCVs are the best characterized type of transport vesicles, mediating cargo delivery to endosomal/lysosomal compartments in most eukaryotic cells. In *G. duodenalis*, the morphology and function of the endosomal/lysosomal system exhibits significant complexity and diversity, although its transport machinery is conserved (Touz et al., 2012). We have previously suggested that this organism retains a very small set of proteins involved in vesicular trafficking mediated by clathrin, with the participation of only two of the five protein adapter complexes described, AP-1 and AP-2, but without the participation of monomeric APs (Rivero et al., 2010; Touz et al., 2004). However, Feliziani et al. (2015) analysed a protein containing a conserved ENTH domain and described a giardial ENTH protein (GlENTHp) involved in protein transport between the endoplasmic reticulum (ER) and the endosomal/lysosomal compartment and in endocytosis in this parasite (Feliziani et al., 2015). Recent results support the hypothesis that the ENTH domain of epsinR is the base of the superfamily, described in very different eukaryotic organisms, from *Homo sapiens* to *G. duodenalis* (De Craene et al., 2012), and is the only representative of the ENTH/ANTH/VHS function in the taxa Chromista (*Toxoplasma gondii*), Euglenosoa (*Trypanosoma brucei*) and Excavata (*G. duodenalis*). The presence of only one member of this superfamily in early divergent organisms may thus indicate that multiple tasks could be performed by unique proteins of the epsinR type (De Craene et al., 2012). GlENTHp has functions and characteristics of both epsin and epsinR in *G. duodenalis*, locating this protein as the origin of the ENTH/ANTH/VHS superfamily, that participates in the organization of differential cellular compartments and that maintains organelle homeostasis in this parasite (Feliziani et al., 2015) (Fig. 2). For instance, GlENTHp interacted with $PI3,4,5P_3$ and PI4P, and this interaction was dependent on the K75 residue of the ENTH domain, similar to what was previously observed in *Dictyostelium* cells and *COS*-7 (Brady et al., 2008; Itoh et al., 2001).

Although PIs have not been described in detail in *Giardia*, it is known that three phosphatidylinositol kinases (PIK) and phosphatidylinositol phosphatases are present in the parasite genome and that PIK genes are expressed throughout the cell cycle (Hernandez et al., 2007). These results suggest that the PIs synthesized can be used by PIK to generate PI3P, PI4P, PI4,5P2 and PI3,4,5P3 for cell signalling (Cox et al., 2006; Hernandez et al., 2007). However, it was not shown until recently that *G. duodenalis* is capable of producing PI3P, PI4P and PI45P_2 (Yichoy et al., 2009). Supporting these new findings, PI4P was detected in the ER and was concentrated around the nuclei in *Giardia* trophozoites, suggesting that this could be the lipid binding GlENTHp at the classification site or ER-exit sites (ERES) (Faso et al., 2013; Zamponi et al., 2017). As for PI3,4,5P_3, it was reported that it is expressed at low levels in the punctate intracellular structures in the cytoplasm and enriched near the PM of trophozoites. Similarly, in *Entamoeba histolytica* and in the non-pathogenic amoeba *Dictyostelium discoideum*, PI3,4,5P_3 is present in the cytosol, PM, and phagosome, suggesting that this lipid may be necessary for continuous nutrient uptake in these lower eukaryotes, a common feature of protozoa including *Giardia* (Byekova et al., 2009; Zhou et al., 1998).

While the N-terminal regions of the proteins containing the ENTH/ANTH/VHS modules are well conserved, the C-terminal motifs are highly divergent, and these are often specific for each family or subfamily (Legendre-Guillemin et al., 2004; Wendland, 2002). Similar observations were done in GlENTHp, which was experimentally shown to bind to clathrin, αAP-2, and ubiquitin (Ub) (Feliziani et al., 2015). However, neither the typical DPW motifs (Asp-Pro-Trp), essential for association with AP-2, nor clathrin binding boxes (LLDLD/LIELE), involved in the interaction with this coatomer, are present in its primary structure (Feliziani et al., 2015; Legendre-Guillemin et al., 2004). Similar to what has been reported in the GlENTHp, the LLDLD/LIELE clathrin boxes were not found in the epsinR sequence of *T. brucei* (TbEpsinR), although it was shown that this protein is associated with TbEpsinR and that this association is required for membrane location of TbEpsinR to the membranes (Gabernet-Castello et al., 2009). However, since the original definition of the clathrin cage motif was defined, several variants of these motifs and new non-canonical union regions have been identified (Lafer, 2002).

Like in epsinR, NPF repeats (Asn-Pro-Phe), which are required for binding to EH domain-containing proteins, such as Eps15, have not been observed in GlENTHp, suggesting that this protein is more distantly related to classical epsins (epsin 1–3) than to epsinR proteins. Although it was experimentally demonstrated that GlENTHp interacts with AP-1, no binding motifs for AP-1/GGA (DFxDF) were found in the GlENTHp sequence (Feliziani et al., 2015; Mills et al., 2003). However, the lack of these motifs is consistent with the absence of GGAs homologous protein in the *Giardia* genome. On the other hand, unlike to what is shown in other organisms in which ENTH proteins interact directly with clathrin through its N-terminal domain of β-helix (Drake et al., 2000; Rosenthal et al., 1999), GlENTHp binds to a sequence of *Giardia* clathrin adjacent to the C-terminal region. It is remarkable that neither the typical clathrin lattices associated with the membrane, nor the emerging coatomer coatings have been detected son far in this parasite. Instead, non-typical coated depressions were observed, closely associated with the endo/lysosomal peripheral vacuoles (PVs) (Lanfredi-Rangel et al., 1998), suggesting that a different clathrin arrangement may occur in this organism (Touz, 2012). Thus, it is possible that the specific interaction of giardial clathrin with GlENTHp (and other adaptor proteins) defines the matrix of a particular complex, where atypical structures may be formed.

Similarly, the interaction of GlENTHp with clathrin, αAP-2 and γAP-1 revealed that the presence of motifs and the conservation of short linear sites are very divergent in evolutionary history in this early branching eukaryotic cell. No classical UIM was detected in the C-terminal region of GlENTHp, although it was experimentally demonstrated that this protein is capable of interacting with Ub. Since no change in the molecular mass of the ~50 kDa band of GlENTHp was observed by immunoblotting and this protein was not identified as a ubiquitinated protein in an in vitro study (Nino et al., 2013), it is likely that the adapter protein under study binds to ubiquitinated receptors rather than being an ubiquitinated protein. Although it remains to be analysed whether GlENTHp is able to bind more than one Ub molecule, the interaction of GlENTHp with Ub suggests that the recruitment of Ub to proteins containing the ENTH domain is not a specific innovation restricted to higher eukaryotes, as recently suggested (Gabernet-Castello et al., 2009).

G. duodenalis lacks endosomes and Golgi apparatus, and there is increasing evidence that the PVs and the ER act as the endosomal/lysosomal compartments and the classification station, respectively (Touz et al., 2012). We observed that GlENTHp is mainly present in the cytosol but it was also detected in the cell with a localization similar to that of epsin, very close to the PM and partially co-localizing with AP-2, as well as with epsinR, in close association with the ER chaperone, BiP. Rivero and colleagues showed that low-density lipoprotein (LDL) and chylomicrons were endocytosed, for nutritional purposes, through a giardial lipoprotein receptor-related protein (LRP) and AP-2 (Rivero et al., 2011), while the soluble acid phosphatase, AcPh, was found to be transported from the ER to the PVs by a Vps-like receptor coupled to AP-1 (Rivero et al., 2012). Regarding these two pathways, functional analysis of GlENTHp showed that, when its expression was reduced, the internalization of LDL was inhibited. The same effect was observed for *glenthk75a* mutant trophozoites (in which the expressed $\text{GlENTH}_{\text{K75A}}$-HA is unable to bind PIs), suggesting that the interaction of GlENTHp with PM is critical to achieve endocytosis mediated by the LDL receptor. On the other hand, the alteration in AcPh activity in these two transgenic cells suggests that this defect could be directly related to the ability of GlENTHp to carry on the vesicular traffic of AcPh, mediated by its receptor and AP-1, from the ER to the PVs. Thus, we propose that GlENTHp performs a double function, either as epsin or as epsinR, depending on the trophozoite requirement for endocytosis (for example, for nutrition, for remodelling of PM composition or the regulation of signalling) or for the classification of lysosomal proteins (for example, for the digestion of molecules).

Previously, it was shown that proteins containing the ENTH module have additional functions in signalling and can carry out other functions in the nucleus (De Camilli et al., 2002). Similar to what was reported for the epsin1 mutant (K76A) in *COS*-7 cells (Itoh et al., 2001), $\text{GlENTH}_{\text{K75A}}$-HA accumulates significantly inside the nucleus (Feliziani et al., 2015). It is possible that the inability of $\text{GlENTH}_{\text{K75A}}$-HA to interact with PIs prevents its retention in the membranes, and consequently it has a greater presence in the nuclei. This indicates a general cytoplasmic but also nuclear distribution of GlENTHp, supporting the observation that epsin-like proteins may also play a role in signalling pathways and links the endocytic machinery with the regulation of nuclear function (Hyman et al., 2000). It has been reported that PI3K signalling plays an important role in cell proliferation and survival (Fresno Vara et al., 2004). The presence of PI3,4,5P_3 in E. *histolytica, D. discoideum* and *G. duodenalis* can therefore also be related to its unicellular nature, since these microorganisms need to divide continuously (Byekova et al., 2009). However, it remains to be defined whether the interaction between the ENTH domain of GlENTHp and PI3,4,5P_3 is essential for signalling in this parasitic organism. Previously, it was shown that incubation of B834 (DE3) cells with leptomycin, a fungal metabolite that inhibits the nuclear export path, leads to the rapid accumulation of epsin in the nucleus, suggesting that the protein carrying the ENTH domain is continuously transported in and out of the nuclear envelope

(Hyman et al., 2000; Vecchi et al., 2001). In *Giardia*, each nucleus uniquely presents a different number of pore complexes, distribution, and grouping (Benchimol, 2004), which could explain the presence of GlENTHp and the accumulation of $GlENTH_{K75A}$-HA preferentially in only one of the two nuclei of the parasite. Although extensive direct passage through the nuclear envelope was shown to occur through nuclear pore complexes (Tran and Wente, 2006), the function of the nuclear envelope in *G. duodenalis* has not yet been completely studied. In addition, differences in the number of chromosomes between the two nuclei appear to occur in certain strains of the parasite (Tumova et al., 2007) and expression of the small nuclear RNA GlsR17 was found to occur mainly in a single nucleolus (Saraiya and Wang, 2008). These observations suggest that the asymmetry of both nuclei gives *Giardia* unique possibilities for the regulation of gene expression, as could be the case of GlENTHp regulation. In any case, the location of GlENTHp in only one of the nuclei is a distinctive feature of this protein.

Another location reported for GlENTHp was the giardial ventral disk, a microtubule structure and the primary organelle of attachment to the cell host (Ebneter and Hehl, 2014). These results significantly differ from the cytoplasmic and nuclear localization reported for GlENTHp (Feliziani et al., 2015). This report did not specify the *Giardia* strain used; thus, it might indicate that the subcellular localisation of GlENTHp differs between strains. In any case, ventral disc localization of GlENTHp may hint at a putative role of GlENTHp in the cytoskeleton structure and function (Hussain et al., 2003).

In eukaryotic cells that diverge late in the evolutionary lineage, there are several protein adapters that are involved in the recognition of specific signals present in the cytosolic domains of transmembrane proteins, directing their transport and destination. The presence of multiple protein adapters provides these cells with the necessary plasticity to allow temporary control even in situations where high levels of protein trafficking occur. In *Giardia* we were able to suggest a model where GlENTHp carries out a double function, as epsin and as epsinR (Feliziani et al., 2015).

As a classical epsin protein, GlENTHp binds to $PI3,4,5P_3$ present in the PM, which leads to the deformation and curvature of the lipid bilayer (Fig. 3). Then, through its C-terminal region, the protein is associated with the ubiquitinated transmembrane LDL receptor (GlLRP), clathrin, and the α-subunit of AP-2, favouring the formation of the vesicle coated with the coatomer. The GlLRP receptor is later associated to the AP-2 complex through a specific motif of internalization present in its cytoplasmic tail and is finally internalized into the cell.

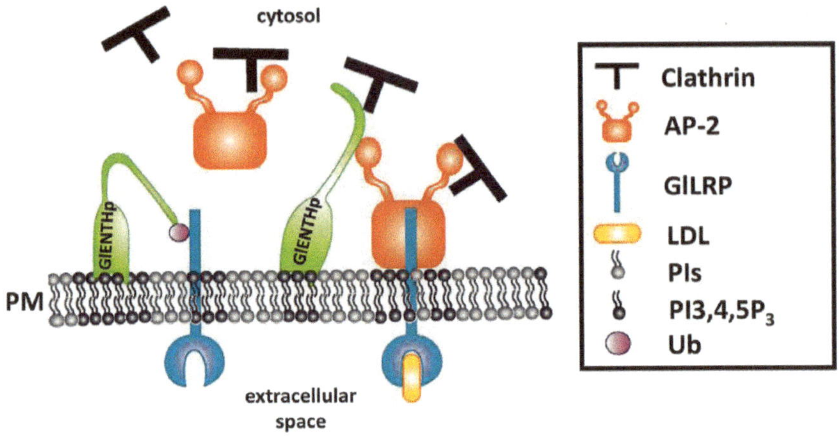

Fig. 3 Proposed model for GlENTHp as a classical epsin in *Giardia duodenalis* in receptor mediated endocytosis. A schematic representation of the molecules involved in LDL internalization is shown, where GlENTHp protein binds to $PI3,4,5P_3$ and the ubiquitinated receptor at PM and, in turn, is associated with the endocytic proteins, AP-2 and clathrin. The LDL receptor, GlLRP, binds the AP-2 complex and the LDL molecule is finally internalized within the cell. *Adapted from Legendre-Guillemin, V., Wasiak, S., Hussain, N. K., Angers, A., Mcpherson, P. S. 2004. ENTH/ANTH proteins and clathrin-mediated membrane budding. J. Cell. Sci. 117, 9–18.*

Like epsinR, GlENTHp is associated with PI4P at the ERES membrane, and is introduced into the lipid bilayer, thus leading to deformation and curvature of the membrane (Fig. 4). Likewise, GlENTHp is able to bind through its carboxyl-terminal region to GlVps, to the γ subunit of AP-1, and to clathrin in the nascent vesicles, which ultimately leads to the transport of AcPh from the ER, where it is synthesized, to the PVs, where it becomes an active enzyme.

Thus, the results obtained suggest a multifunctional role of GlENTHp, consistent with the evidence that *Giardia* has many proteins with combined functions and can be considered as a carrier of a minimal version of the most complex transport machinery present in other eukaryotic organisms.

3. Moonlighting proteins

3.1 Defining moonlighting proteins

There are some requirements to define a protein as moonlighting (Jeffery, 1999):

(i) Its functions must be autonomous. This means that alteration of one of the functions should not affect another.

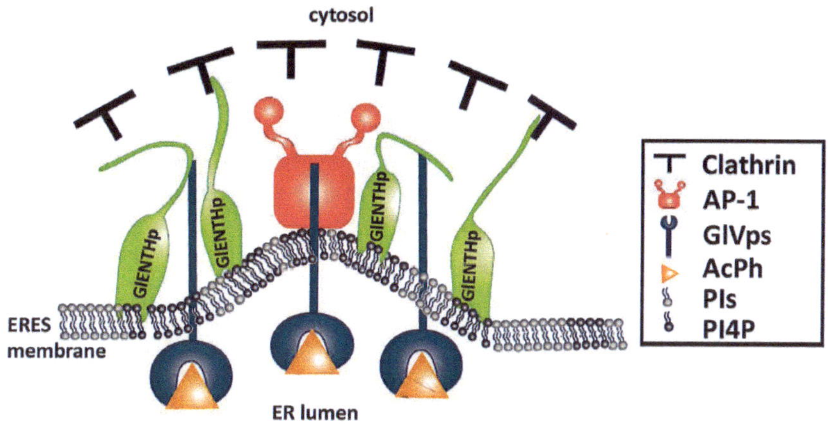

Fig. 4 Proposed Model for GlENTHp as an EpsinR in *Giardia duodenalis*. The mechanism proposed for the assembly of clathrin in the RE mediated by GlENTHp is outlined: The ENTH domain of GlENTHp binds PI4P in the ERES membrane, which leads to the deformation and curvature of the membrane. In addition, GlENTHp is associated with the acid phosphatase receptor (GlVps), AP-1 and clathrin in the nascent vesicles, through its C-terminal region, which leads to the transport of AcPh from the ER to the PVs. *Adapted from Legendre-Guillemin, V., Wasiak, S., Hussain, N. K., Angers, A., Mcpherson, P. S. 2004. ENTH/ANTH proteins and clathrin-mediated membrane budding. J. Cell. Sci. 117, 9–18.*

(ii) Its functions must differ mechanistically (e.g. an enzyme that also functions as a structural protein).

(iii) Multitasking of the protein must not be due to gene fusion (that is why moonlighting proteins were initially named "gene-sharing" proteins) or RNA splicing.

(iv) It must be a multifunctional protein and not a protein that has pleiotropic effects. A pleiotropic protein may be an interaction partner in different pathways or an enzyme acting in different metabolic pathways.

3.2 How did moonlighting evolve?

When the Human Genome Project international consortium published the initial analysis of the human genome sequence, it became clear that the estimated number of genes was lower than predicted. This unexpected result may explain the importance of the alternative splicing of mRNA transcripts in increasing the variety of proteins synthesized. Nowadays, there are more data supporting the role of moonlighting proteins in multiplying the number of protein functions required to maintain life. But how did proteins evolve to a moonlighting phenotype? The most tempting hypothesis is that moonlighting evolved to increase the functional capabilities of an organism without the burden of an expanding genome (Jeffery, 1999). Against that theory is the fact that there seems to be little selection pressure regarding the reduction of genome size, since there is still a large amount of the genome with no apparent function (Gregory, 2005). One explanation for the existence of moonlighting proteins is that the acquisition of a new function is the result of adaptation (Annaert et al., 1997; Gancedo and Flores, 2008). Thus, if the additional protein function results in a benefit to life, this function will be maintained by selection during evolution. It has been proposed that moonlighting is set off only if the protein has some inherent closeness for the novel function, although subsequent mutations should favour the consolidation of this new function and the positive selection (Aharoni et al., 2005). Moonlighting proteins are expressed throughout the evolutionary tree and have attracted scientists because of their role in many processes that are key to life. However, there are still many aspects to be addressed.

3.3 The hallmark of moonlighting proteins

The analysis of already identified moonlighting proteins has shown several common features: in general these are proteins that are constitutively expressed, mostly being highly conserved enzymes, but their functions relay in the conservation of motifs rather than in the protein sequence. The presence of these characteristics in moonlighting proteins may just be a consequence of the ubiquity of these proteins in all species and their key role in the maintenance of cell homeostasis. Thus, new moonlighting proteins may come to light with other characteristics present in particular species. The discovery of as yet undescribed functions of a species-specific protein that belongs to a particular group (e.g. apicomplexa, diplomonae, yeast) may lead to the detection of additional moonlighting proteins in the group and also extend the search to less related species.

3.4 2 × 1: Gene duplication

If moonlighting is having an undeclared second function in addition to a main one, many more moonlighting proteins are likely to be found. The data showed that even a limited number of mutations are enough to introduce a new moonlighting function (Yoshida et al., 2001). Although the discovery of moonlighting proteins revealed improvements in efficiency, sometimes moonlighting function affects the original function of a protein or requires another expression pattern. This may be deleterious or even lethal; therefore, some organisms have carried on gene duplication, thus distributing the original and the moonlighting functions over two genes (Chiou et al., 1991; Piatigorsky et al., 1988).

3.5 When a moonlighting mutation causes or prevents a disease

So far, not many moonlighting proteins have been associated with diseases (Sriram et al., 2005). This may be a consequence of a lack of knowledge about the additional moonlighting functional activities of proteins and to the lack of correlation between genotype and phenotype. Also, since a mutation that affects a moonlighting function may not correlate with a predicted or clear phenotype, the therapy may be more difficult, adding complexity to single-gene disorders. However, blocking moonlighting functions could be a target for future drug design against pathogens since there are examples that link moonlighting proteins with microbicidal drug resistance (Sengupta et al., 2008) and host cell invasion (Pancholi and Fischetti, 1998; Podobnik et al., 2009).

3.6 Searching and serendipity

Classical and novel approaches will be necessary to discover additional moonlighting proteins. However, serendipity has been so far the main source that has provided information on these proteins. These incidental results may be mainly due to the fact that many of the additional functions do not correlated with conserved protein motifs (Babady et al., 2007; Ozimek et al., 2003) and the proteins themselves are not all conserved (Ozimek et al., 2006; Yoshida et al., 2001; Zhao et al., 2009). Still, in the "omic" era, an interrelation of genomic, proteomic, and metabolomics will surely provide new information that will lead to the discovery of new moonlighting proteins. Considering the possibilities of cellular models such as yeasts and microorganisms, it is also possible to use novel strategies to alter the function (or a putative domain) of a protein and to analyse the impact on the metabolism, survival, and virulence of the organism. As moonlight functions generate a whole new level of complexity in the cell, the use of simple organisms could be a good approach to learn more about these proteins.

3.7 Moonlighting, pathogenic microorganisms, and *Giardia*

An overview of the moonlighting proteins of important human pathogen microorganisms shows that this phenomenon is not restricted to bacteria

(Henderson and Martin, 2011) but rather increasing data are been reported from studies in pathogen yeast (Kapteyn et al., 2000; Nombela et al., 2006) and protozoa parasites (Jewett and Sibley, 2003; Pal-Bhowmick et al., 2007). Like in other species, the majority of the moonlighting proteins described in microorganisms have been associated with enzymes (Henderson and Martin, 2011). However, a direct correlation between effects associated with the alteration of enzyme expression and changes in its metabolism with unpredicted phenotypes, has not yet been reported. Thus, new findings beyond changes in the metabolite profile of an organism are important to the discovery of new moonlighting proteins.

Since whole sequence identity between moonlighting proteins is not a requirement, one approach that will lead to their identification in other organisms is searching for proteins with similar canonical function. In the case of *G. duodenalis*, no moonlighting proteins have been described per se but there are several candidates that may meet the requirements, opening a new field of research in the role of these proteins in parasite biology and in the cause of disease. Early divergent organisms, like *G. duodenalis*, show clearly reductive evolution from a structurally complex ancestor, probably as a result of adaptation to their parasitic lifestyle. Reductive evolution is a process that involves the loss of genes, organelles, and functions that commonly occur in many parasites, in which the host renders some structures and functions redundant (Koonin, 2010). Thus moonlighting proteins are expected to be present in *G. duodenalis*. A selection of moonlighting proteins described in different species including animals, yeast, bacteria, and protozoa parasites, that may help in the search for moonlighting proteins in *G. duodenalis* is presented in Table 1. This selection was based on the fact that the protein was present in the GiardiaDB (https://giardiadb.org) and its canonical function has been experimentally proved. Based on these facts some putative giardial moonlighting proteins and their potential role in the development of the disease are described.

*3.7.1 ERK2: UniProtKB—Q8IS81/*Giardia *gene ID GL50803_22850*

The homologous member of the mitogen-activated protein kinase (MAPK) family, ERK2, has been identified in *G. duodenalis* trophozoites as a protein of 41-kDa with catalytic activity (Ellis et al., 2003). ERK1 and 2 are extracellular signal transducers that link the stimulation of membrane-bound receptors with changes in cell function (Robinson and Cobb, 1997; Roux and Blenis, 2004). In mammalian cells, ERK1 and -2 are cytoplasmic proteins that phosphorylate multiple substrates in all cellular compartments.

Table 1 Selected moonlighting proteins.

Protein name	Organism	NCBI code	UniProt code	Canonical function	Moonlighting function	References
ERK2	*Homo sapiens*	AAA58459	P28482	MAP kinase	Transcriptional repressor	Hu et al. (2009)
Aldolase	*Saccharomyces cerevisiae*	DN59849	A6ZZQ6	Splits the fructose 1,6-bisphosphate, into dihydroxyacetone phosphate & glyceraldehyde 3-phosphate (Glycolysis)	V-ATPase assembly	Lu et al. (2007)
	Plasmodium Vivax	ADX87407	Q968V9		Host cell invasion	Bosch et al. (2007)
	Toxoplasma gondii	XP_002368989	B9PW35		Host cell invasion	Starnes et al. (2009)
	Streptococcus pneumoniae	P0A4S2	P0A4S2		Cell surface lectin which binds host cadherin receptor	Blau et al. (2007)
Enolase	*Saccharomyces cerevisiae*	AAA88712	P00924	Conversion of 2-phosphoglycerate to phosphoenolpyruvate (Glycolysis)	Homotypic vacuole fusion; mitochondrial tRNA import	Decker and Wickner (2006)
	Rattus norvegicus (& Homo sapiens)	NP_647541	P07323		Neurotrophic and neuroprotective effects in the central nervous system	Hattori et al. (1995)
	Plasmodium falciparum	AAA18634	Q27727		Blood cell invasion; food vacuole formation	Bhowmick et al. (2009)

Continued

Table 1 Selected moonlighting proteins.—cont'd

Protein name	Organism	NCBI code	UniProt code	Canonical function	Moonlighting function	References
	Trichomonas vaginalis	AAW78351	Q5EFD8		Plasminogen binding	Mundodi et al. (2008)
	Streptococcus pneumoniae	YP_003876656	E0SZH7		Plasminogen binding; heat shock protein; cytoskeletal/ chromatin structure binding	Pancholi and Fischetti (1998)
Clathrin	*Homo sapiens*	NP004850	Q00610	Membrane trafficking protein	Stabilize michrotubules in kinetochore fibers.	Royle et al. (2005)
					Nuclear function	Enari et al. (2006)
Clathrin adaptor AP-2	*Homo sapiens*	Q96CW1	Q96CW1	Adaptor for clathrin-mediated endocytosis	Activity in MitosisRNAi gives mitotic phenotype	Cayrol et al. (2002)
						Boucrot and Kirchhausen (2007)
Dynamin	*Homo sapiens*	AAA88025	P50570	Membrane fission	Dynamic instability of microtubules in interphase	Tanabe and Takei (2009)
					Centrosome cohesion	Thompson et al. (2004)
					Role in cytokinesis	Thompson et al. (2002) Kazazic et al. (2009)
					Actin polymerization	Gu et al. (2010)

Epsin	*Homo sapiens*	AAH44651	Q9Y6I3	Generating membrane curvature	Organize mitotic membranes Signalling	Liu and Zheng (2009)
						Vecchi et al. (2001)
						Kazazic et al. (2009) and Chen et al. (2009)
						Aguilar et al. (2006)
ESCRT-II complex	*Drosophila melanogaster*	NP_610398	Q8SY83	Sorting ubiquitinated endosomal proteins into internal vesicles	Bicoid mRNA localization	Irion and St Johnston (2007)
Actin	*Homo sapiens*	P60709	P60709	Cytoskeletal	Host cell invasion	Backert et al. (2008)

Upon phosphorylation in the cytoplasm, they translocate to the nucleus, where they activate specific transcription factors (Liu et al., 2002; Widmann et al., 1999). ERK1 and 2 were also found in association with tubulin, participating in the spindle assembly checkpoint (Wang et al., 1997), and a moonlighting function of ERK2 was described as a transcriptional repressor by direct binding of ERK2 to DNA (Profiling the human protein–DNA interactome reveals ERK2 as a transcriptional repressor of interferon signalling). In *G. duodenalis*, ERK2 localized to the cytoplasm, plasma membrane, nuclei, and anterior and caudal flagella, suggesting a canonical interaction with microtubule-associated proteins in cytoskeletal structures (Ellis et al., 2003). Since the ERK cascade plays a crucial role in multiple cellular processes such as cell differentiation and survival, the finding of the role of ERK2 during trophozoite growth and differentiation into cyst was expected. Its function was speculatively linked to its enzymatic activity; further experiments are necessary to validate its targets and related function. As ERK2 was defined as a moonlighting protein acting directly on DNA, additional experiments such as chromatin immunoprecipitation (ChIP) and site-directed mutagenesis may disclose whether this is also the case for the giardia ERK2. Also, based on its association with the cytoskeleton, it will be important to carry on yeast-two hybrid assays and immunoprecipitation (IPP) assays, among other techniques, to test protein-protein interactions.

*3.7.2 Aldolase: (ALD): UniProtKB—A8B2U2/*Giardia *gene ID GL50803_11043*

The fructose-bisphosphate aldolase, often called aldolase, is a glycolytic enzyme that catalyses the conversion of fructose 1-6-diphosphate to glyceraldehyde 3-phosphate and dihydroxy-acetone phosphate via the glycolysis metabolic pathway. In *G. duodenalis*, the generation of ATP via the glycolytic pathway is fundamental since it lacks mitochondria and the components of oxidative energy metabolism (Jarroll et al., 1989). Giardial ALD is a cytoplasmic protein that was found to be secreted following interaction with intestinal epithelial cells (Ma'ayeh et al., 2017). The release of glycolytic enzymes has also been reported in other protozoa parasites including *T. vaginalis*, *T. brucei* and *Leishmania donovani* (Gomez-Arreaza et al., 2014) and has been associated with virulence (Collingridge et al., 2010). However, it was demonstrated in *Plasmodium vivax* and *T. gondii* that ALD also plays a critical role in parasite invasion of host cells and it is therefore described as a moonlighting protein in these intracellular protozoa parasites as well (Bosch et al., 2007; Starnes et al., 2009). In the case of *Giardia*, although ALD has been found in the excretory-secretory products (ESPs) of trophozoites, the possibility that ALD is localized in the surface of the trophozoite or in the host cell surface when it is secreted, has not been examined and, therefore, whether giardial ALD may possess a moonlighting structural function requires further investigation.

*3.7.3 Enolase: UniProtKB—E2RTS6/*Giardia *gene ID GL50803_11118*

2-phosphoglycerate hydrolase or enolase is a metalloenzyme that catalyses the reversible elimination of water from 2-phosphoglycerate to form phosphoenolpyruvate during glycolysis. Giardial enolase was located in the cytosol of trophozoites, associated with the plasma membrane, and as part of the cell wall in mature cysts (Castillo-Romero et al., 2012). In other pathogenic species, enolase was present on the cell wall, cell membranes, and in the cell nucleus and has been recognized as a moonlighting protein (Bhowmick et al., 2009; Mundodi et al., 2008). For instance, in *P. falciparum*, enolase was associated with red blood cell invasion, food vacuole formation and/or development, and transcription, depending on its subcellular localisation (Bhowmick et al., 2009). A similar moonlighting function of enolase was suggested for *T. gondii*, since enolase translocation to the nuclei was linked with nuclear activity and the control of gene regulation during the parasite cell cycle (Ferguson et al., 2002). A moonlighting function of enolase is likely to occur in *Giardia* and may depend on different roles performed at distinct subcellular locations and on its release to the medium in the presence of intestinal epithelial cells. However, whether giardial enolase is associated to the trophozoite plasma membrane or cyst wall to interact with host cells remains to be defined.

Collingridge et al. (2010) reviewed and tested potential moonlighting enzymes present in parasitic protozoa, among which the secreted giardial metabolic enzymes, ADI and ornithine carbamoyl transferase (OCT), as well as enolase, were mentioned as possible moonlighting proteins. Many more studies, addressed earlier in this chapter, have been performed to disclose the function of ADI. However, an interesting question is how these cytosolic enzymes are secreted, since they contain no N-terminal signal to be incorporated into the vesicular transport pathways. How metabolic enzymes are secreted is clearly a non-conventional function which may be interesting to study. In the last decade, the discovery of the multitasking function of extracellular vesicles produced by almost all analysed cell types revealed that some of these enzymes were present inside those vesicles

(Perez-Hernandez et al., 2013; Raikar et al., 2006). Recently, ADI and OCT were found as part of the proteome recovered from enriched micro vesicles shed from the plasma membrane in *G. duodenalis* (Evans-Osses et al., 2017). However, a process of vesicle secretion, discharge and association of the enzymes to the cell surface should occur, as has been suggested for the surface-bound enolase of *T. vaginalis* (Mundodi et al., 2008). Therefore, it may be possible that, as was demonstrated for mast cells, the giardial ADI has a direct role on immune cells that would add a novel function of this enzyme in addition to L-Arg starvation, thus it may be considered as a putative moonlight protein.

*3.7.4 Clathrin: Clathrin heavy chain UniProtKB—A8B515/*Giardia *gene ID GL50803_102108*

The first examples of a moonlighting protein included cytosolic enzymes with an extra function independent of their enzymatic activity (Jeffery, 1999). Nevertheless, reports of new proteins with moonlighting functions are now available; these include ribosome and proteasome proteins, chaperones, receptors, ion channels, and membrane trafficking proteins (Copley, 2012; Jeffery, 2003; Royle, 2011). In the case of clathrin, its moonlighting function was mainly related to mitosis, which is independent of its role in membrane trafficking (Maro et al., 1985; Okamoto et al., 2000; Royle, 2006; Royle et al., 2005). Another moonlighting function of clathrin has been proposed in the nucleus, where it facilitates p53-mediated transcription (Enari et al., 2006; Ohata et al., 2009; Ohmori et al., 2008). These findings are still under discussion since these involve clathrin as a monomeric protein. More controversial results have arisen from the analysis of the clathrin function in *G. duodenalis*. First of all, the typical CCV are absent in this parasite, although participation in canonical protein trafficking has been shown, at least for the clathrin heavy chain (CHC) (Feliziani et al., 2015; Hernandez et al., 2007; Touz et al., 2004). So far, monomeric clathrin is not thought to be present in cells, as CHC is an obligate trimer that forms a triskelion shape composed of three CHC and three clathrin light chains (CLC) (Brodsky, 1985). Moreover, while it is not clear that CLC lies free in the cells (Hoffmann et al., 2010), the fact that CCVs were never observed in *Giardia* suggests that (at least in this parasite) each chain may function separately, in a combination that differs from the triskelion. In a recent work, a non-canonical function of clathrin was suggested for *Giardia* (Zumthor et al., 2016). Pull-down assays using CHC-HA fusion proteins expressed in *Giardia* trophozoites showed CHC interaction with a highly diverged giardial CLC, the α and β subunits of the endocytic complex AP-2, and dynamin. Together with structural and functional data, this indicates that clathrin still possesses a conserved function in endocytosis in this parasite. Interestingly, novel CHC interactors were also reported in this study, suggesting that CHC may directly or indirectly play other roles beyond protein trafficking (Zumthor et al., 2016). These findings need to be confirmed and extended before a moonlighting function for clathrin can consider in this parasite.

3.7.5 Clathrin adaptor AP-2

Subunit	UniProtKB	*Giardia* gene ID
beta adaptin	A8B9U8	GL50803_21423
alpha adaptin	A8BAR6	GL50803_1730
mu adaptin	E2RTN5	GL50803_8917
sigma adaptin	Q8T4M9	GL50803_5328

The analysis of the moonlighting function of AP-2 showed a novel participation in cell division (Boucrot and Kirchhausen, 2007). The best indication of a moonlighting function was discovered between the beta subunit of AP-2 and mitotic checkpoint kinase BubR1 (Cayrol et al., 2002). Interestingly, IPP using α and β subunits of *G. duodenalis* suggested an association of AP-2 with the predicted metabolically inactive NEK kinase (Zumthor et al., 2016). In this work, also several unknown giardial proteins were found to be associated with AP-2 subunits and CHC and related with their function in protein trafficking (Zumthor et al., 2016). These assays provide data that may be the "tip of the iceberg" for discovering moonlighting functions for membrane trafficking proteins in this parasite and other cells.

3.7.6 Dynamin: UniProtKB—E2RU04/Giardia gene ID GL50803_14373

The GTPase dynamin was first described as a microtubule-binding protein (Paschal et al., 1987) but later, data supporting its participation in membrane fission were reported (Shpetner and Vallee, 1989). In mammalian cells, closely related isoforms and splice variants of GTPase dynamin have been detected and identified in distinct tissues and at different cellular locations (Urrutia et al., 1997). Its moonlighting functions have been connected to mitosis, since it was found in proteomic analyses of purified mitotic spindles (Sauer et al., 2005). Dynamin was found to be fundamental in cytokinesis in a variety of organisms (Konopka et al., 2006; Thompson et al., 2002). While dynamin function in cytokinesis may be associated with its primary role, the direct interaction of dynamin-1 and actin has been proved. Interestingly, dynamin-1 mutants with altered binding to actin showed no inhibition of clathrin-mediated endocytosis (Gu et al., 2010), suggesting a real moonlighting function for dynamin in its interplay with the actin cytoskeleton. The giardial dynamin was initially reported as a dynamin-like protein (DLP) because it lacks the pleckstrin homology (PH) domain, implicated in lipid membrane binding (Gaechter et al., 2008). However, later it was suggested that it is a member of the dynamin family, since it is formed by other domains, like the GTPase domain, the proline-rich domain (PRD), which contains several SH3-binding sites, and the C-terminal GTPase effector domain (GED) (Gaechter et al., 2008). This single member of the dynamin family plays a classical role in endocytosis of plasma membrane proteins but not in fluid-phase endocytosis into PVs and it has also been linked to secretory vesicle maturation during trophozoite differentiation into cysts (Gaechter et al., 2008). It would be interesting, however, to test its participation in cytokinesis, as has been observed in other eukaryotes (Masud Rana et al., 2013). Unfortunately, the mutant giardial dynamin was expressed under a promoter that is induced only with encystation and, thus, is not appropriate for testing the role of dynamin during cell division (Gaechter et al., 2008). The presence of the PRD domain indicated a direct interaction of dynamin with actin in this parasite. Affinity chromatography, using TwinStrep-Actin fusion protein as bait, showed around 57 interacting proteins including dynamin (Paredez et al., 2014). Nevertheless, it was not possible to validate the dynamin-acting direct interaction by reciprocal immunoprecipitation using a C-terminal triple HA-tagged dynamin (Paredez et al., 2014). This may be explained by the interference of the C-terminal tag that was added to dynamin in this work, and this may also be the case for the negative results obtained when HA-tagged dynamin and clathrin were used as bait in another work (Zumthor et al., 2016). Although this interaction needs to be confirmed, it is possible that dynamin may not participate in the canonical coated pit formation driven by actin-mediated deformation of the plasma membrane, explaining the absence of classical CCV in this parasite. However, it may participate together with actin in cell division that depends on the actin cytoskeleton (Pollard and Cooper, 2009). Additionally, the role of dynamin in receptor-mediated endocytosis can be addressed as was demonstrated for actin, AP-2, and epsin in this parasite (Feliziani et al., 2015; Paredez et al., 2014; Rivero et al., 2010). Further it will be interesting to determine whether the dynamin functions remain independent as has been shown in other cells. *Giardia* may be a good model for this, since endocytosis and cell division can be analysed in genetically manipulated healthy cells (Feliziani et al., 2015, Paredez et al., 2014, Rivero et al., 2010).

3.7.7 Epsin: EH domain binding protein epsin 2 UniProtKB—A8BIK9/ Giardia gene ID GL50803_3256

Epsins are a conserved family of endocytic monomeric clathrin adaptor proteins, which main function was associated with the recognition of ubiquitinated membrane receptors at the plasma membrane, favouring membrane bending and clathrin-coated pit formation (Itoh et al., 2001). Besides this initial function, other roles have been described. For instance, epsins play a fundamental role in signalling, participating in the regulation of the EGFR (epidermal growth factor receptor) (Kazazic et al., 2009), notch (Chen et al., 2009), and RhoGTPase (Aguilar et al., 2006) pathways. Also, another function was disclosed in transcription regulation after using a nuclear export inhibitor (Hyman et al., 2000; Vecchi et al., 2001). The interaction of epsin with proteins of the cytoskeleton revealed its involvement in the organization of membranes during mitosis (Liu and Zheng, 2009) and the participation in concert with tubulin in the formation of endocytic vesicles (Hussain et al., 2003). Although epsin has been described as a moonlighting protein, all the functions described require conservation of the NH2-terminal homology (ENTH) domain directly involved in producing membrane curvature. Thus, the participation of this domain and its function remains to be defined. In *G. duodenalis*, the multifunctional role of an epsin-like protein (GlENTHp) has been extensively studied (Ebneter and Hehl, 2014; Feliziani et al., 2015; Feliziani et al., 2016) (see Section 2.2.6). These studies are consistent with data showing that *Giardia* has proteins with multiple functions and that have a minimal version of a more complex machinery present in other eukaryotes. Similarly, all the functions described for GlENTHp were dependent on the ENTH domain but further studies using *Giardia* as a model may provide insights on possible moonlighting functions for epsin.

3.7.8 ESCRT-II Complex

Subunit	UniProtKB	*Giardia* gene ID
GlVps22	A8BDI6	Gl50803_90710
GlVps25	A8BH59	GL50803_8329

The ESCRT (endosomal sorting complex required for transport) complex is conserved from Archaea to animals (Gruenberg and Stenmark, 2004; Hurley, 2008). These evolutionarily conserved proteins are assembled into four multiprotein subcomplexes: (ESCRT) -0, -I, -II and -III, which are associated with accessory proteins. It is now known that they have functions that go beyond participation in the biogenesis of multivesicular bodies (MVBs) (Katzmann et al., 2001), such as their role in cell division in mammals (Carlton and Martin-Serrano, 2007) and in a subset of the Archaea (Lindas et al., 2008; Samson and Bell, 2009), and the finding that the HIV and other viruses involved sequester ESCRTs to the budding of the plasma membrane of infected cells (Garrus et al., 2001; Martin-Serrano et al., 2001). In particular, the ESCRT-II subcomplex, formed by the Vps22p, Vps25p, and Vps36p subunits, was shown to participate also in the anterior localisation of *bicoid* mRNA in *Drosophila* eggs (Irion and St Johnston, 2007), which is independent of its role in endosomal protein sorting, since mutations in ESCRT-I and III subcomplexes showed no effect on *bicoid* mRNA targeting. A search in the complete genome database of *G. duodenalis* showed that there is a huge reduction in the number of ESCRT components in this parasite. In an analysis of the evolution of the components of the ESCRT complex and the presence of MVBs, Field and Dacks (2009) showed that, although the genus *Giardia* has an extreme evolutionary divergence and often results in the lack of recovery of orthologous candidates, this does not explain the complete failure to detect ESCRT I coding sequences, suggesting that the minimal ESCRT/MVBs machinery is probably the result of the presence of an unusual endocytic system in this parasite (Field and Dacks, 2009). Recently, Saha et al. (2018) described the minimal ESCRT machinery of *G. duodenalis* (Saha et al., 2018). Functional analysis is required to disclose whether the reduced ESCRT machinery of *Giardia* is participating in endo/lysosomal trafficking. Interestingly, *Giardia* lacks MVBs and contains little of the necessary ESCRT machinery to form them (Table 2). However, the finding of a reduced number of proteins from a conserved complex is not surprising, since *G. duodenalis* has a small number of genes and proteins and conserves many proteins with more than one function, possibly due to a process adaptive to its parasitic lifestyle (Ropolo and Touz, 2010; Touz and Zamponi, 2017; Touz et al., 2012). In any case, further studies are needed to define canonical and moonlighting functions of the ESCRT complex in this parasite.

Table 2 Subunits of the ESCRT complex and accessory proteins present in yeast, metazoan and *Giardia*.

Subcomplex	Yeast	Metazoa	*Giardia*
ESCRT-0	Vps27	Hrs	GlVPS27
	Hse1	STAM1,2	–
ESCRT-I	Vps23	VPS23	–
	Vps28	VPS28	–
	Vps37	VPS37	–
	Mvb12	MVB12a	–
ESCRT-II	Vps22	VPS22	GlVPS22
	Vps25	VPS25	GlVPS25
	Vps36	VPS36	–
ESCRT-III	Vps2	VPS2	GlVPS2
	Vps20	VPS20	–
	Vps24	VPS24	GlVPS24
	Snf7	SNF7	–
	Vps60	VPS60	–
	Did2	DID2	VPS46/Did2
		IST1	–
VPS4-VTA1	Vps4	VPS4	VPS4
	Vta1	VTA1	–
Bro1/ALIX	Bro1	ALIX	–

*3.7.9 Actin: UniProtKB—A8BV70/*Giardia *gene ID GL50803_40817*

Actin participates in fundamental cellular events such as cell division, adhesion, migration, and polarity through the transition between G-actin (monomeric) and F-actin (filamentous), which depend on nucleotide hydrolysis, ions, and a substantial number of actin-binding proteins (ABPs) (Dos Remedios et al., 2003). Among the multiple functions described for actin, an established moonlighting function was described for this abundant protein during *Shigella* invasion (Backert et al., 2008) (Table 3). *Giardia* lacks canonical ABPs and is the most divergent eukaryotic actin-related protein described

Table 3 Actin functions and accessory actin proteins.

Function	Associated proteins	*Giardia* data	Known *Giardia* associated proteins
Actin nucleation (Campellone and Welch, 2010)	Arp2/3, formin, spire, Cobl, leiomodin	–	–
Actin signalling (Ladwein and Rottner, 2008)	Rho, Rac, Cdc42	GiRac signalling regulates the actin cytoskeleton (Paredez et al., 2011). Although the mechanisms seemed to be conserved, the ABPs linking GlRac to actin are not found in *Giardia*.	giRac Rho, Rac, Cdc42
Downstream of G protein (Ladwein and Rottner, 2008)	PAK, cofilin, myosin, formin, Arp2/3, gelsolin	–	PAK
Endocytosis (Kaksonen et al., 2006)	Clathrin, dynamin, Wasp, Wasp regulators, Arp2/3, Arp2/3	Some studies showed the participation of actin in *Giardia* clathrin-mediated endocytosis (Hernandez et al., 2007, Paredez et al., 2011)	Clathrin, dynamin
Cytokinesis (contractile) (Eggert et al., 2006)	Rho, myosin, formin, annilin, cofilin, capping protein	–	
Cytokinesis (Baluska et al., 2006)	Dynamin, Sec1, Snap, CDC48, Rab11	The G protein, giRac, modified the actin cytoskeleton of Giardia, in the absence of canonical ABPs (Paredez et al., 2011); (Paredez et al., 2014) giRab11 participated in the progress of trophozoite differentiation to cyst by regulating the actin-mediated transport of secretory vesicles towards the periphery(Castillo-Romero et al., 2010). Alteration of the giardial 14-3-3 protein resulted in defects in cell polarity and cytokinesis, strongly suggesting that 14-3-3 has a role in regulating the organization of actin and tubulin cytoskeletal. (Krtkova et al., 2017)	Dynamin, Sec1, Snap, CDC48, Rab11 14.3.3
Flagella (inner arm dynein) (Yanagisawa and Kamiya, 2001)	Actin, p28, centrin	–	giActin, p28, centrin

(Paredez et al., 2011). In the absence of bona fide ABPs, giardial actin still possesses evolutionarily conserved functions (Paredez et al., 2011). In Table 3, the known functions of actin in other eukaryotic cells are included, together with associated proteins involved in these functions, as well as similar actin functions reported in *Giardia*, and the identified and putative giardial actin-associated proteins. The information reported in this table considers the data described by Paredez et al. (2011), in which the authors conclude that, although the origin of the actin regulation in this parasite it is not yet clear, the specific recruitment and regulation of giActin throughout the *Giardia* life cycle favour the presence of some not yet identified regulatory actin-interacting proteins. Thus, the discovery of novel accessory proteins linked to actin in *Giardia* may reveal still undisclosed moonlighting functions for this protein.

4. Conclusions and perspectives

The multifunctional role of gADI and GlENTHp is compatible with evidences showing that *Giardia* possesses many proteins with combined functions. On one hand, during the trophozoite growth, gADI participates in ATP production and antigenic variation. It also has a role during encystation by controlling the expression of the CWPs. In addition, when released, gADI regulates the host immune response. On the other hand, the finding that GlENTHp acts indiscriminately as a classical epsin and as an epsinR is another example of a giardial protein playing more than one function. However, whether these proteins behave as moonlighting proteins is still undefined. In a near future it is likely that more multifunctional properties of conserved proteins will be discovered.

In the omics era, new discoveries of moonlighting proteins are promising. Although most of the moonlighting functions were found unexpectedly, now it is feasible to confirm that proteins can develop unrelated multitasking functions. Thus, the search for moonlighting functions can be addressed using diverse and complementary approaches. From the evolutionary perspective, analysis of the secondary and tertiary structures of proteins would be very helpful to understand how moonlighting functions have evolved. Thus, complete genome sequences of organisms as distant as bacteria and humans may allow to define, based on data-mining and prediction of orthologous proteins, the presence of proteins with the same canonical functions and putative moonlighting functions. However, the fact that a protein could be defined as a moonlighting protein does not mean that all of its orthologues would have moonlighting (or at least the same) functions. Thus, a combination of genomics, proteomics, and metabolomics approaches may help to clarify the function(s) of the many proteins. Further, data from mass spectrometry, yeast two-hybrid, and gene knock-(out, -in, -down) are likely to lead to the identification of more moonlighting proteins. In many cases, unexpected findings from a large proteome project may lead to the discovery of unpredicted functions for a protein.

There are two available databases for moonlighting proteins: Moonprot 2.0 (Chen et al., 2018) and MultitaskProtDB-II (Franco-Serrano et al., 2018), which present information of around 400 experimentally verified moonlighting proteins. Like in any database, a critical point is the quality of annotations thus these should include only well-documented moonlighting functions, discriminating among moonlighting, pleiotropy, and the secondary metabolic effects of a protein.

Unicellular organisms that can be genetically modified, like bacteria, yeast, and protozoa parasites, may be very useful in determining, for instance, whether the cellular function of metabolic enzymes may extend beyond classic roles in metabolism. The implication of moonlighting proteins from pathogenic organisms has added new information on their participation in host cell invasion. In *Giardia*, due to the fact that its protein sequences are highly divergent despite keeping canonical functions, it could be possible to block proteins with a critical role in survival by attacking the second moonlighting function, likely residing within the divergent domain. Thus there is stilla gap in the knowledge on moonlighting proteins and their modes of action that still remains to be filled up. Nevertheless, current and future studies may help for a better understanding of their role in human diseases as well as to allow the design of more effective therapeutic strategies, skipping side effects.

Acknowledgments

We are grateful to Dr. Adriana Lanfredi-Rangel and Dr. Nahuel Zamponi for collaboration in scanning electron microscopy images. The authors'work in this chapter was supported in part by the Agencia Nacional para la Promoción de la Ciencia y Tecnología (FONCyT-PICT 2015-0154, PICT2017-2435).

References

Aggarwal, A., Nash, T.E., 1988. Antigenic variation of Giardia lamblia in vivo. Infect. Immun. 56, 1420–1423.

Aguilar, R.C., Longhi, S.A., Shaw, J.D., Yeh, L.Y., Kim, S., Schon, A., Freire, E., Hsu, A., McCormick, W.K., Watson, H.A., Wendland, B., 2006. Epsin N-terminal homology domains perform an essential function regulating Cdc42 through binding Cdc42 GTPase-activating proteins. Proc. Natl. Acad. Sci. U. S. A. 103, 4116–4121.

Aguilar, R.C., Watson, H.A., Wendland, B., 2003. The yeast Epsin Ent1 is recruited to membranes through multiple independent interactions. J. Biol. Chem. 278, 10737–10743.

Aharoni, A., Gaidukov, L., Khersonsky, O., Mc, Q.G.S., Roodveldt, C., Tawfik, D.S., 2005. The 'evolvability' of promiscuous protein functions. Nat. Genet. 37, 73–76.

Ahle, S., Ungewickell, E., 1986. Purification and properties of a new clathrin assembly protein. EMBO J. 5, 3143–3149.

Alderton, W.K., Cooper, C.E., Knowles, R.G., 2001. Nitric oxide synthases: structure, function and inhibition. Biochem. J. 357, 593–615.

Alican, I., Kubes, P., 1996. A critical role for nitric oxide in intestinal barrier function and dysfunction. Am. J. Phys. 270, G225–G237.

Andersson, J.O., Sjogren, A.M., Horner, D.S., Murphy, C.A., Dyal, P.L., Svard, S.G., Logsdon Jr., J.M., Ragan, M.A., Hirt, R.P., Roger, A.J., 2007. A genomic survey of the fish parasite Spironucleus salmonicida indicates genomic plasticity among diplomonads and significant lateral gene transfer in eukaryote genome evolution. BMC Genomics 8, 51.

Annaert, W.G., Partoens, P., Slembrouck, D., Bakker, A., Jacob, W., De Potter, W.P., 1997. Rab3 dissociation and clathrin-mediated endocytosis, two key steps in the exo-endocytotic pathway of large dense-cored vesicles in primary cultures of superior cervical ganglia. Eur. J. Cell Biol. 74, 217–229.

Anzilotti, C., Pratesi, F., Tommasi, C., Migliorini, P., 2010. Peptidylarginine deiminase 4 and citrullination in health and disease. Autoimmun. Rev. 9, 158–160.

Babady, N.E., Pang, Y.P., Elpeleg, O., Isaya, G., 2007. Cryptic proteolytic activity of dihydrolipoamide dehydrogenase. Proc. Natl. Acad. Sci. U. S. A. 104, 6158–6163.

Backert, S., Feller, S.M., Wessler, S., 2008. Emerging roles of Abl family tyrosine kinases in microbial pathogenesis. Trends Biochem. Sci. 33, 80–90.

Baluska, F., Menzel, D., Barlow, P.W., 2006. Cytokinesis in plant and animal cells: endosomes' shut the door'. Dev Biol 294, 1–10.

Banik, S., Renner Viveros, P., Seeber, F., Klotz, C., Ignatius, R., Aebischer, T., 2013. Giardia duodenalis arginine deiminase modulates the phenotype and cytokine secretion of human dendritic cells by depletion of arginine and formation of ammonia. Infect. Immun. 81, 2309–2317.

Benchimol, M., 2004. Giardia lamblia: behavior of the nuclear envelope. Parasitol. Res. 94, 254–264.

Bhattacharya, S.K., Crabb, J.S., Bonilha, V.L., Gu, X., Takahara, H., Crabb, J.W., 2006. Proteomics implicates peptidyl arginine deiminase 2 and optic nerve citrullination in glaucoma pathogenesis. Invest. Ophthalmol. Vis. Sci. 47, 2508–2514.

Bhowmick, I.P., Kumar, N., Sharma, S., Coppens, I., Jarori, G.K., 2009. Plasmodium falciparum enolase: stage-specific expression and sub-cellular localization. Malar. J. 8, 179.

Biagini, G.A., Yarlett, N., Ball, G.E., Billetz, A.C., Lindmark, D.G., Martinez, M.P., Lloyd, D., Edwards, M.R., 2003. Bacterial-like energy metabolism in the amitochondriate protozoon Hexamita inflata. Mol. Biochem. Parasitol. 128, 11–19.

Blau, K., Portnoi, M., Shagan, M., Kaganovich, A., Rom, S., Kafka, D., Chalifa Caspi, V., Porgador, A., Givon-Lavi, N., Gershoni, J.M., Dagan, R., Mizrachi Nebenzahl, Y., 2007. Flamingo cadherin: a putative host receptor for Streptococcus pneumoniae. J Infect Dis 195, 1828–1837.

Bogdan, C., 2001. Nitric oxide and the immune response. Nat. Immunol. 2, 907–916.

Bosch, J., Buscaglia, C.A., Krumm, B., Ingason, B.P., Lucas, R., Roach, C., Cardozo, T., Nussenzweig, V., Hol, W.G., 2007. Aldolase provides an unusual binding site for thrombospondin-related anonymous protein in the invasion machinery of the malaria parasite. Proc. Natl. Acad. Sci. U. S. A. 104, 7015–7020.

Boucrot, E., Kirchhausen, T., 2007. Endosomal recycling controls plasma membrane area during mitosis. Proc. Natl. Acad. Sci. U. S. A. 104, 7939–7944.

Brady, R.J., Wen, Y., O'halloran, T.J., 2008. The ENTH and C-terminal domains of Dictyostelium epsin cooperate to regulate the dynamic interaction with clathrin-coated pits. J. Cell Sci. 121, 3433–3444.
Brodsky, F.M., 1985. Clathrin structure characterized with monoclonal antibodies. II. Identification of in vivo forms of clathrin. J. Cell Biol. 101, 2055–2062.
Brodsky, F.M., Chen, C.Y., Knuehl, C., Towler, M.C., Wakeham, D.E., 2001. Biological basket weaving: formation and function of clathrin-coated vesicles. Annu. Rev. Cell Dev. Biol. 17, 517–568.
Bronte, V., Zanovello, P., 2005. Regulation of immune responses by L-arginine metabolism. Nat. Rev. Immunol. 5, 641–654.
Brown, D.M., Upcroft, J.A., Edwards, M.R., Upcroft, P., 1998. Anaerobic bacterial metabolism in the ancient eukaryote Giardia duodenalis. Int. J. Parasitol. 28, 149–164.
Byekova, Y.A., Powell, R.R., Welter, B.H., Temesvari, L.A., 2009. Localization of phosphatidylinositol (3,4,5)-trisphosphate to phagosomes in entamoeba histolytica achieved using glutathione S-transferase- and green fluorescent protein-tagged lipid biosensors. Infect. Immun. 78, 125–137.
Campellone, K.G., Welch, M.D., 2010. A nucleator arms race: cellular control of actin assembly. Nat Rev Mol Cell Biol 11, 237–251.
Carlton, J.G., Martin-Serrano, J., 2007. Parallels between cytokinesis and retroviral budding: a role for the ESCRT machinery. Science 316, 1908–1912.
Castillo-Romero, A., Davids, B.J., Lauwaet, T., Gillin, F.D., 2012. Importance of enolase in Giardia lamblia differentiation. Mol. Biochem. Parasitol. 184, 122–125.
Cayrol, C., Cougoule, C., Wright, M., 2002. The beta2-adaptin clathrin adaptor interacts with the mitotic checkpoint kinase BubR1. Biochem. Biophys. Res. Commun. 298, 720–730.
Cendan, J.C., Souba, W.W., Copeland, E.M., 3RD & Lind, D. S., 1995. Characterization and growth factor stimulation of L-arginine transport in a human colon cancer cell line. Ann. Surg. Oncol. 2, 257–265.
Clark, I.A., Rockett, K.A., 1996. Nitric oxide and parasitic disease. Adv. Parasitol. 37, 1–56.
Collingridge, P.W., Brown, R.W., Ginger, M.L., 2010. Moonlighting enzymes in parasitic protozoa. Parasitology 137, 1467–1475.
Conner, S.D., Schmid, S.L., 2003a. Differential requirements for AP-2 in clathrin-mediated endocytosis. J. Cell Biol. 162, 773–779.
Conner, S.D., Schmid, S.L., 2003b. Regulated portals of entry into the cell. Nature 422, 37–44.
Copley, S.D., 2012. Moonlighting is mainstream: paradigm adjustment required. Bioessays 34, 578–588.
Cox, S.S., Van Der Giezen, M., Tarr, S.J., Crompton, M.R., Tovar, J., 2006. Evidence from bioinformatics, expression and inhibition studies of phosphoinositide-3 kinase signalling in Giardia intestinalis. BMC Microbiol. 6, 45.
Cunin, R., Glansdorff, N., Pierard, A., Stalon, V., 1986. Biosynthesis and metabolism of arginine in bacteria. Microbiol. Rev. 50, 314–352.
Cuthbert, G.L., Daujat, S., Snowden, A.W., Erdjument-Bromage, H., Hagiwara, T., Yamada, M., Schneider, R., Gregory, P.D., Tempst, P., Bannister, A.J., Kouzarides, T., 2004. Histone deimination antagonizes arginine methylation. Cell 118, 545–553.
Chang, X., Fang, K., 2010. PADI4 and tumourigenesis. Cancer Cell Int. 10, 7.
Chen, C., Zabad, S., Liu, H., Wang, W., Jeffery, C., 2018. MoonProt 2.0: an expansion and update of the moonlighting proteins database. Nucleic Acids Res. 46, D640–D644.
Chen, H., Fre, S., Slepnev, V.I., Capua, M.R., Takei, K., Butler, M.H., Di Fiore, P.P., De Camilli, P., 1998. Epsin is an EH-domain-binding protein implicated in clathrin-mediated endocytosis. Nature 394, 793–797.

Chen, H., Ko, G., Zatti, A., Di Giacomo, G., Liu, L., Raiteri, E., Perucco, E., Collesi, C., Min, W., Zeiss, C., De Camilli, P., Cremona, O., 2009. Embryonic arrest at midgestation and disruption of Notch signaling produced by the absence of both epsin 1 and epsin 2 in mice. Proc. Natl. Acad. Sci. U. S. A. 106, 13838–13843.

Chiou, S.H., Lo, C.H., Chang, C.Y., Itoh, T., Kaji, H., Samejima, T., 1991. Ostrich crystallins. Structural characterization of delta-crystallin with enzymic activity. Biochem. J. 273 (Pt 2), 295–300.

Daubener, W., SchmidT, S.K., Heseler, K., Spekker, K.H., Mackenzie, C.R., 2009. Antimicrobial and immunoregulatory effector mechanisms in human endothelial cells. Indoleamine 2,3-dioxygenase versus inducible nitric oxide synthase. Thromb. Haemost. 102, 1110–1116.

De Camilli, P., Chen, H., Hyman, J., Panepucci, E., Bateman, A., Brunger, A.T., 2002. The Enth domain. FEBS Lett. 513, 11–18.

De Craene, J.O., Ripp, R., Lecompte, O., Thompson, J.D., Poch, O., Friant, S., 2012. Evolutionary analysis of the Enth/ANTH/VHS protein superfamily reveals a coevolution between membrane trafficking and metabolism. BMC Genomics 13, 297.

Decker, B.L., Wickner, W.T., 2006. Enolase activates homotypic vacuole fusion and protein transport to the vacuole in yeast. J Biol Chem 281, 14523–14528.

Dos Remedios, C.G., Chhabra, D., Kekic, M., Dedova, I.V., Tsubakihara, M., Berry, D.A., Nosworthy, N.J., 2003. Actin binding proteins: regulation of cytoskeletal microfilaments. Physiol. Rev. 83, 433–473.

Drake, M.T., Downs, M.A., Traub, L.M., 2000. Epsin binds to clathrin by associating directly with the clathrin-terminal domain. Evidence for cooperative binding through two discrete sites. J. Biol. Chem. 275, 6479–6489.

Ebneter, J.A., Hehl, A.B., 2014. The single epsin homolog in Giardia lamblia localizes to the ventral disk of trophozoites and is not associated with clathrin membrane coats. Mol. Biochem. Parasitol. 197, 24–27.

Eckmann, L., Laurent, F., Langford, T.D., Hetsko, M.L., Smith, J.R., Kagnoff, M.F., Gillin, F.D., 2000. Nitric oxide production by human intestinal epithelial cells and competition for arginine as potential determinants of host defense against the lumen-dwelling pathogen Giardia lamblia. J. Immunol. 164, 1478–1487.

Edwards, M.R., Schofield, P.J., O'sullivan, W.J., Costello, M., 1992. Arginine metabolism during culture of Giardia intestinalis. Mol. Biochem. Parasitol. 53, 97–103.

Eggert, U.S., Mitchison, T.J., Field, C.M., 2006. Animal cytokinesis: from parts list to mechanisms. Annu Rev Biochem 75, 543–566.

Ellis, J.G.T., Davila, M., Chakrabarti, R., 2003. Potential involvement of extracellular signal-regulated kinase 1 and 2 in encystation of a primitive eukaryote, Giardia lamblia. Stage-specific activation and intracellular localization. J. Biol. Chem. 278, 1936–1945.

Enari, M., Ohmori, K., Kitabayashi, I., Taya, Y., 2006. Requirement of clathrin heavy chain for p53-mediated transcription. Genes Dev. 20, 1087–1099.

Espinosa-Cantu, A., Ascencio, D., Barona-Gomez, F., Deluna, A., 2015. Gene duplication and the evolution of moonlighting proteins. Front. Genet. 6, 227.

Esposito, G., Vitale, A.M., Leijten, F.P., Strik, A.M., Koonen-Reemst, A.M., Yurttas, P., Robben, T.J., Coonrod, S., Gossen, J.A., 2007. Peptidylarginine deiminase (PAD) 6 is essential for oocyte cytoskeletal sheet formation and female fertility. Mol. Cell. Endocrinol. 273, 25–31.

Evans-Osses, I., Mojoli, A., Monguio-Tortajada, M., Marcilla, A., Aran, V., Amorim, M., Inal, J., Borras, F.E., Ramirez, M.I., 2017. Microvesicles released from Giardia intestinalis disturb host-pathogen response in vitro. Eur. J. Cell Biol. 96, 131–142.

Faso, C., Konrad, C., Schraner, E.M., Hehl, A.B., 2013. Export of cyst wall material and Golgi organelle neogenesis in Giardia lamblia depend on endoplasmic reticulum exit sites. Cell. Microbiol. 15, 537–553.

Feliziani, C., Valdez Taubas, J., Moyano, S., Quassollo, G., Poprawski, J.E., Wendland, B., Touz, M.C., 2016. Vestiges of Ent3p/Ent5p function in the giardial epsin homolog. Biochim. Biophys. Acta 1863, 749–759.
Feliziani, C., Zamponi, N., Gottig, N., Ropolo, A.S., Lanfredi-Rangel, A., Touz, M.C., 2015. The giardial Enth protein participates in lysosomal protein trafficking and endocytosis. Biochim. Biophys. Acta 1853, 646–659.
Ferguson, D.J., Parmley, S.F., Tomavo, S., 2002. Evidence for nuclear localisation of two stage-specific isoenzymes of enolase in Toxoplasma gondii correlates with active parasite replication. Int. J. Parasitol. 32, 1399–1410.
Field, M.C., Dacks, J.B., 2009. First and last ancestors: reconstructing evolution of the endomembrane system with ESCRTs, vesicle coat proteins, and nuclear pore complexes. Curr. Opin. Cell Biol. 21, 4–13.
Ford, M.G., Mills, I.G., Peter, B.J., Vallis, Y., Praefcke, G.J., Evans, P.R., McMahon, H.T., 2002. Curvature of clathrin-coated pits driven by epsin. Nature 419, 361–366.
Franco-Serrano, L., Hernandez, S., Calvo, A., Severi, M.A., Ferragut, G., Perez-Pons, J., Pinol, J., Pich, O., Mozo-Villarias, A., Amela, I., Querol, E., Cedano, J., 2018. MultitaskProtDB-Ii: an update of a database of multitasking/moonlighting proteins. Nucleic Acids Res. 46, D645–D648.
Fresno Vara, J.A., Casado, E., De Castro, J., Cejas, P., Belda-Iniesta, C., Gonzalez-Baron, M., 2004. PI3K/Akt signalling pathway and cancer. Cancer Treat. Rev. 30, 193–204.
Gabernet-Castello, C., Dacks, J.B., Field, M.C., 2009. The single Enth-domain protein of trypanosomes; endocytic functions and evolutionary relationship with epsin. Traffic 10, 894–911.
Gaechter, V., Schraner, E., Wild, P., Hehl, A.B., 2008. The single dynamin family protein in the primitive protozoan Giardia lamblia is essential for stage conversion and endocytic transport. Traffic 9, 57–71.
Gancedo, C., Flores, C.L., 2008. Moonlighting proteins in yeasts. Microbiol. Mol. Biol. Rev. 72, 197–210. table of contents.
Garrus, J.E., Von Schwedler, U.K., Pornillos, O.W., Morham, S.G., Zavitz, K.H., Wang, H.E., Wettstein, D.A., Stray, K.M., Cote, M., Rich, R.L., Myszka, D.G., Sundquist, W.I., 2001. Tsg101 and the vacuolar protein sorting pathway are essential for HIV-1 budding. Cell 107, 55–65.
Geiss-Friedlander, R., Melchior, F., 2007. Concepts in sumoylation: a decade on. Nat. Rev. Mol. Cell Biol. 8, 947–956.
Gomez-Arreaza, A., Acosta, H., Quinones, W., Concepcion, J.L., Michels, P.A., Avilan, L., 2014. Extracellular functions of glycolytic enzymes of parasites: unpredicted use of ancient proteins. Mol. Biochem. Parasitol. 193, 75–81.
Gregory, T.R., 2005. Synergy between sequence and size in large-scale genomics. Nat. Rev. Genet. 6, 699–708.
Gruenberg, J., Stenmark, H., 2004. The biogenesis of multivesicular endosomes. Nat. Rev. Mol. Cell Biol. 5, 317–323.
Gu, C., Yaddanapudi, S., Weins, A., Osborn, T., Reiser, J., Pollak, M., Hartwig, J., Sever, S., 2010. Direct dynamin-actin interactions regulate the actin cytoskeleton. EMBO J. 29, 3593–3606.
Hattori, T., Takei, N., Mizuno, Y., Kato, K., Kohsaka, S., 1995. Neurotrophic and neuro-protective effects of neuron-specific enolase on cultured neurons from embryonic rat brain. Neurosci Res 21, 191–198.
Henderson, B., Martin, A., 2011. Bacterial virulence in the moonlight: multitasking bacterial moonlighting proteins are virulence determinants in infectious disease. Infect. Immun. 79, 3476–3491.

Hernandez, Y., Castillo, C., Roychowdhury, S., Hehl, A., Aley, S.B., Das, S., 2007. Clathrin-dependent pathways and the cytoskeleton network are involved in ceramide endocytosis by a parasitic protozoan, Giardia lamblia. Int. J. Parasitol. 37, 21–32.

Hicke, L., Riezman, H., 1996. Ubiquitination of a yeast plasma membrane receptor signals its ligand-stimulated endocytosis. Cell 84, 277–287.

Hinners, I., Tooze, S.A., 2003. Changing directions: clathrin-mediated transport between the Golgi and endosomes. J. Cell Sci. 116, 763–771.

Hirst, J., Motley, A., Harasaki, K., Peak Chew, S.Y., Robinson, M.S., 2003. EpsinR: an ENTH domain-containing protein that interacts with AP-1. Mol. Biol. Cell 14, 625–641.

Hodel, M.R., Corbett, A.H., Hodel, A.E., 2001. Dissection of a nuclear localization signal. J. Biol. Chem. 276, 1317–1325.

Hoffmann, A., Dannhauser, P.N., Groos, S., Hinrichsen, L., Curth, U., Ungewickell, E.J., 2010. A comparison of GFP-tagged clathrin light chains with fluorochromated light chains in vivo and in vitro. Traffic 11, 1129–1140.

Hu, S., Xie, Z., Onishi, A., Yu, X., Jiang, L., Lin, J., Rho, H.S., Woodard, C., Wang, H., Jeong, J.S., Long, S., He, X., Wade, H., Blackshaw, S., Qian, J., Zhu, H., 2009. Profiling the human protein-DNA interactome reveals ERK2 as a transcriptional repressor of interferon signaling. Cell 139, 610–622.

Hurley, J.H., 2008. ESCRT complexes and the biogenesis of multivesicular bodies. Curr. Opin. Cell Biol. 20, 4–11.

Hussain, N.K., Yamabhai, M., Bhakar, A.L., Metzler, M., Ferguson, S.S., Hayden, M.R., McPherson, P.S., Kay, B.K., 2003. A role for epsin N-terminal homology/AP180 N-terminal homology (ENTH/ANTH) domains in tubulin binding. J. Biol. Chem. 278, 28823–28830.

Hyman, J., Chen, H., Di Fiore, P.P., De Camilli, P., Brunger, A.T., 2000. Epsin 1 undergoes nucleocytosolic shuttling and its eps15 interactor NH(2)-terminal homology (ENTH) domain, structurally similar to Armadillo and HEAT repeats, interacts with the transcription factor promyelocytic leukemia Zn(2)+ finger protein (PLZF). J. Cell Biol. 149, 537–546.

Irion, U., St Johnston, D., 2007. bicoid RNA localization requires specific binding of an endosomal sorting complex. Nature 445, 554–558.

Ishigami, A., Ohsawa, T., Hiratsuka, M., Taguchi, H., Kobayashi, S., Saito, Y., Murayama, S., Asaga, H., Toda, T., Kimura, N., Maruyama, N., 2005. Abnormal accumulation of citrullinated proteins catalyzed by peptidylarginine deiminase in hippocampal extracts from patients with Alzheimer's disease. J. Neurosci. Res. 80, 120–128.

Itoh, T., Koshiba, S., Kigawa, T., Kikuchi, A., Yokoyama, S., Takenawa, T., 2001. Role of the ENTH domain in phosphatidylinositol-4,5-bisphosphate binding and endocytosis. Science 291, 1047–1051.

James, S.L., 1995. Role of nitric oxide in parasitic infections. Microbiol. Rev. 59, 533–547.

Jarroll, E.L., Manning, P., Berrada, A., Hare, D., Lindmark, D.G., 1989. Biochemistry and metabolism of Giardia. J Protozool 36, 190–197.

Jeffery, C.J., 1999. Moonlighting proteins. Trends Biochem. Sci. 24, 8–11.

Jeffery, C.J., 2003. Moonlighting proteins: old proteins learning new tricks. Trends Genet. 19, 415–417.

Jeffery, C.J., 2015. Why study moonlighting proteins? Front. Genet. 6, 211.

Jewett, T.J., Sibley, L.D., 2003. Aldolase forms a bridge between cell surface adhesins and the actin cytoskeleton in apicomplexan parasites. Mol. Cell 11, 885–894.

Kaksonen, M., Toret, C.P., Drubin, D.G., 2006. Harnessing actin dynamics for clathrin-mediated endocytosis. Nat Rev Mol Cell Biol 7, 404–414.

Kalthoff, C., Alves, J., Urbanke, C., Knorr, R., Ungewickell, E.J., 2002a. Unusual structural organization of the endocytic proteins AP180 and epsin 1. J. Biol. Chem. 277, 8209–8216.

Kalthoff, C., Groos, S., Kohl, R., Mahrhold, S., Ungewickell, E.J., 2002b. Clint: a novel clathrin-binding ENTH-domain protein at the Golgi. Mol. Biol. Cell 13, 4060–4073.

Kapteyn, J.C., Hoyer, L.L., Hecht, J.E., Muller, W.H., Andel, A., Verkleij, A.J., Makarow, M., Van Den Ende, H., Klis, F.M., 2000. The cell wall architecture of Candida albicans wild-type cells and cell wall-defective mutants. Mol. Microbiol. 35, 601–611.

Katzmann, D.J., Babst, M., Emr, S.D., 2001. Ubiquitin-dependent sorting into the multivesicular body pathway requires the function of a conserved endosomal protein sorting complex, ESCRT-I. Cell 106, 145–155.

Kazazic, M., Bertelsen, V., Pedersen, K.W., Vuong, T.T., Grandal, M.V., Rodland, M.S., Traub, L.M., Stang, E., Madshus, I.H., 2009. Epsin 1 is involved in recruitment of ubiquitinated EGF receptors into clathrin-coated pits. Traffic 10, 235–245.

Knodler, L.A., Edwards, M.R., Schofield, P.J., 1994. The intracellular amino acid pools of Giardia intestinalis, Trichomonas vaginalis, and Crithidia luciliae. Exp. Parasitol. 79, 117–125.

Knodler, L.A., Schofield, P.J., Edwards, M.R., 1995. L-arginine transport and metabolism in Giardia intestinalis support its position as a transition between the prokaryotic and eukaryotic kingdoms. Microbiology 141 (Pt 9), 2063–2070.

Konopka, C.A., Schleede, J.B., Skop, A.R., Bednarek, S.Y., 2006. Dynamin and cytokinesis. Traffic 7, 239–247.

Koonin, E.V., 2010. Preview. The incredible expanding ancestor of eukaryotes. Cell 140, 606–608.

Ladwein, M., Rottner, K., 2008. On the Rho'd: the regulation of membrane protrusions by Rho-GTPases. FEBS Lett 582, 2066–2074.

Lafer, E.M., 2002. Clathrin-protein interactions. Traffic 3, 513–520.

Lanfredi-Rangel, A., Attias, M., De Carvalho, T.M., Kattenbach, W.M., De Souza, W., 1998. The peripheral vesicles of trophozoites of the primitive protozoan Giardia lamblia may correspond to early and late endosomes and to lysosomes. J. Struct. Biol. 123, 225–235.

Legendre-Guillemin, V., Wasiak, S., Hussain, N.K., Angers, A., McPherson, P.S., 2004. ENTH/ANTH proteins and clathrin-mediated membrane budding. J. Cell Sci. 117, 9–18.

Lindas, A.C., Karlsson, E.A., Lindgren, M.T., Ettema, T.J., BernandeR, R., 2008. A unique cell division machinery in the Archaea. Proc. Natl. Acad. Sci. U. S. A. 105, 18942–18946.

Liu, F., Austin, D.A., Mellon, P.L., Olefsky, J.M., Webster, N.J., 2002. GnRH activates ERK1/2 leading to the induction of c-fos and LHbeta protein expression in LbetaT2 cells. Mol. Endocrinol. 16, 419–434.

Liu, G.Y., Liao, Y.F., Chang, W.H., Liu, C.C., Hsieh, M.C., Hsu, P.C., Tsay, G.J., Hung, H.C., 2006. Overexpression of peptidylarginine deiminase IV features in apoptosis of haematopoietic cells. Apoptosis 11, 183–196.

Liu, Z., Zheng, Y., 2009. A requirement for epsin in mitotic membrane and spindle organization. J. Cell Biol. 186, 473–480.

Lu, M., Ammar, D., Ives, H., Albrecht, F., Gluck, S.L., 2007. Physical interaction between aldolase and vacuolar H+-ATPase is essential for the assembly and activity of the proton pump. J Biol Chem 282, 24495–24503.

Lujan, H.D., Mowatt, M.R., Byrd, L.G., Nash, T.E., 1996. Cholesterol starvation induces differentiation of the intestinal parasite Giardia lamblia. Proc. Natl. Acad. Sci. U. S. A. 93, 7628–7633.

Ma'ayeh, S.Y., Liu, J., Peirasmaki, D., Hornaeus, K., Bergstrom Lind, S., Grabherr, M., Bergquist, J., Svard, S.G., 2017. Characterization of the Giardia intestinalis secretome during interaction with human intestinal epithelial cells: The impact on host cells. PLoS Negl. Trop. Dis. 11, e0006120.

Mailliard, M.E., Stevens, B.R., Mann, G.E., 1995. Amino acid transport by small intestinal, hepatic, and pancreatic epithelia. Gastroenterology 108, 888–910.

Maro, B., Johnson, M.H., Pickering, S.J., Louvard, D., 1985. Changes in the distribution of membranous organelles during mouse early development. J. Embryol. Exp. Morpholog. 90, 287–309.

Martin-Serrano, J., Zang, T., Bieniasz, P.D., 2001. HIV-1 and Ebola virus encode small peptide motifs that recruit Tsg101 to sites of particle assembly to facilitate egress. Nat. Med. 7, 1313–1319.

Masud Rana, A.Y., Tsujioka, M., Miyagishima, S., Ueda, M., Yumura, S., 2013. Dynamin contributes to cytokinesis by stabilizing actin filaments in the contractile ring. Genes Cells 18, 621–635.

McGraw, W.T., Potempa, J., Farley, D., Travis, J., 1999. Purification, characterization, and sequence analysis of a potential virulence factor from Porphyromonas gingivalis, peptidylarginine deiminase. Infect. Immun. 67, 3248–3256.

McPherson, P.S., Kay, B.K., Hussain, N.K., 2001. Signaling on the endocytic pathway. Traffic 2, 375–384.

Melchior, F., 2000. SUMO—nonclassical ubiquitin. Annu. Rev. Cell Dev. Biol. 16, 591–626.

Mills, I.G., Praefcke, G.J., Vallis, Y., Peter, B.J., Olesen, L.E., Gallop, J.L., Butler, P.J., Evans, P.R., McMahon, H.T., 2003. EpsinR: an AP1/clathrin interacting protein involved in vesicle trafficking. J. Cell Biol. 160, 213–222.

Moncada, S., Palmer, R.M., Higgs, E.A., 1991. Nitric oxide: physiology, pathophysiology, and pharmacology. Pharmacol. Rev. 43, 109–142.

Morgan, J.R., Prasad, K., Hao, W., Augustine, G.J., Lafer, E.M., 2000. A conserved clathrin assembly motif essential for synaptic vesicle endocytosis. J. Neurosci. 20, 8667–8676.

Moscarello, M.A., Mastronardi, F.G., Wood, D.D., 2007. The role of citrullinated proteins suggests a novel mechanism in the pathogenesis of multiple sclerosis. Neurochem. Res. 32, 251–256.

Motley, A.M., Berg, N., Taylor, M.J., Sahlender, D.A., Hirst, J., Owen, D.J., Robinson, M.S., 2006. Functional analysis of AP-2 alpha and mu2 subunits. Mol. Biol. Cell 17, 5298–5308.

Mundodi, V., Kucknoor, A.S., Alderete, J.F., 2008. Immunogenic and plasminogen-binding surface-associated alpha-enolase of Trichomonas vaginalis. Infect. Immun. 76, 523–531.

Nash, T.E., 2002. Surface antigenic variation in Giardia lamblia. Mol. Microbiol. 45, 585–590.

Nash, T.E., Aggarwal, A., 1986. Cytotoxicity of monoclonal antibodies to a subset of Giardia isolates. J. Immunol. 136, 2628–2632.

Nino, C.A., Chaparro, J., Soffientini, P., Polo, S., Wasserman, M., 2013. Ubiquitination dynamics in the early-branching eukaryote Giardia intestinalis. MicrobiologyOpen 2, 525–539.

Nombela, C., Gil, C., Chaffin, W.L., 2006. Non-conventional protein secretion in yeast. Trends Microbiol. 14, 15–21.

Novak, L., Zubacova, Z., Karnkowska, A., Kolisko, M., Hroudova, M., Stairs, C.W., Simpson, A.G., Keeling, P.J., Roger, A.J., Cepicka, I., Hampl, V., 2016. Arginine deiminase pathway enzymes: evolutionary history in metamonads and other eukaryotes. BMC Evol. Biol. 16, 197.

Ohata, H., Ota, N., Shirouzu, M., Yokoyama, S., Yokota, J., Taya, Y., Enari, M., 2009. Identification of a function-specific mutation of clathrin heavy chain (CHC) required for p53 transactivation. J. Mol. Biol. 394, 460–471.

Ohmori, K., Endo, Y., Yoshida, Y., Ohata, H., Taya, Y., Enari, M., 2008. Monomeric but not trimeric clathrin heavy chain regulates p53-mediated transcription. Oncogene 27, 2215–2227.

Okamoto, C.T., McKinney, J., Jeng, Y.Y., 2000. Clathrin in mitotic spindles. Am. J. Phys. Cell Physiol. 279, C369–C374.

Orgovan, G., Noszal, B., 2011. The complete microspeciation of arginine and citrulline. J. Pharm. Biomed. Anal. 54, 965–971.

Ozimek, P., Kotter, P., Veenhuis, M., Van Der Klei, I.J., 2006. Hansenula polymorpha and Saccharomyces cerevisiae Pex5p's recognize different, independent peroxisomal targeting signals in alcohol oxidase. FEBS Lett. 580, 46–50.

Ozimek, P., Van Dijk, R., Latchev, K., Gancedo, C., Wang, D.Y., Van Der Klei, I.J., Veenhuis, M., 2003. Pyruvate carboxylase is an essential protein in the assembly of yeast peroxisomal oligomeric alcohol oxidase. Mol. Biol. Cell 14, 786–797.

Pal-Bhowmick, I., Vora, H.K., Jarori, G.K., 2007. Sub-cellular localization and post-translational modifications of the Plasmodium yoelii enolase suggest moonlighting functions. Malar. J. 6, 45.

Palm, J.E., Weiland, M.E., Griffiths, W.J., Ljungstrom, I., Svard, S.G., 2003. Identification of immunoreactive proteins during acute human giardiasis. J. Infect. Dis. 187, 1849–1859.

Pan, M., Stevens, B.R., 1995. Protein kinase C-dependent regulation of L-arginine transport activity in Caco-2 intestinal cells. Biochim. Biophys. Acta 1239, 27–32.

Pancholi, V., Fischetti, V.A., 1998. alpha-enolase, a novel strong plasmin(ogen) binding protein on the surface of pathogenic streptococci. J. Biol. Chem. 273, 14503–14515.

Paredez, A.R., Assaf, Z.J., Sept, D., Timofejeva, L., Dawson, S.C., Wang, C.J., Cande, W.Z., 2011. An actin cytoskeleton with evolutionarily conserved functions in the absence of canonical actin-binding proteins. Proc. Natl. Acad. Sci. U. S. A. 108, 6151–6156.

Paredez, A.R., Nayeri, A., Xu, J.W., Krtkova, J., Cande, W.Z., 2014. Identification of obscure yet conserved actin-associated proteins in Giardia lamblia. Eukaryot. Cell 13, 776–784.

Paschal, B.M., Shpetner, H.S., Vallee, R.B., 1987. MAP 1C is a microtubule-activated ATPase which translocates microtubules in vitro and has dynein-like properties. J. Cell Biol. 105, 1273–1282.

Peranzoni, E., Marigo, I., Dolcetti, L., Ugel, S., Sonda, N., Taschin, E., Mantelli, B., Bronte, V., Zanovello, P., 2007. Role of arginine metabolism in immunity and immunopathology. Immunobiology 212, 795–812.

Perez-Hernandez, D., Gutierrez-Vazquez, C., Jorge, I., Lopez-Martin, S., Ursa, A., Sanchez-Madrid, F., Vazquez, J., Yanez-Mo, M., 2013. The intracellular interactome of tetraspanin-enriched microdomains reveals their function as sorting machineries toward exosomes. J. Biol. Chem. 288, 11649–11661.

Piatigorsky, J., O'brien, W.E., Norman, B.L., Kalumuck, K., Wistow, G.J., Borras, T., Nickerson, J.M., Wawrousek, E.F., 1988. Gene sharing by delta-crystallin and argininosuccinate lyase. Proc. Natl. Acad. Sci. U. S. A. 85, 3479–3483.

Podobnik, M., Tyagi, R., Matange, N., Dermol, U., Gupta, A.K., Mattoo, R., Seshadri, K., Visweswariah, S.S., 2009. A mycobacterial cyclic AMP phosphodiesterase that moonlights as a modifier of cell wall permeability. J. Biol. Chem. 284, 32846–32857.

Polo, S., Sigismund, S., Faretta, M., Guidi, M., Capua, M.R., Bossi, G., Chen, H., De Camilli, P., Di Fiore, P.P., 2002. A single motif responsible for ubiquitin recognition and monoubiquitination in endocytic proteins. Nature 416, 451–455.

Pollard, T.D., Cooper, J.A., 2009. Actin, a central player in cell shape and movement. Science 326, 1208–1212.

Raikar, L.S., Vallejo, J., Lloyd, P.G., Hardin, C.D., 2006. Overexpression of caveolin-1 results in increased plasma membrane targeting of glycolytic enzymes: the structural basis for a membrane associated metabolic compartment. J. Cell. Biochem. 98, 861–871.

Ringqvist, E., Palm, J.E., Skarin, H., Hehl, A.B., Weiland, M., Davids, B.J., Reiner, D.S., Griffiths, W.J., Eckmann, L., Gillin, F.D., Svard, S.G., 2008. Release of metabolic enzymes by Giardia in response to interaction with intestinal epithelial cells. Mol. Biochem. Parasitol. 159, 85–91.

Ritter, B., McPherson, P.S., 2006. There's a Gap in the ENTH domain. Proc. Natl. Acad. Sci. U. S. A. 103, 3953–3954.

Rivero, M.R., Miras, S.L., Feliziani, C., Zamponi, N., Quiroga, R., Hayes, S.F., Ropolo, A.S., Touz, M.C., 2012. Vacuolar protein sorting receptor in Giardia lamblia. PLoS One 7 e43712.

Rivero, M.R., Miras, S.L., Quiroga, R., Ropolo, A.S., Touz, M.C., 2011. Giardia lamblia low-density lipoprotein receptor-related protein is involved in selective lipoprotein endocytosis and parasite replication. Mol. Microbiol. 79, 1204–1219.

Rivero, M.R., Vranych, C.V., Bisbal, M., Maletto, B.A., Ropolo, A.S., Touz, M.C., 2010. Adaptor protein 2 regulates receptor-mediated endocytosis and cyst formation in Giardia lamblia. Biochem. J. 428, 33–45.

Robinson, M.J., Cobb, M.H., 1997. Mitogen-activated protein kinase pathways. Curr. Opin. Cell Biol. 9, 180–186.

Ropolo, A.S., Touz, M.C., 2010. A lesson in survival, by Giardia lamblia. ScientificWorldJournal 10, 2019–2031.

Rosenthal, J.A., Chen, H., Slepnev, V.I., Pellegrini, L., Salcini, A.E., Di Fiore, P.P., De Camilli, P., 1999. The epsins define a family of proteins that interact with components of the clathrin coat and contain a new protein module. J. Biol. Chem. 274, 33959–33965.

Roux, P.P., Blenis, J., 2004. ERK and p38 MAPK-activated protein kinases: a family of protein kinases with diverse biological functions. Microbiol. Mol. Biol. Rev. 68, 320–344.

Royle, S.J., 2006. The cellular functions of clathrin. Cell. Mol. Life Sci. 63, 1823–1832.

Royle, S.J., 2011. Mitotic moonlighting functions for membrane trafficking proteins. Traffic 12, 791–798.

Royle, S.J., Bright, N.A., Lagnado, L., 2005. Clathrin is required for the function of the mitotic spindle. Nature 434, 1152–1157.

Saha, N., Dutta, S., Datta, S.P., Sarkar, S., 2018. The minimal ESCRT machinery of Giardia lamblia has altered inter-subunit interactions within the ESCRT-II and ESCRT-III complexes. Eur. J. Cell Biol. 97, 44–62.

Salusso, A., Zlocowski, N., Mayol, G.F., Zamponi, N., Ropolo, A.S., 2017. Histone methyltransferase 1 regulates the encystation process in the parasite Giardia lamblia. FEBS J. 284, 2396–2409.

Salzman, A., Denenberg, A.G., Ueta, I., O'connor, M., Linn, S.C., Szabo, C., 1996. Induction and activity of nitric oxide synthase in cultured human intestinal epithelial monolayers. Am. J. Physiol. 270, G565–G573.

Samson, R.Y., Bell, S.D., 2009. Ancient ESCRTs and the evolution of binary fission. Trends Microbiol. 17, 507–513.

Saraiya, A.A., Wang, C.C., 2008. snoRNA, a novel precursor of microRNA in Giardia lamblia. PLoS Pathog. 4, e1000224.

Sauer, G., Korner, R., Hanisch, A., Ries, A., Nigg, E.A., Sillje, H.H., 2005. Proteome analysis of the human mitotic spindle. Mol. Cell. Proteomics 4, 35–43.

Scott, K.G., Logan, M.R., Klammer, G.M., Teoh, D.A., Buret, A.G., 2000. Jejunal brush border microvillous alterations in Giardia muris-infected mice: role of T lymphocytes and interleukin-6. Infect. Immun. 68, 3412–3418.

Schofield, P.J., Edwards, M.R., Matthews, J., Wilson, J.R., 1992. The pathway of arginine catabolism in Giardia intestinalis. Mol. Biochem. Parasitol. 51, 29–36.

Seeler, J.S., Dejean, A., 2003. Nuclear and unclear functions of SUMO. Nat. Rev. Mol. Cell Biol. 4, 690–699.

Sengupta, S., Ghosh, S., Nagaraja, V., 2008. Moonlighting function of glutamate racemase from Mycobacterium tuberculosis: racemization and DNA gyrase inhibition are two independent activities of the enzyme. Microbiology 154, 2796–2803.

Shirai, H., Blundell, T.L., Mizuguchi, K., 2001. A novel superfamily of enzymes that catalyze the modification of guanidino groups. Trends Biochem. Sci. 26, 465–468.

Shpetner, H.S., Vallee, R.B., 1989. Identification of dynamin, a novel mechanochemical enzyme that mediates interactions between microtubules. Cell 59, 421–432.

Slack, J.L., Jones Jr., L.E., Bhatia, M.M., Thompson, P.R., 2011. Autodeimination of protein arginine deiminase 4 alters protein-protein interactions but not activity. Biochemistry 50, 3997–4010.

Slepnev, V.I., De Camilli, P., 2000. Accessory factors in clathrin-dependent synaptic vesicle endocytosis. Nat. Rev. Neurosci. 1, 161–172.

Sonda, S., Morf, L., Bottova, I., Baetschmann, H., Rehrauer, H., Caflisch, A., Hakimi, M.A., Hehl, A.B., 2010. Epigenetic mechanisms regulate stage differentiation in the minimized protozoan Giardia lamblia. Mol. Microbiol. 76, 48–67.

Sriram, G., Martinez, J.A., McCabe, E.R., Liao, J.C., Dipple, K.M., 2005. Single-gene disorders: what role could moonlighting enzymes play? Am. J. Hum. Genet. 76, 911–924.

Stadelmann, B., Merino, M.C., Persson, L., Svard, S.G., 2012. Arginine consumption by the intestinal parasite Giardia intestinalis reduces proliferation of intestinal epithelial cells. PLoS One 7 e45325.

Starnes, G.L., Coincon, M., Sygusch, J., Sibley, L.D., 2009. Aldolase is essential for energy production and bridging adhesin-actin cytoskeletal interactions during parasite invasion of host cells. Cell Host Microbe 5, 353–364.

Svard, S.G., Meng, T.C., Hetsko, M.L., Mccaffery, J.M., Gillin, F.D., 1998. Differentiation-associated surface antigen variation in the ancient eukaryote Giardia lamblia. Mol. Microbiol. 30, 979–989.

Takei, K., Haucke, V., 2001. Clathrin-mediated endocytosis: membrane factors pull the trigger. Trends Cell Biol. 11, 385–391.

Tanabe, K., Takei, K., 2009. Dynamic instability of microtubules requires dynamin 2 and is impaired in a Charcot-Marie-Tooth mutant. J Cell Biol 185, 939–948.

Thompson, H.M., Skop, A.R., Euteneuer, U., Meyer, B.J., Mcniven, M.A., 2002. The large GTPase dynamin associates with the spindle midzone and is required for cytokinesis. Curr. Biol. 12, 2111–2117.

Thompson, H.M., Cao, H., Chen, J., Euteneuer, U., Mcniven, M.A., 2004. Dynamin 2 binds gamma-tubulin and participates in centrosome cohesion. Nat Cell Biol 6, 335–342.

Touz, M.C., 2012. The unique endosomal/lysosomal system of Giardia lamblia. In: Ceresa, B. (Ed.), Molecular Regulation of Endocytosis. InTech, Croatia.

Touz, M.C., Kulakova, L., Nash, T.E., 2004. Adaptor protein complex 1 mediates the transport of lysosomal proteins from a Golgi-like organelle to peripheral vacuoles in the primitive eukaryote Giardia lamblia. Mol. Biol. Cell 15, 3053–3060.

Touz, M.C., Rivero, M.R., Miras, S.L., Bonifacino, J.S., 2012. Lysosomal protein trafficking in Giardia lamblia: common and distinct features. Front Biosci 4, 1898–1909.

Touz, M.C., Ropolo, A.S., Rivero, M.R., Vranych, C.V., Conrad, J.T., Svard, S.G., Nash, T.E., 2008. Arginine deiminase has multiple regulatory roles in the biology of Giardia lamblia. J. Cell Sci. 121, 2930–2938.

Touz, M.C., Zamponi, N., 2017. Sorting without a Golgi complex. Traffic 10, 637–645.

Tran, E.J., Wente, S.R., 2006. Dynamic nuclear pore complexes: life on the edge. Cell 125, 1041–1053.

Traub, L.M., 2003. Sorting it out: AP-2 and alternate clathrin adaptors in endocytic cargo selection. J. Cell Biol. 163, 203–208.

Trejo-Soto, P.J., Aguayo-Ortiz, R., Yepez-Mulia, L., Hernandez-Campos, A., Medina-Franco, J.L., Castillo, R., 2016. Insights into the structure and inhibition of Giardia intestinalis arginine deiminase: homology modeling, docking, and molecular dynamics studies. J. Biomol. Struct. Dyn. 34, 732–748.

Tumova, P., Hofstetrova, K., Nohynkova, E., Hovorka, O., Kral, J., 2007. Cytogenetic evidence for diversity of two nuclei within a single diplomonad cell of Giardia. Chromosoma 116, 65–78.

Tutturen, A.E., Holm, A., Jorgensen, M., Stadtmuller, P., Rise, F., Fleckenstein, B., 2010. A technique for the specific enrichment of citrulline-containing peptides. Anal. Biochem. 403, 43–51.

Urrutia, R., Henley, J.R., Cook, T., Mcniven, M.A., 1997. The dynamins: redundant or distinct functions for an expanding family of related GTPases? Proc. Natl. Acad. Sci. U. S. A. 94, 377–384.

Vecchi, M., Polo, S., Poupon, V., Van De Loo, J.W., Benmerah, A., Di Fiore, P.P., 2001. Nucleocytoplasmic shuttling of endocytic proteins. J. Cell Biol. 153, 1511–1517.

Vossenaar, E.R., Nijenhuis, S., Helsen, M.M., Van Der Heijden, A., Senshu, T., Van Den Berg, W.B., Van Venrooij, W.J., Joosten, L.A., 2003a. Citrullination of synovial proteins in murine models of rheumatoid arthritis. Arthritis Rheum. 48, 2489–2500.

Vossenaar, E.R., Zendman, A.J., Van Venrooij, W.J., 2004. Citrullination, a possible functional link between susceptibility genes and rheumatoid arthritis. Arthritis Res Ther 6, 1–5.

Vossenaar, E.R., Zendman, A.J., Van Venrooij, W.J., Pruijn, G.J., 2003b. PAD, a growing family of citrullinating enzymes: genes, features and involvement in disease. Bioessays 25, 1106–1118.

Vranych, C.V., Rivero, M.R., Merino, M.C., Mayol, G.F., Zamponi, N., Maletto, B.A., Pistoresi-Palencia, M.C., Touz, M.C., Ropolo, A.S., 2014. SUMOylation and deimination of proteins: two epigenetic modifications involved in Giardia encystation. Biochim. Biophys. Acta 1843, 1805–1817.

Wang, X.M., Zhai, Y., Ferrell Jr., J.E., 1997. A role for mitogen-activated protein kinase in the spindle assembly checkpoint in XTC cells. J. Cell Biol. 137, 433–443.

Wang, Y., Wysocka, J., Sayegh, J., Lee, Y.H., Perlin, J.R., Leonelli, L., Sonbuchner, L.S., McDonald, C.H., Cook, R.G., Dou, Y., Roeder, R.G., Clarke, S., Stallcup, M.R., Allis, C.D., Coonrod, S.A., 2004. Human PAD4 regulates histone arginine methylation levels via demethylimination. Science 306, 279–283.

Wang, Y.J., Wang, J., Sun, H.Q., Martinez, M., Sun, Y.X., Macia, E., Kirchhausen, T., Albanesi, J.P., Roth, M.G., Yin, H.L., 2003. Phosphatidylinositol 4 phosphate regulates targeting of clathrin adaptor AP-1 complexes to the Golgi. Cell 114, 299–310.

Wasiak, S., Legendre-Guillemin, V., Puertollano, R., Blondeau, F., Girard, M., De Heuvel, E., Boismenu, D., Bell, A.W., Bonifacino, J.S., McPherson, P.S., 2002. Enthoprotin: a novel clathrin-associated protein identified through subcellular proteomics. J. Cell Biol. 158, 855–862.

Wendland, B., 2002. Epsins: adaptors in endocytosis? Nat. Rev. Mol. Cell Biol. 3, 971–977.

Widmann, C., Gibson, S., Jarpe, M.B., Johnson, G.L., 1999. Mitogen-activated protein kinase: conservation of a three-kinase module from yeast to human. Physiol. Rev. 79, 143–180.

Wu, G., Morris Jr., S.M., 1998. Arginine metabolism: nitric oxide and beyond. Biochem. J. 336 (Pt 1), 1–17.

Yanagisawa, H.A., Kamiya, R., 2001. Association between actin and light chains in Chlamydomonas flagellar inner-arm dyneins. Biochem Biophys Res Commun 288, 443–447.

Yarlett, N., Lindmark, D.G., Goldberg, B., Moharrami, M.A., Bacchi, C.J., 1994. Subcellular localization of the enzymes of the arginine dihydrolase pathway in Trichomonas vaginalis and Tritrichomonas foetus. J. Eukaryot. Microbiol. 41, 554–559.

Yepez-Mulia, L., Montano-Escalona, C., Fonseca-Linan, R., Munoz-Cruz, S., Arizmendi-Puga, N., Boireau, P., Ortega-Pierres, G., 2009. Differential activation of mast cells by antigens from Trichinella spiralis muscle larvae, adults, and newborn larvae. Vet. Parasitol. 159, 253–257.

Yichoy, M., Nakayasu, E.S., Shpak, M., Aguilar, C., Aley, S.B., Almeida, I.C., Das, S., 2009. Lipidomic analysis reveals that phosphatidylglycerol and phosphatidylethanolamine are newly generated phospholipids in an early-divergent protozoan, Giardia lamblia. Mol. Biochem. Parasitol. 165, 67–78.

Ying, S., Dong, S., Kawada, A., Kojima, T., Chavanas, S., Mechin, M.C., Adoue, V., Serre, G., Simon, M., Takahara, H., 2009. Transcriptional regulation of peptidylarginine deiminase expression in human keratinocytes. J. Dermatol. Sci. 53, 2–9.

Yoshida, N., Oeda, K., Watanabe, E., Mikami, T., Fukita, Y., Nishimura, K., Komai, K., Matsuda, K., 2001. Protein function. Chaperonin turned insect toxin. Nature 411, 44.

Zamponi, N., Zamponi, E., Mayol, G.F., Lanfredi-Rangel, A., Svard, S.G., Touz, M.C., 2017. The ER is the sorting core facility in the Golgi-lacking protozoan Giardia lamblia. Traffic 9, 604–621.

Zhao, B., Lei, L., Vassylyev, D.G., Lin, X., Cane, D.E., Kelly, S.L., Yuan, H., Lamb, D.C., Waterman, M.R., 2009. Crystal structure of albaflavenone monooxygenase containing a moonlighting terpene synthase active site. J. Biol. Chem. 284, 36711–36719.

Zhou, K., Pandol, S., Bokoch, G., Traynor-Kaplan, A.E., 1998. Disruption of Dictyostelium PI3K genes reduces [32P]phosphatidylinositol 3,4 bisphosphate and [32P]phosphatidylinositol trisphosphate levels, alters F-actin distribution and impairs pinocytosis. J. Cell Sci. 111 (Pt 2), 283–294.

Zumthor, J.P., Cernikova, L., Rout, S., Kaech, A., Faso, C., Hehl, A.B., 2016. Static clathrin assemblies at the peripheral vacuole-plasma membrane interface of the parasitic protozoan Giardia lamblia. PLoS Pathog. 12, e1005756.

Zuniga, M., Perez, G., Gonzalez-Candelas, F., 2002. Evolution of arginine deiminase (ADI) pathway genes. Mol. Phylogenet. Evol. 25, 429–444.

CHAPTER TWO

The protein 14-3-3: A functionally versatile molecule in *Giardia duodenalis*

Marco Lalle[a,*], Annarita Fiorillo[b]
[a]Department of Infectious Diseases, European Union Reference Laboratory for Parasites, Istituto Superiore di Sanità, Rome, Italy
[b]Department of Biochemical Sciences "A. Rossi Fanelli", Sapienza University of Rome, Rome, Italy
*Corresponding author: e-mail address: marco.lalle@iss.it

Contents

Abstract

Giardia duodenalis is a cosmopolitan zoonotic protozoan parasite causing giardiasis, one of the most common diarrhoeal diseases in human and animals. Beyond its public health relevance, *Giardia* represents a valuable and fascinating model microorganism. The deep-branching phylogenetic position of *Giardia*, its simple life cycle and its minimalistic genomic and cellular organization provide a unique opportunity to define basal and "ancestral" eukaryotic functions. The eukaryotic 14-3-3 protein family

Advances in Parasitology, Volume 106
ISSN 0065-308X
https://doi.org/10.1016/bs.apar.2019.08.002

represents a distinct example of phosphoserine/phosphothreonine-binding proteins. The extended network of protein-protein interactions established by 14-3-3 proteins place them at the crossroad of multiple signalling pathways that regulate physiological and pathological cellular processes. Despite the remarkable insight on 14-3-3 protein in different organisms, from yeast to humans, so far little attention was given to the study of this protein in protozoan parasites. However, in the last years, research efforts have provided evidences on unique properties of the single 14-3-3 protein of *Giardia* and on its association in key aspects of *Giardia* life cycle. In the first part of this chapter, a general overview of the features commonly shared among 14-3-3 proteins in different organisms (i.e. structure, target recognition, mode of action and regulatory mechanisms) is included. The second part focus on the current knowledge on the biochemistry and biology of the *Giardia* 14-3-3 protein and on the possibility to use this protein as target to propose new strategies for developing innovative antigiardial therapy.

1. Introduction

Giardia duodenalis (syn. *lamblia* or *intestinalis*) is a cosmopolitan zoonotic enteroparasite. This flagellated protist colonizes and proliferates in the upper part of the small intestine of mammals and it is the most common gastrointestinal protozoan parasite of humans (Lalle and Hanevik, 2018). Up to now, eight genetic groups (designated assemblages A-H) are recognized in *Giardia*, with differences in host distribution and host specificity. Assemblages A and B are associated with human infections, but display capacity for zoonotic infection (Cacciò et al., 2018). In the human host, infection can be asymptomatic or cause giardiasis, an acute self-limited diarrhoeal disease. With almost 300 million cases reported annually, giardiasis contributes substantially to the global burden of diarrhoeal disease, especially in children living in regions with poor hygiene (Lalle and Hanevik, 2018). *Giardia* infection can become chronic and, in immunologically naïve patients, has been associated with the development of post-infection gut dysfunctions (Lalle and Hanevik, 2018). In addition to its public health relevance, *Giardia* represents a valuable and fascinating model microorganism. This parasite has a direct life cycle, that can be reproduced *in vitro* as well as in animal models, which has two main stages: (i) the trophozoite, a pear-shaped binucleated cell which colonizes the host intestine and reproduces through binary fission, and (ii) the cyst, an infective stage which is able to survive in the external environment (Cacciò et al., 2018). Once the cysts are ingested, they pass through the stomach where excystation initiates and then each cyst releases two trophozoites in the proximal small intestine. In the jejunum, exposure to external stimuli, such as increase in biliary content and pH, induces trophozoite differentiation and encystation and then cysts are expelled to the environment through the faeces (Argüello-Garciá et al., 2009). *Giardia* has been considered for long an early branching organism, a "missing link" in eukaryotic evolutionary lineage. However, since the complete genome sequence from different reference isolates are now available, *Giardia* is now recognized as "deep-branching" and simplified organism (Thompson and Monis, 2012). The adoption of a parasitic life style has likely driven a process leading to genomic minimalism, with a compact genome largely lacking introns (Morrison et al., 2007), and reduce biological complexity. Several eukaryotic organelles (i.e. peroxisomes and lysosomes) are absent in *Giardia* and others are profoundly modified (Faso and Hehl, 2011). The reduction in complexity thus reflects a reduced gene repertoire. *Giardia* is an excellent model system to dissect complex basic eukaryotic processes, including cell differentiation, signal transduction, cell division and intracellular transport, from a simplified perspective (Ankarklev et al., 2010). At the same time, *Giardia* is also a valuable pathogen model that can be studied both *in vitro* and *in vivo* (Lauwaet et al., 2007). *Giardia* establishes a complex relation with its host and has developed various adaptations to survive in the hostile gastrointestinal tract and to cope with environmental conditions within and outside the host that may induce mutations (Allain et al., 2017). Transient regulated protein-protein interactions (PPI) are universal mechanisms for cells to respond and adapt rapidly to intracellular and extracellular stimuli. Protein post-translational modifications such as phosphorylation/dephosphorylation on serine, threonine or tyrosine residues, regulate many PPIs dynamic (Jin and Pawson, 2012). Phosphorylation provides the docking platform for proteins containing phospho-binding domain to promote the assembly of multiprotein complexes (Roque and Lowe, 2005). The 14-3-3 protein family represents a distinct example of phosphoserine/phosphothreonine (pSer/pThr)-binding protein with an exceptional network of interacting proteins. The 14-3-3 proteins can potentially comprise around 0.6% of the human proteome (Jin et al., 2004). These are small dimeric proteins originally identified at the end of 60s (Moore and Perez, 1968) as highly abundant proteins in bovine brain and their name was given by the combination of the number of the eluted fraction in DEAE-cellulose chromatography (14th fraction) and the position in which these proteins migrate in starch-gel electrophoresis (position 3.3). In the late 80s the first functional role as activators of both tryptophan 5-monooxygenase (TPH) and tyrosine 3-monooxygenase was assigned to

14-3-3s (Ichimura et al., 1987) and the reliance on TPH phosphorylation for 14-3-3 binding was assessed (Furukawa et al., 1993). After these initial observations, the expression of 14-3-3 proteins in tissue other than the brain, the existence of multiple isoforms capable to form homo and heterodimers, and the ubiquitous presence of 14-3-3 in all eukaryotic kingdoms were documented (Aitken, 2006; Rosenquist et al., 2000). 14-3-3 proteins are now considered as the core for integrating controlling of diverse physiological processes (i.e. cell cycle, differentiation, apoptosis, protein trafficking, signals transduction and metabolism) in evolutionary distant organisms, as well as for contributing in several diseases and pathologies (Lozano-Durán and Robatzek, 2015; Pennington et al., 2018). 14-3-3 "client" proteins include enzymes as well as transcriptional factors and structural proteins (Paul et al., 2009; van Heusden, 2005). The ancient and essential role of 14-3-3 proteins was clearly demonstrated by the capacity of 14-3-3 proteins from *Arabidopsis thaliana* to rescue the lethal double 14-3-3 genes deletion phenotype in the yeast *Saccharomyces cerevisiae* (van Heusden et al., 1995). Thus, the study of the 14-3-3 protein in *Giardia* provides an opportunity to define basal and "ancestral" functions of this class of regulatory molecules.

In the first part of this chapter, we provide a general overview of the characteristics commonly shared by each 14-3-3 protein (i.e. structure, target recognition, mode of action and regulatory mechanisms), and in the second part we describe the current knowledge on the biochemistry and biology of 14-3-3 protein in *Giardia duodenalis*.

2. General overview of 14-3-3 proteins

2.1 Evolution and structure of 14-3-3 proteins

The 14-3-3 are small soluble and acidic proteins, with an approximate molecular mass of 30 kDa, and a pI of 4–5 (Yaffe, 2002). Until recently, the presence of genes encoding for 14-3-3 was restricted to the eukaryotic kingdom thereafter, as the number of available genomes increased, sequence mining of bacterial databases have allowed to retrieve several hypothetical proteins with high similarity in sequence and structure to 14-3-3, particularly in *Gammaproteobacteria bacterium*, thus challenging the evolutionary origin of 14-3-3 (McGowan et al., 2017). It is well established that unicellular and lower eukaryotes have either one or two 14-3-3s, e.g., the slime mold *Dictyostelium discoideum* has one, the yeast *Saccharomyces cerevisiae* and the nematode *Caenorhabditis elegans* have two. However, there are exceptions (Hirt et al., 2011; Rosenquist et al., 2000). In higher eukaryotes multiple isoforms are found, and mammals, including *Homo sapiens*, have seven 14-3-3 genes (i.e. β, γ, ε, σ, ζ, τ, η), while plants have the largest number of 14-3-3 genes, e.g., 15 genes in *A. thaliana* (χ, ω, ψ, ϕ, υ, λ, ν, κ, μ, ε, ο, ι, π) (Rosenquist et al., 2000).

Overall, 14-3-3s have a significant degree of sequence conservation sharing about 50% identity among amino acids both within and across species (Rosenquist et al., 2000). Most of the 14-3-3s fall into four major groups largely overlapping the eukaryotic kingdoms, Viridiplantae (plants), Fungi, Alveolata, and Metazoa (animals), although most unicellular and parasite 14-3-3 proteins cluster separately (McGowan et al., 2017; Rosenquist et al., 2000). Considering an evolutionary perspective, the 14-3-3 epsilon isoform is recognized as the closest to the ancestral 14-3-3 (McGowan et al., 2017; Rosenquist et al., 2000). 14-3-3 proteins exist mainly as dimers, and self-assemble into homo- or heterodimers, although under particular conditions they can be found as monomers (Denison et al., 2014). The dimeric and highly helical nature of 14-3-3 proteins was first elucidated upon the determination of the crystal structures of the mammalian 14-3-3 isoforms ξ and τ (Liu et al., 1995; Xiao et al., 1995). Up to February 2019, 187 structures of 14-3-3 proteins have been deposited in the Protein Data Bank (PDB), more than half in the last 4 years, indicating the increasing interest in these proteins. The most of them (166) belongs to the human isoforms, while only 9 are from eukaryotic single-celled microorganisms, namely, yeasts, *Cryptosporidium parvum* and *Giardia*, and the remaining are from plant isoforms. The available 14-3-3 structures are either in apo forms or in binary complexes with phosphopeptides, in which the binding site of the partner protein is present while in only few cases the larger part of the partner protein is observed (serotonin N-acetyltransferase, florigen Hd3a, small heat shock protein HSPB6, and the yeast neutral trehalase Nth1) (Alblova et al., 2017; Gardino et al., 2006; Obsil et al., 2001; Sluchanko et al., 2017; Taoka et al., 2011). All isoforms largely share a very similar organization. (Fig. 1).

In each monomer a bundle of nine antiparallel α-helices (α1–α9) connected by short loops are found. Monomers interact through the N-terminal domain to form the dimeric molecule. The 14-3-3 dimer exhibits a clamp-like shape with a large central channel (approximatively 35 Å broad, 35 Å wide and 20 Å deep) composed of highly invariable residues among isoforms, whereas the outer convex surface has higher sequence variability. Dimerization occurs on multiple widely conserved hydrophobic and polar contacts together with variable salt bridges established between

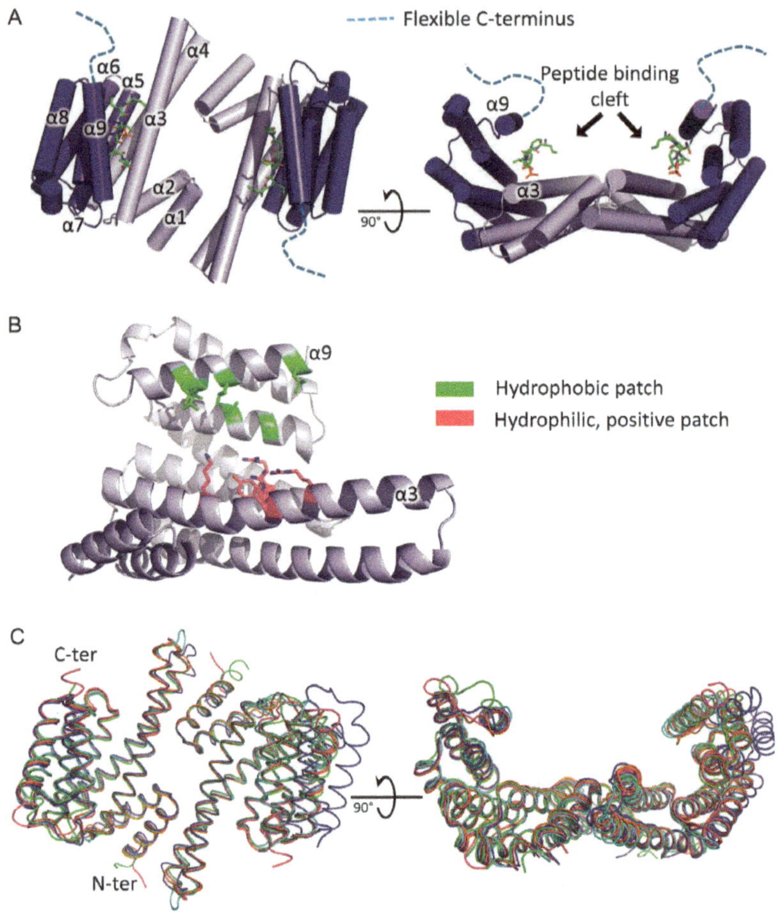

Fig. 1 Structure of 14-3-3 proteins. (A) Two views of the dimer of human 14-3-3ε (N-terminal domain light blue, C-terminal domain dark blue) in complex with phosphopeptide (green) (pdb code: 2BR9). (B) Monomer of human 14-3-3ε in which hydrophobic and hydrophilic residues that characterize the binding cleft are highlighted. (C) Superimposition of representative 14-3-3 proteins from different sources, namely, *Cryptosporidium parvum* (pdb 2NPM, green), *Saccharomyces cerevisiae* (pdb 5N6N, cyan), *Nicotiana tabacum* (pdb 5NWI, magenta), human β (pdb 2BQ0, blue), human ε (pdb 2BR9, orange).

α-helices α1 and α2 from one monomer and between the α3 and the α4 from the other monomer (Gardino et al., 2006). Small sequence variations within the dimer interface determine the number of inter-subunit salt bridges and explains the different propensity of individual 14-3-3 isoforms to form homo- or heterodimers (Chaudhri et al., 2003). The dimer composition is functionally relevant as it contributes to determine the range of

14-3-3 interacting client proteins (Aitken, 2006). A concave surface in each monomer contains highly conserved residues that compose an amphipathic ligand binding groove formed by α3 and α5, enriched in polar and positively charged residues, and the α7 and α9, enriched in hydrophobic residues. Instead, a high degree of sequence divergence and size variation occurs within 14-3-3 isoforms in the C-terminal highly acidic stretch. This unstructured region does not display any electron density in the crystal structures indicating a remarkable structural flexibility (Gardino et al., 2006). Some specific and different functions have been assigned to the C-terminal stretch of some 14-3-3 isoforms, particularly in the regulation of the binding properties (Truong et al., 2002; Shen et al., 2003).

2.2 14-3-3 Target recognition and binding mechanism(s)

After the discovery of the first phosphoserine 14-3-3 binding sequence, RQRSTS$_{259}$TP, in the Raf-1 protein kinase (Muslin et al., 1996), two major consensus binding sequences (or motifs) were defined, and, namely, mode-1, R[S/Ar][+/Ar]p(S/T)[L/E/A/M]P, and mode-2, RX[S/Ar][+]p(S/T)[L/E/A/M]P. In these, the p(S/T) are either phosphorylated serine or threonine residues, Ar indicates an aromatic residue, + a basic residue, and X any amino acid except cysteine (Muslin et al., 1996; Yaffe, 2002). Later on, a third consensus motif, named mode-3, XXpS/pTX$_{1-2}$COOH (where X is any amino acid except proline), was defined (Coblitz et al., 2006). Whereas mode-3 motifs are always located at the extreme C-terminus of the target proteins (Coblitz et al., 2006), the majority of the high-affinity 14-3-3 binding motifs are found within structural disorder regions, suggesting the relevance of these regions in 14-3-3 proteins binding (Bustos, 2012). However, the characterization of a large number of target sites has clearly proven the occurrence of several phosphorylated binding sequences that do not adjust to the consensus motifs (Tinti et al., 2014). The suboptimal binding sequences, to which the 14-3-3 proteins might show a lower affinity, are physiologically preferable to ensure a dynamic regulation of the 14-3-3 target interaction. Noteworthy, many 14-3-3 target proteins possess more than one binding site, so that two binding sites can regulate the protein affinity in dimeric 14-3-3 proteins and promote a more stable interaction by modulation of the phosphorylation status of each binding sequence (Yaffe, 2002). In addition, the 14-3-3 proteins can interact with non-phosphorylated targets, such as binding the LDSLDL sequence in the ADP-ribosyltransferase ExoS of *Pseudomonas aeruginosa*

(Henriksson et al., 2002) or the synthetic peptide R18, containing the WLDLE sequence (Petosa et al., 1998). In any case, primary interaction is mediated by residues located in the ligand binding groove of each 14-3-3 monomer. Co-crystallization studies of 14-3-3 proteins in complex with phosphorylated synthetic peptides demonstrated that the peptides adopt an extended conformation within the ligand binding groove (Obsil and Obsilova, 2011). The primary binding force is provided by the electrostatic interactions between the phosphate group on the peptide and a cluster of highly conserved positively charged residues, such as the triad Lys49, Arg56 and Arg127, along with Tyr-128 (human 14-3-3ζ numbering). The peptide backbone interacts with an hydrophobic patch and the side chains of Asn-173 and Asn-224 (Coblitz et al., 2006; Rittinger et al., 1999). Mutations of residues of the positively charged triad and/or the hydrophobic cluster hamper the association of 14-3-3 proteins with targets (Petosa et al., 1998). Non-phosphorylated targets bind to 14-3-3 proteins in the same ligand binding groove, however with remarkable differences. R18 binding occurs in an amphipathic conformation by establishing both electrostatic interactions, between the aspartic and glutamic acids of the WLDLE sequence and the positively charged triad of 14-3-3 proteins, and hydrophobic interactions, with the two leucine residues making contacts with the hydrophobic side chains of the binding groove. In comparison to consensus motif, R18 extends further down the groove, contacting residues from α7 (Petosa et al., 1998). Nevertheless, 14-3-3-target interaction can also occur outside the amphipathic groove, thus contributing to stabilize the 3D configuration and to modulate the target conformation (Obsil and Obsilova, 2011). Structural evidences indicate that the 14-3-3 region encompassing the α-8 and α-9 can be important in this respect (Alblova et al., 2017; Obsil and Obsilova, 2011; Sluchanko et al., 2017; Taoka et al., 2011). Although these secondary contacts may not be sufficient to establish an effective binding to 14-3-3 proteins in the absence of phosphopeptides, these can contribute to explain the variable affinity that different 14-3-3 isoforms might have for the same target and the ability of 14-3-3 to distinguish target vs non-target proteins (Parua et al., 2014). So far, the exact mechanism involved in the binding of the diverse 14-3-3 interactions is unclear. This is mainly due to a limited number of high-resolution structures of the 14-3-3 in complex with relatively large target protein fragments as well as to the lack of information on the kinetic process of binding itself. Molecular dynamics simulation together with structural data provided evidence that 14-3-3ζ move from an open conformation in the apo form towards a wide-opened conformation when a phosphopeptide enters the binding site, to finally shift into a closed conformation after phosphopeptide binding (Nagy et al., 2017).

2.3 Mode of action and regulatory mechanisms

Up to date, no enzymatic activity has been clearly define for 14-3-3 proteins. Experimental evidence indicates that the 14-3-3 function is almost based on PPIs. Due to the presence in each 14-3-3 dimer of two phosphopeptide binding sites, 14-3-3 can simultaneously bind either two independent targets or two portions of the same target. Indeed, evidence is scarce to support a prominent role of 14-3-3 as an adaptor/scaffold protein able to mediate the formation of ternary complexes between proteins that otherwise could not interact (Chalupska et al., 2019; Chatterjee et al., 2016). Conversely, in accordance to the "molecular anvil" hypothesis, the very rigid structure of the 14-3-3 dimer by binding to two different sites within the same target can function as a clamp that forces the target molecule to conformational changes (Yaffe, 2002) or, as recently suggested, restrains the target structural flexibility (Sluchanko, 2018). This is consistent with a "disorder-to-order" transition induced by 14-3-3 binding, as the paired binding sites are commonly contained within disordered regions and/or straddle either side of functional domains (Bustos, 2012). In multiple proteins, plasticity of disorder regions has been shown to enable the binding diversity to 14-3-3. As consequence, 14-3-3 binding can hide or reveal an active site in target protein, a ligand-binding region or specific motifs that in turn impact on target stability, catalytic activity, localization, interaction with other proteins, accessibility to modifying enzymes (e.g. kinases, phosphatases, proteases, etc.) (Fig. 2).

The primary mechanism that regulates 14-3-3 interactions is characterized by the phosphorylation status of the target. Commonly, 14-3-3 binding sites overlap with motifs that are phosphorylated by basophilic protein kinases such as AGC (protein kinase A/protein kinase G/protein kinase C family) and CaMK ($Ca2+$/calmodulin-dependent protein kinase) (Johnson et al., 2010). Another level of regulation occurs in the presence of multiple binding sites in the same target. Selective phosphorylation of the 14-3-3 client protein in more than one 14-3-3 binding sites, as the results of different protein kinases in response to disparate stimuli, can result in alternative 14-3-3-binding configurations that might improve the 14-3-3 affinity for the target or in allowing 14-3-3 to exert different effect on

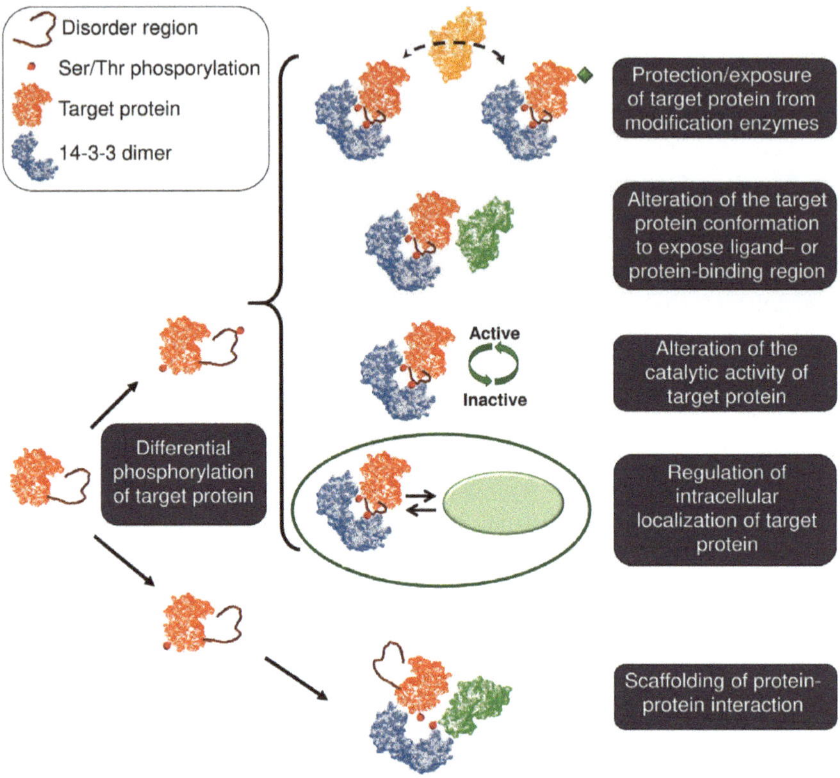

Fig. 2 Modes of action of 14-3-3 proteins. The 14-3-3 protein dimer generally interacts with client proteins upon phosphorylation of two 14-3-3 binding sequences, often located in disordered regions of the client protein. 14-3-3 Protein binding can induce conformational changes in the client that has the following properties: (i) to protect or to expose client protein domain from modification enzymes; (ii) to allow client protein to establish interaction with ligands or other proteins; (iii) to modify the catalytic activity of the client protein; (iv) to affect intracellular localization of the client protein. In a limited number of cases, the 14-3-3 protein dimer can bind simultaneously two client proteins, one for each binding groove, thus acting as scaffold protein.

the target. In an attempt to improve the definition of the dynamics that regulate 14-3-3 PPIs, the presence of 14-3-3 "sinks" mechanism that exclude 14-3-3 away from binding partners has been proposed (Pennington et al., 2018). In this model, removal of 14-3-3 from the binding target is further enhanced through docking 14-3-3 to alternative "parking" sites in abundant proteins, such as keratin and vimentin (Sluchanko et al., 2017), thus creating at the same time a "constant" pool of 14-3-3 available to engage in more specific interactions as needed. A further regulatory mechanism directly involves 14-3-3 post-translational modifications (PTMs) including phosphorylation, acetylation, methylation, s-nitrosylation, ubiquitination and proteolytic cleavage (Aitken, 2011). However, only for few of these PTMs, in particular for phosphorylation, a clear function was assigned.

3. 14-3-3 Protein in *Giardia*

As for other unicellular eukaryotes, a single 14-3-3 gene (*g14-3-3*; GL50803_6430) is present in the genome of the *Giardia* reference isolate WBC6 (Assemblage AI; Lalle et al., 2006), as well as in the isolates ADH (Assemblage AII), GS/M (Assemblage B) and P15 (Assemblage E) (https://giardiadb.org), and it was also cloned from Assemblage C and D isolates (Marco Lalle et al., unpublished). The *g14-3-3* gene does not contain introns and encodes for a protein of 248 amino acids with a predicted molecular weight of 28.5 kDa and a Ip of 5.1, almost identical in all the Assemblages. *Giardia* 14-3-3 shares a 60% of protein sequence identity with the ε subgroup of Metazoan 14-3-3s (Lalle et al., 2006), consistent with the general notion that ε isoform is the most closely related to the ancestral 14-3-3 protein and the evolutionary position of *Giardia* in the deep-branching group of *Excavata* (Fig. 3).

3.1 Functional and structural characterization of the g14-3-3

Functional characterization of g14-3-3 has been carried out using both recombinant and native protein from *Giardia* WBC6 isolate (Lalle et al., 2006, 2010). The g14-3-3 is able to form homodimers as proven by both overlay technique (also known as far western blot), using γ^{32}P-labelled recombinant g14-3-3 as bait and filter immobilized recombinant g14-3-3 as prey (Lalle et al., 2006), and polyacrylamide gel electrophoresis either in native condition or following *in vitro* cross-linking (Fiorillo et al., 2014). *In vivo* g14-3-3 is exclusively dimeric. N-terminally FLAG-tagged g14-3-3 expressed in *Giardia*, under its own promoter, co-immunopurifies with endogenous g14-3-3, even after complete removal of any binding partners by means of a competing phosphopeptide reproducing 14-3-3 consensus motif (Lalle et al., 2010).

The structure of the recombinant g14-3-3 has been solved both in the apo form and in complex with the mode-1 octapeptide A8Ap, reproducing a mode-1 consensus motif (Cau et al., 2015; Fiorillo et al., 2014). Structural analysis confirmed that the g14-3-3 protein has many of the features common to the other 14-3-3 family members but even relevant distinctive traits. The classical N-terminal dimerization interface, relying on residues largely

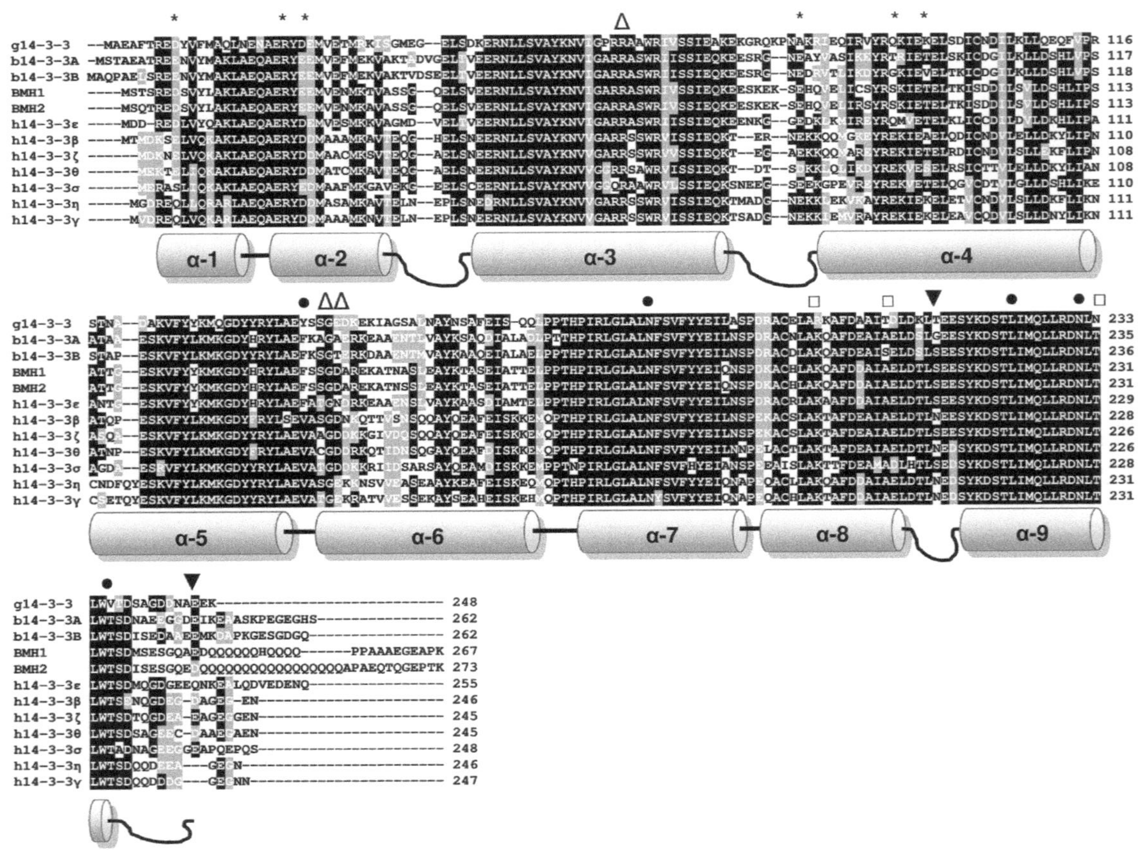

Fig. 3 See legend on opposite page.

conserved among the 14-3-3 family members. Dimer formation involves three pairs of salt bridges, Asp9-Lys82, Arg22-Glu97, and Glu25-Lys93 (Asp9, Arg22, and Glu25 in α-helices 1 and 2 of one monomer, Glu97, Lys82, Lys93 in α-helix 4 of the other monomer) (Fig. 4). This suggests that g14-3-3 homodimers are highly stable and less prone, eventually, to heterodimerise as compared to human 14-3-3ε or the ε-like Cp14e from the protozoan parasite *Cryptosporidium parvum*, in which only the first salt bridge (Arg19-Glu92 in h14-3-3ε and Arg43-Glu119 in ε-like Cp14e, respectively) is formed. The preference to form homodimers is supported by heterologous expression of g14-3-3 in *Drosophila melanogaster*, or vice-versa. A moderate g14-3-3 heterodimerization was shown with D14-3-3ζ (LeoII) isoform but never with D14-3-3ε (Lalle et al., 2013). LeoII/g14-3-3 heterodimers can eventually be stabilized via the same salt bridges, gAsp9-dArg77, gArg22-dGlu92 and gGlu25-dArg88 (where g indicates *Giardia* and d *Drosophila*). Only one salt bridge, gArg22-dGlu92, can be form between the D14-3-3ε and g14-3-3, whereas gAsp9-dGlu77 pairing results in charge repulsion between the two molecules (Lalle et al., 2013). Since the occurrence of three salt bridges in the dimer interface is a feature that the g14-3-3 shares with the 14-3-3ζ, it may be argued that the *Giardia* protein possesses features of both epsilon (higher sequence homology) and zeta isoforms (stable homodimerization). This is consistent with the need for a single 14-3-3 protein to recapitulate properties that, during 14-3-3 proteins evolution, have been allocated to different isoforms when multiple 14-3-3 proteins are present in the same organism.

Fig. 3 Multiple alignment of g14-3-3 protein with plant, yeast and mammalian 14-3-3 isoforms. *Ordeum vulgaris* b14-3-3A, accession number P29305.1, and b14-3-3B, Q43470.1, representing an epsilon-like and one non-epsilon plant 14-3-3 subgroups, respectively, *Saccharomyces cerevisiae* yeast isoforms BMH1, P29311.4 and BMH2, P34730.3, human 14-3-3 isoforms h14-3-3β, NP_647539.1, h14-3-3θ, NP_006817.1, h14-3-3γ, NP_003396.1, h14-3-3ζ, NP_003397.1, h14-3-3γ, NP_036611.2, h14-3-3σ, NP_006133.1, h14-3-3ε, NP_006752.1. Black boxed: identical residues; grey boxed; similar residues; unboxed; divergent residues. Dashes indicate gaps. Key residues for N-terminal dimerization (*); residues contacting the phosphate moiety in the target phosphopeptide (Δ); other residues taking contact with the target phosphopeptide backbone and lateral chains (●). Referring to the sole g14-3-3, Thr214 and Glu246 (▲) and residues Arg200, Thr208, and Asn233 forming intermolecular hydrogen bound in the C-terminal dimer interface (□). The secondary structure, α-helices and loops, are included and numbered. *Adapted with permission and originally published in PLoS One (Fiorillo, A., di Marino, D., Bertuccini, L., Via, A., Pozio, E., Camerini, S., Ilari, A., Lalle, M., 2014. The crystal structure of* Giardia duodenalis *14-3-3 in the apo form: when protein post-translational modifications make the difference. PLoS One 9 (3), e92902).*

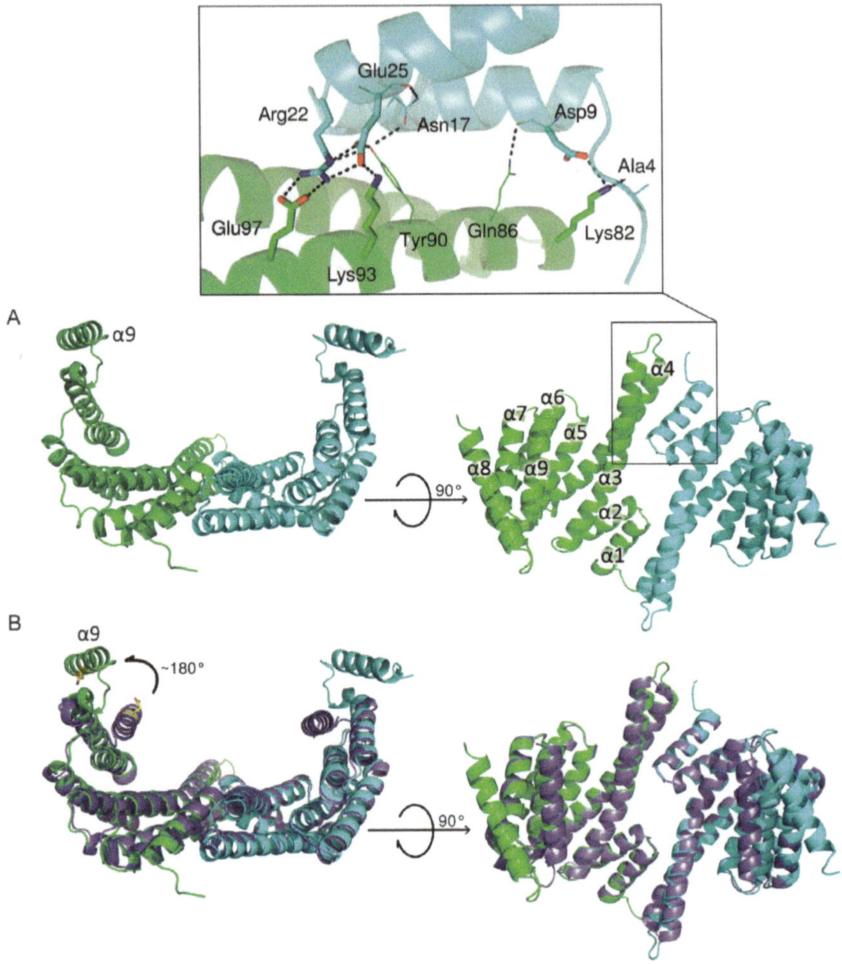

Fig. 4 Structure of g14-3-3. (A) Two views of the apo, open conformation of the g14-3-3. Secondary structure elements are indicated. The zoom shows the residues involved in the N-terminal, canonical dimerization. (B) Superimposition with the structure of human 14-3-3ε (pdb 2BR9, violet) emphasizes the open conformation of the g14-3-3. *Originally published in PLoS One (Fiorillo, A., di Marino, D., Bertuccini, L., Via, A., Pozio, E., Camerini, S., Ilari, A., Lalle, M., 2014. The crystal structure of* Giardia duodenalis *14-3-3 in the apo form: when protein post-translational modifications make the difference. PLoS One 9 (3), e92902).*

In the absence of ligands, the g14-3-3 adopts an "extended" open conformation where the C-terminal helix α9 is rotated of about 180° around helix α8 with respect to canonical conformation, implying a substantial rearrangement of the loop connecting helices α8 and α9 (α8-α9 loop) that acts as a hinge (Fig. 4). A milder degree of flexibility for the region encompassing helices α7 and α9 has been also described for human 14-3-3, likely allowing the accommodation of different types of partners (Yang et al., 2006). The displacement of helix α9 in the g14-3-3 gives rise to a new C-terminal dimerization interface that, together with the usual N-terminal dimerization, causes the formation of filaments by the swapping of helices α9 among adjacent functional dimers (Fiorillo et al., 2014). Interestingly, this assembly reconstitutes the peptide-binding groove, but requires the rearrangement of the α8-α9 loop (Fig. 5).

These fibrillar assemblies, further confirmed by transmission electron microscopy (Fig. 5), are not observed for endogenous g14-3-3 that is exclusively dimeric in solution (Fiorillo et al., 2014). As discussed later, this is associated to constitutive post-translational modifications located in the C-terminus of g14-3-3.

The target binding mechanism are well conserved in the g14-3-3. When the g14-3-3 was crystallized in the presence of the model phosphopeptide A8Ap, the protein adopts the canonical closed conformation supporting a "open-to-closed" conformational rearrangement (Cau et al., 2015). All the residues known to be involved in the phosphopeptide binding are conserved in g14-3-3 (Figs 3 and 4) (Cau et al., 2015; Fiorillo et al., 2014),

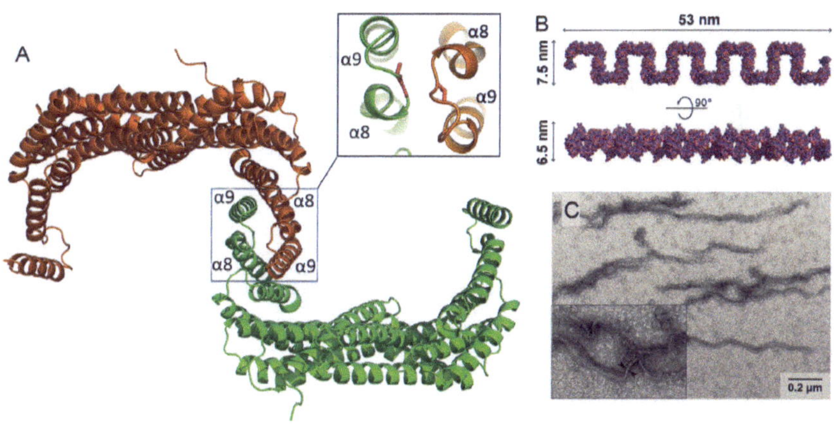

Fig. 5 C-terminal dimerization and fibrils formation. (A) The open extended conformation of apo g14-3-3 gives rise to a new C-terminal dimerization interface. The magnification shows a detail of the loop connecting helices α8 and α9 where Thr214 (red), the phosphorylable residue, is located. (B) The combination of N-terminal and C-terminal dimerization give rise to endless fibres in the crystal. (C) Fibres compatible with crystallographic results are found in solution by TEM imaging. *Originally published in PLoS One (Fiorillo, A., di Marino, D., Bertuccini, L., Via, A., Pozio, E., Camerini, S., Ilari, A., Lalle, M., 2014. The crystal structure of* Giardia duodenalis *14-3-3 in the apo form: when protein post-translational modifications make the difference. PLoS One 9 (3), e92902).*

including the positive charged triad Arg60, Arg135 and Tyr136, that establishes H-bonds with the phosphate moiety as well as residues Lys53 and Arg64, Asn180, and Asn23 (Cau et al., 2015). Indeed mutations in the ligand binding groove of g14-3-3, such as charge reversion of Lys53 (K53E) or introduction of a negative charge instead of the hydrophobic residue Val184 (V184D), strongly hamper or even abolish the capacity of recombinant g14-3-3 to bind *in vitro* to both phosphopeptides reproducing consensus motifs and the prototype phosphorylation independent of the interactor difopein, a synthetic polypeptide containing a tandem repeat of the WLDLE sequence (Lalle et al., 2006, 2010; Masters and Fu, 2001).

3.2 *Giardia* 14-3-3 post-translational modifications

As previously anticipated, the g14-3-3 undergoes extensive PTMs. The first evidence came from the observation that the apparent molecular size (MW) of the g14-3-3 in *Giardia* trophozoites was higher compared to the recombinant protein expressed in bacteria (Lalle et al., 2006) and that multiple spots, with different MW and pI, were resolved after 2D gel electrophoresis (2D-PAGE) as detected by a specific anti-g14-3-3 antibody (Marco Lalle et al., unpublished). A further variation was observed in trophozoites undergoing encystation, mainly after 12h from stimulation, with the appearance of a second g14-3-3 band at lower molecular size associated with a different pattern of spot after 2D-PAGE (Lalle et al., 2006; Marco Lalle et al., unpublished). The nature of such PTM was defined using a highly purified endogenous g14-3-3. This was achieved by designing an affinity purification strategy to pull-down endogenous 14-3-3 from *Giardia* protein lysate of trophozoite and encysting parasites taking advantage of the general property of difopein (Lalle et al., 2006). Indeed, one molecule of difopein strongly interact with any 14-3-3 by covering simultaneously both ligand binding sites of a single 14-3-3 dimer and thus competing with and displacing natural binding partners. By a combination of MALDI-MS and LC-MS/MS analysis, two PTMs were detected at the same time on the g14-3-3, phosphorylation of residue Thr214 and polyglycylation of residue Glu246 (Lalle et al., 2006, 2010).

Phosphorylation of Thr214 is an extensive g14-3-3 post-translational modification detectable in almost all g14-3-3 molecules and likely occurring concomitantly to protein synthesis, both in the trophozoites and in the encysting cells. *In vitro* protein kinase assay using trophozoite lysate and, as a control, an unphosphorylatable recombinant T214A mutant

(Lalle et al., 2006), as well as the expression in *Giardia* of a FLAG-tagged T214A mutant (Lalle et al., 2010), indicate that Thr214 is the unique phosphorylated site on g14-3-3. In a limited phosphoproteomic study, phosphorylated g14-3-3 was also detected during excystation, although the phosphorylation site was not reported (Alvarado and Wassermann, 2010). Altogether, these evidences point out on a crucial function of Thr214 phosphorylation. To date, the g14-3-3 represents the first, and yet unique, example of constitutively phosphorylated 14-3-3 protein (Aitken, 2011). The phosphorylation site slightly resembles that of the acidophilic serine/threonine kinase group (such as casein kinase1/2), also present in *Giardia* (Manning et al., 2011), although the protein kinase responsible for Thr214 phosphorylation has not yet been identified. Since Thr214 is located in the highly flexible loop between α-helices 8 and 9, introduction of a negative charge following phosphorylation can alter the local conformation and in turn affecting g14-3-3-binding properties. Molecular dynamics (MD) simulations performed on the crystallographic open structure confirmed that unmodified g14-3-3 is highly flexible and never achieves geometric convergence (Fig. 6). In particular, the C-terminus, encompassing the α8-α9 loop and helix α9, does not assume a definite conformation but fluctuates continuously (Cau et al., 2015; Fiorillo et al., 2014). On the contrary, both phosphorylation and phosphomimetic mutation on Thr214, modelled in silico (pThr or Glu), induces a remarkable dihedral angles conformational restraint and a large-scale structural rearrangement that has the effect of stiffening the loop and both systems evolve towards an "open-to-closed" conformational transition with g14-3-3 moving towards the canonical W-like shaped binding conformation, thus most likely favouring the binding kinetic process (Cau et al., 2015; Fiorillo et al., 2014). The effect of this favourable binding conformation was supported by 14-3-3-phopshopetide overlay experiments. In comparison to either wild type g14-3-3 or the Thr214 to Ala replacement, the substitution of Thr214 with the negative charged glutamic acid enhances the *in vitro* binding efficiency of recombinant g14-3-3 with a subset of synthetic phosphopeptides reproducing mode-1 consensus motif with no effect on phosphopeptides selectivity (Lalle et al., 2010).

Polyglycylation of the g14-3-3 was detected in MALDI-MS spectra as a series of peaks differing by multiples of 57 Da, corresponding to mass increases of the protein extreme C-terminal peptide $_{230}$DNLNLWVTDSAGDDNAEEK2$_{48}$ due to successive additions of glycine residues (Lalle et al., 2006) (Fig. 7). Polyglycylation (together with polyglutamylation) is a rare polymeric post-translational modification

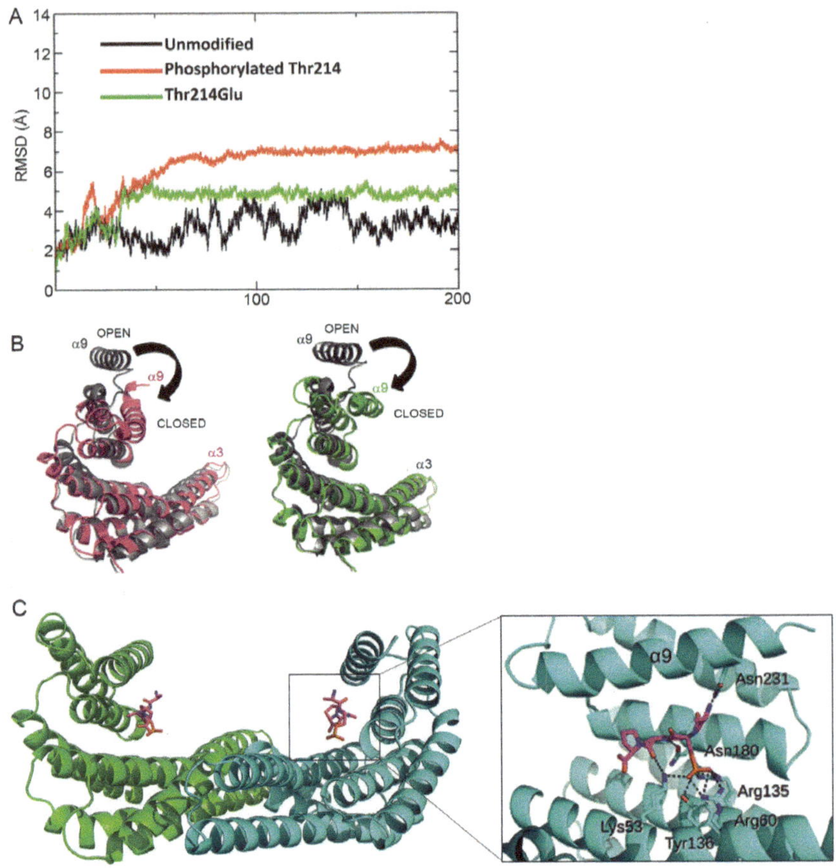

Fig. 6 The effect of Thr214 phosphorylation analysed by molecular dynamics (MD). (A) Plot of root mean square deviation (RMSD) of MD trajectories for 200 ns simulations. The trend of RMSD shows that phosphorylated and phosphomimetic variants of the g14-3-3 reach stable but different conformations. (B) Conformation of phosphorylated (pink) and phosphomimetic (green) compared to unmodified g14-3-3. (D) Structure of g14-3-3 in complex with phosphopeptide A8Ap (pink). The structure assumes the canonical closed conformation. The residues that interact with the peptide are shown, including the conserved triad directly binding the phosphate moiety. *Reprinted and adapted with permission from Cau, Y., Fiorillo, A., Mori, M., Ilari, A., Botta, M., Lalle, M. 2015. Molecular dynamics simulations and structural analysis of* Giardia duodenalis *14-3-3 protein-protein interactions. J. Chem. Inf. Model 55, 2611–2622. Copyright 2015 American Chemical Society.*

(or polymodification) first discovered and commonly reported at the C-terminus of α- and β-tubulins that consists in the covalent addition of one (glycylation) or multiple (polyglycylation) glycines to the γ-carboxyl groups of specific glutamic acids in the target protein (Yu et al., 2015). The

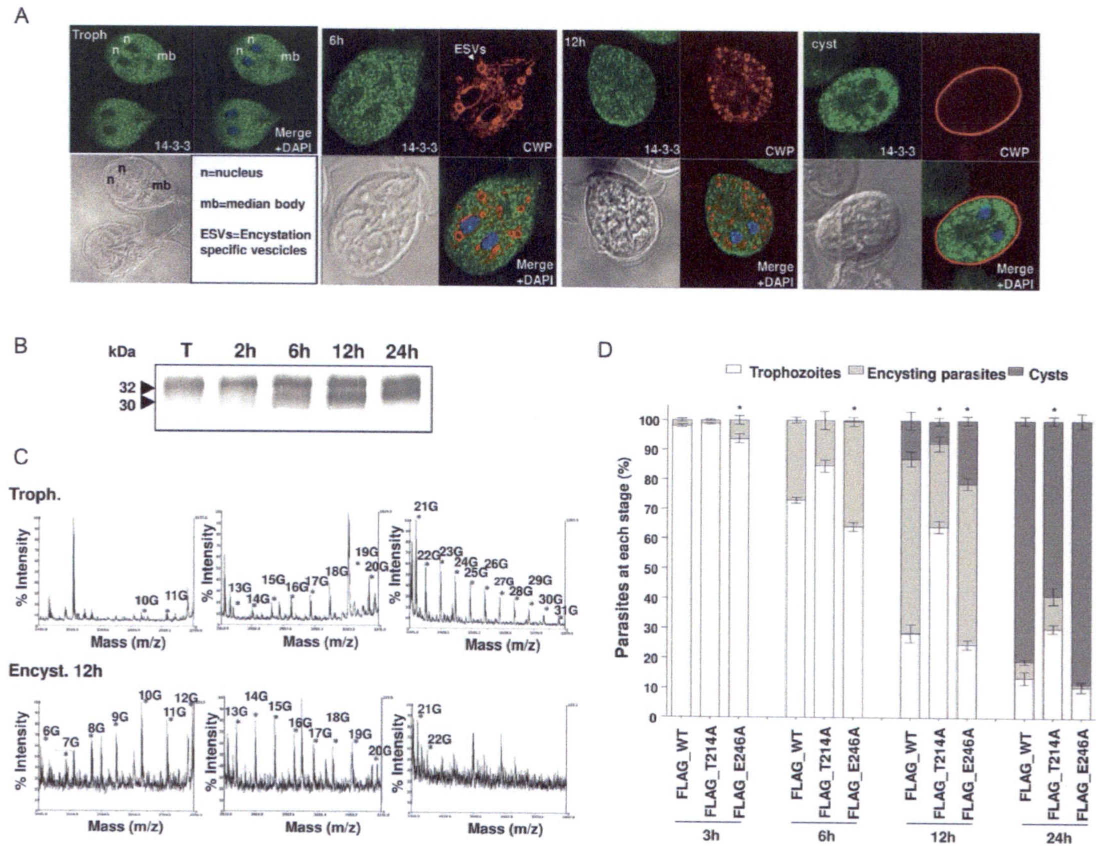

Fig. 7 See legend on next page.

first glycine is attached via a γ-linked isopeptide bond, whereas the other glycines are added by conventional peptide bond. Glycylation and polyglycylation occur almost exclusively in ciliary and flagellar tubulins and are important for the stability, length, and function of motile cilia, and participate in proliferation control in ciliated and flagellated cells and organisms (Yu et al., 2015). It has been proposed that tubulin polymodifications influence microtubule dynamics indirectly, by regulating the interaction of motor proteins and microtubule-interacting proteins with the microtubule (Yu et al., 2015). In *Giardia*, polyglycylation has also been detected as the main post-translational modification of tubulins, but the glutamic acids involved are unknown (Weber et al., 1997). Of the two glutamic acid residues in the C-terminus of the g14-3-3 (Glu246 and Glu247), only the residue 246 is subject to polyglycylation, as proved by the lack of detectable polyglycine chain in the mutant E246A expressed in *Giardia* (Lalle et al., 2010). As for Thr214 phosphorylation, polyglycylation also appears to be a constitutive PTM of the g14-3-3, although regulated in a timely and stage dependent fashion (Fig. 7). In the early phase of encystation, the polyglycine chain undergoes an average length reduction (but without being

Fig. 7 The g14-3-3 protein in *Giardia*. (A) Subcelluar immunolocalization of the g14-3-3 in *Giardia* trophozoites, encysting parasite (6-12 h) and cyst. Parasites were stained with a rabbit anti-g14-3-3 polyclonal serum (14-3-3), a mouse anti CWP2 mAb (cyst wall protein, CWP) and DAPI. Microphotographs obtained by optical microscopy are also shown. (B) Expression of the g14-3-3 protein in trophozoites (T) and during different time points following encystation induction (6–24 h). Arrows indicate two bands (30 and 32 kDa), representing high and low polyglycylated g14-3-3. (C) Mass spectrometry analysis of affinity purified g14-3-3 from trophozoites (T) or 12 h encysting parasites (12 h). MALDI-MS spectra shows and compares the distribution of glycylated species in the two protein preparations. Polyglycylated peptides (*); the numbers of glycine residues are included. (D) Effect of 14-3-3 point mutants on encystation. Bar graph of the percentage of trophozoites, encysting parasites and cysts in transgenic parasites expressing in FLAG-tagged wild type g14-3-3 and in the g14-3-3 mutants T214A, non-phosphorylatable, and E246A, non-polyglycylatable after 3, 6, 12 and 24 h following encysting induction. The error is expressed as standard deviation. The asterisk denotes statistically significant differences ($P < 0.05$). Panels (A)–(C) *are reprinted and adapted, with permission from research originally published in Journal of Biological Chemistry: Lalle, M., Salzano, A.M., Crescenzi, M., Pozio, E. 2006. The* G. duodenalis *14-3-3 protein is post-translationally modified by phosphorylation and polyglycylation of the C-terminal tail. J. Biol. Chem. 281, 5137–5148 (©) the American Society for Biochemistry and Molecular Biology.* Panel (B) *is reprinted and adapted from Lalle M, Bavassano C, Fratini F, Cecchetti S, Boisguerin P, Crescenzi M, Pozio E. 2010. Involvement of 14-3-3 protein post-translational modifications in* G. duodenalis *encystation. Int. J. Parasitol 40, 201–213.*

completely removed) from 20 down to 10 residues to finally reverts at the original length at the end of the process (Lalle et al., 2006, 2010). The length of the polyglycine chain has been functionally linked to a partial intracellular re-localization of the g14-3-3 during encystation (Fig. 7). In *Giardia* trophozoites, the g14-3-3 is largely cytoplasmatic and excluded from nuclei, but it can be visualized also in the nuclei in early and late encysting cells but not in cysts (Lalle et al., 2006). Indeed, the g14-3-3 holding the mutation E246A is also detectable in the nuclei of trophozoites, cysts as well as encysting parasites, confirming the function of polyglycylation in intracellular localization regulatory mechanism (Lalle et al., 2010). In the proposed model, the C-terminal polyglycine chain acts as a "molecular tie" that keeps the g14-3-3, and eventually its targets, in the cytoplasm without altering the g14-3-3-binding properties (Lalle et al., 2010). However, the evidence that physiologically the g14-3-3 does not exist in unpolyglycylated form, independently from the chain length, suggests an additional role of polyglycylation. Indeed, polyglycylation has been shown to provide a mechanism to prevent the g14-3-3 oligomerization (Fiorillo et al., 2014). Recombinant human isoforms 14-3-3β and 14-3-3ζ migrate as homodimers in native PAGE, whereas recombinant unmodified g14-3-3 easily forms oligomers. This phenomenon does not occur with native polyglycylated g14-3-3 and can be partially prevented by mutating the g14-3-3 to encode an additional stretch of 10 or 20 glycine residues at the C-terminus, thus mimicking both the presence and the length variation of the polyglycine chain during encystation (Fiorillo et al., 2014). Furthermore, the mutants encoding the additional stretch of glycines are also incapable to form fibrils, as observed for the recombinant unmodified g14-3-3 (Fiorillo et al., 2014). Noteworthy, despite Thr214 is located in a region (the hinge of the "closed to open" transition) potentially affecting the flexibility of the g14-3-3 and its oligomerization capability, the phosphomimiking mutant T214E does not affect the aggregation state *in vitro*.

The reason behind the evolutionary conservation of a post-translational modification that potentially "regulates" the g14-3-3 oligomerization is yet unclear but it might indicate that specific unknown function could be performed only by the g14-3-3 in its oligomeric state. Indeed, despite C-terminal swapping, the conformation of the residues involved in the recognition and binding to target motif is conserved in the g14-3-3 structure (Fiorillo et al., 2014). It has been shown that *in vitro* oligomerization of the h14-3-3ζ occurs in presence of arachidonic acid, also known to favour the polymerization of both tau and synuclein (Brock, 2008). A speculative hypothesis is that, ancestral 14-3-3 proteins could experience a C-terminal-mediated oligomerization and that this tendency has been evolutionary regulated in multiple ways; i.e., by post-translational polyglycylation, by encoding a C-terminal polyglutamine stretch (as in the yeast isoforms), or allowing the C-terminus tail to fold within the binding groove in the absence of ligands (as in mammalian and plant 14-3-3).

The enzymes responsible for the addition and removal of the glycine chain to the g14-3-3 have been characterized in *Giardia* (Lalle et al., 2011). Polyglycylation is accomplish by gTTLL3, a member of the tubulin tyrosine ligase-like family, and likely to a minor extent by gTTLL1 (Lalle et al., 2011). Giardial gTTLL3 function, as both initiating and elongating enzyme, is able to catalyse both the addition of the first glycine and the subsequent elongation of the polyglycine chain on the C-terminus of the g14-3-3, and likely tubulin (Lalle et al., 2011). This occurs also in *Drosophila*, where mono- and polyglycylation are accompolished by TTLL3A on tubulin and by TTLL3B on non-tubulin proteins (Rogowski et al., 2009). In vertebrates, polyglycylation occurs by a two-step mechanism requiring the initiating activity of TTLL3/8 enzymes and the elongase activity of TTLL10 (Yu et al., 2015). Intriguingly, despite bi-functional TTLL3 exists both in *Giardia* and *Drosophila*, the g14-3-3 expressed in the fruit fly cannot be polyglycylated whereas Dm14-3-3ε was polyglycylated to a limited extent in *Giardia* background, suggesting that polyglycylation signature can be different between unrelated organisms (Lalle et al., 2013). Deglycylation of the g14-3-3 is performed by two enzymes, gDIP1 and gDIP2, both members of metallopeptidase MH clan, subfamily M20C (Lalle et al., 2011). These enzymes are able to shorten, but not to completely remove, the polyglycine chain of the g14-3-3, and possibly tubulins, both *in vivo* and *in vitro* (Lalle et al., 2011). Individual overexpression in *Giardia* of both enzymes results in a comparable shortening of the g14-3-3 polyglycine chain (as evaluated by MALDI-MS analysis); however, a nuclear re-localization of the g14-3-3 and a lower polyglycine staining in the cytoplasm associate only to the gDIP2 overexpression, suggesting that the latter enzyme has a higher specificity towards the g14-3-3 (Lalle et al., 2011).

4. Multiple biological roles of 14-3-3 in *Giardia*

The significant role of both Thr214 phosphorylation and Glu246 polyglycylation to support a functional g14-3-3 comes from the observation that the unmodified protein is unable to complement *D. melanogaster* deletion mutants for either the endogenous D14-3-3ε or the DLeoII (a 14-3-3ζ isoform) (Lalle et al., 2013). Indeed, the first biological role of g14-3-3 in *Giardia* was discovered studying g14-3-3 mutants defective in each of the two post-translational modifications. An opposite effect on *Giardia* encystation occurs in relation to the polyglycylation and phosphorylation condition of g14-3-3 (Lalle et al., 2010, 2011) (Fig. 7). During the encystation process *Giardia* undergoes extensive remodelling of the cytoskeleton, changes in genome ploidy as well as metabolic adjustments necessary to covert the tear-shaped, binucleate and flagellated trophozoites into an immotile, round and tetra-nucleated cysts. *Co*-expression in *Giardia* of the unphosphorylatable (but polyglycylated) FLAG-tagged T214A mutant decreases the responsiveness of the parasite to *in vitro* encystation stimuli, markedly delays trophozoites differentiation into cysts and results in a higher percentage of cysts with nuclei replication defects. As the phosphorylation positively affects g14-3-3-binding to target proteins, the heterodimerization that occurs between the wild type g14-3-3 and the mutant would overall decrease the binding efficiency with protein involved in encystation as well in DNA replication and/or nuclear division (Lalle et al., 2010). Contrary, a higher responsiveness of parasites to encystation stimuli (as early as 3h post induction), with a faster differentiation of trophozoites into cysts, occurs when the unpolyglycylatable (but phosphorylated) FLAG-tagged E246A mutant is co-expressed (Lalle et al., 2010). The g14-3-3 nuclear localization at trophozoite stage in parasites expressing the E246A mutant has been associated to a promoting effect on encystation. The mutation likely favours an early association of g14-3-3 with nuclear protein or an early nuclear re-localization of g14-3-3 client proteins. Nevertheless, overexpression of any of the two deglycylases in *Giardia* (in particularly gDIP2), despite shorts down the g14-3-3 polyglycine chain, also results in a broad reduction of intracellular polyglycylation level that strongly hampers cyst formation and the expression of the cyst wall proteins (Lalle et al., 2011). The role(s) that polyglycylation plays in *Giardia* encystation is evidently not limited to g14-3-3 and likely affects microtubules dynamics.

In addition to the role of the g14-3-3 in encystation, the general biological relevance of this protein in *Giardia* has been highlighted by conditional knockdown experiments using antisense translation-blocking morpholino (Krtková et al., 2017). In *Giardia* trophozoites, 14-3-3 is a constitutively and highly transcribed gene both *in vitro* and *in vivo* (Pham et al., 2017), with 14-3-3 protein accounting for approximatively 1% of the *Giardia* proteome

(Krtková et al., 2017). Depletion of 14-3-3 transcript, although for a short time, remarkably hampers cell proliferation leading to reduction of parasite growth associated to defects in cell polarity, increment of nuclear size, abnormal flagellar positioning and accumulation of multinucleate cells (Krtková et al., 2017). In agreement with this phenotype and with a general pleiotropic role, g14-3-3 has been detected in the proteomes of different organelles and cellular compartments of *Giardia*, such as encystation specific vesicles (ESV), peripheral vesicles (PV) and mitosome (Jedelský et al., 2011; Wampfler et al., 2014), and basal body enriched fractions (Lauwaet et al., 2011). At transcriptional level, up-regulation of *g14-3-3* gene has been reported in WBC6 isolate early during *in vitro* induced encystation (Einarsson et al., 2016; Lalle et al., 2006; Morf et al., 2010), but also during *in vitro* interaction of Assemblage A and B isolates with intestinal epithelial cell IEC-6 (Ma'ayeh and Brook-Carter, 2012). Quantitative proteomic studies partially overlap with the transcription data. Expression of g14-3-3 protein increases in WBC6 isolate at 4 h following induction of encystation, but it drops down later, as well as in *in vivo* formed cysts (Faso et al., 2013; Lingdan et al., 2012). Protein up-regulation also occurs during *in vitro* interaction of WBC6 with different intestinal epithelial cell lines (Emery et al., 2016). Microvesicles released by *Giardia* trophozoites and encysting parasite have been also described to contain g14-3-3 (Evans-Osses et al., 2017). 14-3-3 proteins are commonly identified in the proteome of exosomes isolated from different sources and associated to exosome-mediate protein secretion and disease induction (Kaplan et al., 2017). Proteomic and transcriptomic data overall support the involvement of *Giardia* 14-3-3 in response to environmental stress (including encystation) as well as in pathogenesis and disease induction. Additionally, by using an antibody against a consensus serine phosphorylated 14-3-3 binding motif, changes in the phosphorylated 14-3-3 substrate network have been observed between isogenic MTZ sensitive *Giardia* strains vs laboratory induced MTZ tolerant stains, without significant changes in the abundance of the majority of potential 14-3-3 substrates (Emery et al., 2018). Although a specific role of g14-3-3 in drug resistance cannot be envisaged (Emery et al., 2018), the reported observation strengthens the involvement of 14-3-3 PPIs in response to stresses.

A further step in deciphering the involvement of g14-3-3 in the wide range of *Giardia* processes come from the characterization of the protein interaction network (interactome) in trophozoites and encysting parasite of the WBC6 isolate (Lalle et al., 2012). 14-3-3-protein complexes formed in *Giardia* were purified by an affinity chromatography approach by means of overexpression of a FLAG-tagged g14-3-3 and protein identification by LC-MS/MS (Lalle et al., 2012). A total of 296 proteins (54% identified with more than one peptide) and 50 proteins (27% assigned with more than one peptide) were identified in the IPs from trophozoites and parasites at 12 h of encystation, respectively, with a subset of 33 proteins common to both datasets (Lalle et al., 2012). Since a significant percentage of identified proteins (24% and 17.5%, respectively) have unknown function or belongs to protein 21.1, a *Giardia* protein family with ankyrin-repeat domains, the significance, if any, of their interaction with g14-3-3 cannot be inferred. Likewise to other described 14-3-3 interactomes (Kjarland et al., 2006), subunits of well characterized and stable multiprotein complexes (i.e. ribosomes) were part of the g14-3-3 interactome, indicating also that indirect interactors were included. Despite these limitations, the characterized 14-3-3 interactome was highly enriched (>90%) in protein containing at least one, or multiple putative 14-3-3-binding motifs if compared with the whole *Giardia* proteome, with >25% of the detected motifs predicted to be within disordered regions, a feature common to most of the 14-3-3 ligands (Bustos, 2012). As the proteome of trophozoites and 12 h encysting parasites do not significantly differ in relative abundance (Faso et al., 2013), the remarkable size difference observed between the two interactomes is likely the result of the overall decrease in protein Ser/Thr phosphorylation level as reported in late encystation (Lalle et al., 2012). However, the intersection with *Giardia* phosphoproteome data, once available, will be necessary to confirm or not the existence of a heavy down-regulation of 14-3-3 targets for phosphorylation during encystation. An equal distribution of proteins into general function/process categories has been reported between the two interactomes, although proteins associated to metabolic and energy-related processes were relatively enriched in the interactome of encysting parasite (Lalle et al., 2012). A significant proportion of proteins experimentally defined as 14-3-3 interactors or affinity purified with 14-3-3 in other organisms were also present in the g14-3-3 interactome, thus confirming that the involvement of 14-3-3 proteins in certain biological processes has been well conserved throughout eukaryotic evolution. However, distinct 14-3-3 targets were not found, either reflecting different regulatory mechanisms or due to the absence of their counterpart in *Giardia*. A clear example of the latter case could be represented by class II histone deacetylases (HDACs) (Paul et al., 2009) absent in *Giardia* (Sonda et al., 2010).

Based on the proteins identified in the g14-3-3 interactome (Lalle et al., 2012) the possible functions of this protein in different biological processes in *Giardia* are presented and discussed in the following sections.

4.1 The g14-3-3 in protein synthesis and degradation

Histones and other proteins turnover can be regulated via lysine ubiquitination. In trophozoites, the g14-3-3 co-purifies with three ubiquitin-E3 ligases (two putative) and two ubiquitin carboxyl-terminal hydrolase, one of them (GL50803_8189) belongs to *Giardia* proteasome, whereas only a different ubiquitin carboxyl-terminal hydrolase was affinity captured during encystation (Lalle et al., 2012). Ubiquitin conjugation requires the ubiquitin-activating enzymes (E1), ubiquitin-conjugating enzymes (E2), and ubiquitin ligases (E3), whereas removal is achieved by specialized deubiquitinating enzymes (DUBs) (Ohtake and Tsuchiya, 2017). Ubiquitination profile of proteins changes during encystation being maximal in trophozoites and minimal late in the process (12–24h) as the result of different availability of the substrates or reduced activity of ubiquitinating enzymes (Niño et al., 2013). Indeed, only histone H2A is ubiquitinated in trophozoites, whereas all histones are modified during encystation (Niño et al., 2013). Interaction of the g14-3-3 with ubiquitination-related enzymes is compatible with a role in influencing both enzyme target specificity and enzyme accessibility to target, by affecting intracellular localization, in particular by regulating the access to the nucleus during encystation. For example, in the signalling cascade that suppresses the non-homologous-end-joining (NHEJ) repairing mechanism for DSBs, 14-3-3β binding to phosphorylated XLF causes XLF cytoplasmic retention and degradation through ubiquitination and proteasome degradation (Liu et al., 2015). Similar, the function of p53 E3 ubiquitin ligase COP1 is prevented by 14-3-3 interaction and sequestration in the cytoplasm following DNA damage signalling (Su et al., 2010). Several human 14-3-3 isoforms can interact and inhibit the phosphorylated deubiquitinating enzyme UBPY/USP8, a regulator of cargo sorting and membrane traffic at early endosomes (Mizuno et al., 2007). Another possibility is that g14-3-3 is itself substrate for ubiquitination. Indeed, both gTTLL3 and gDIP2, known to modify g14-3-3 but to not be its ligands, were present in the g14-3-3 interactome (Lalle et al., 2012). In response to oestrogen-dependent cell proliferation signalling, human 14-3-3σ isoform is targeted by the RING finger-dependent ubiquitin ligase (E3) and directed to proteolysis, thus promoting cell proliferation and releasing the G2 arrest mediated by cytosolic sequestration of cyclin B1-CDC2 complexes bound to 14-3-3 (Urano et al., 2002). Indeed, the same mechanism could be conserved in *Giardia*. In the early phase of encystation (6 h), but not later, the g14-3-3 is polyubiquitinated through the Lys48 residue of ubiquitin and likely targeted to proteasome for degradation (Niño et al., 2013). Noteworthy, exit of *Giardia* trophozoites from canonical cell cycle to differentiate into a cyst takes place in the G2 phase (Reiner et al., 2008).

In addition to the interaction with ubiquitination machinery and similarly to what has been reported in other organisms (Paul et al., 2009), the g14-3-3 seems to be involved in the protein degradation processes as proved by co-purification with subunits of the 19S regulatory cap of the 26S proteasome in trophozoites (Lalle et al., 2012). Conversely, the g14-3-3 seems also involved in protein synthesis. The experimentally defined g14-3-3 network also includes component of the translation machinery, such as subunits of the eukaryotic translational initiation factor 2 (eIF2) and several aminoacyl-tRNA synthetases (Lalle et al., 2012). In mammalian hippocampal neurons, it has been described that the non-phosphorylated form of eEF-2 is efficiently exported in the cytoplasm, where it can support constitutive levels of protein synthesis. On the contrary, it's the phosphorylated form eEF-2 binds to 14-3-3 proteins, although both in the nucleus and cytoplasm, suggesting that 14-3-3 proteins can work in eEF-2 subcellular compartmentalization (Argüelles et al., 2013). In yeast, a suboptimal 14-3-3 protein activity leads to an overall decrease of proteins associated with amino acid synthesis and translation (Bruckmann et al., 2007). Additionally, plant 14-3-3 proteins participate in a phosphorylation-dependent nutrient-sensing pathway controlling the cleavage of many targets including glutamyl-tRNA synthetase (GluRS). 14-3-3-binding protects partners from protease-specific degradation but lost of 14-3-3 interaction under nutrient starvation leads to target degradation to enhance cell survival. Glutamyl-tRNA synthetase, as well as other tRNA synthetases, co-purifies with the g14-3-3 in the trophozoite but not in the encystation stage (Lalle et al., 2012), despite this protein category is enriched in encystation proteome (Faso et al., 2013). Indeed, the parasite in the late encystation stage gets ready to enter dormancy, associated with a down-regulation of genes associated to the translation processes at this stage (Einarsson et al., 2016). In addition to gene down-regulation, it is reasonable to propose that the g14-3-3 could contribute to the gradual decrease of protein synthesis by affecting stability of protein synthesis components, as well as in response to nutrient deprivation eventually occurring in the gut during starving condition.

Autophagy is an evolutionarily conserved and regulated pathway and generally occurs during physiological and pathological processes being critical for microorganisms in response to nutrient starvation and stress. Portions of the cytoplasm become randomly surrounded by a cup-shaped structure formed as a double-membrane that develops in autophagosomes in which, following fusion with lysosomes, sequestered material is digested and then transported back to the cytosol. Nucleation of autophagosomes requires membranes enrichment with phosphatidylinositol 3-phosphate by the activity of the vacuolar membrane-associated class III phosphatidylinositol 3-kinase (PtdIns3K) complex comprising in the core VPS34 (the PtnIns3K) and VPS15 (a Ser/Thr protein kinase), as well as several factors termed AuTophaGy-related proteins, such as ATG6 (Brennand et al., 2011). 14-3-3 proteins can inhibit or promote autophagy at different levels by direct interaction with autophagy-related proteins. In particular, autophagy is inhibited by phosphorylation-dependent sequestration of ATG6 via the formation of the ATG6/14-3-3/vimentin complex or inhibiting phosphatidylinositol 3-kinase activity following 14-3-3 interaction with hVPS34 (Jia et al., 2017). It has been shown that very few genes associate with autophagy are detectable in the *Giardia* genome, including the core components required for initiation of autophagy and expansion of the autophagosome. Further, the parasite lacks many ATG proteins, and nutrient starvation induces in the parasite changes that resemble autophagy, producing punctate staining with monodansylcadaverine (Bagchi et al., 2012; Brennand et al., 2011). Remarkably, the g14-3-3 co-precipitates with both VPS34 and VPS15 in trophozoites (Lalle et al., 2012) strongly suggesting that, under normal condition, control of autophagy by 14-3-3-dependent inhibition of VPS34 activity is conserved in *Giardia*. The fact that such association was missing in encysting parasites, together with the observation that autophagosomal-like vesicles are associated with encystation induction (Maia et al., 2007), indicates the involvement of the g14-3-3 in *Giardia* differentiation into cyst possibly also via autophagy.

4.2 The g14-3-3 in transcription and RNA metabolism

Regulation of gene(s) expression by 14-3-3 proteins is well-documented in different eukaryotes and occurs at different levels. A prominent role of 14-3-3 proteins in transcriptional regulation is supported by the identification of several transcription factors as 14-3-3 binding partners as well as via 14-3-3 interaction with upstream regulators of transcription factors

(Bridges and Moorhead, 2005; de Boer et al., 2013). Although no specific transcriptional factors were found in the g14-3-3 interactome, subunits of the RNA polymerase II complex and elongation factors were co-purified with the g14-3-3, providing evidence of participation in transcriptional process too (Lalle et al., 2012). In yeast, transcriptional regulation in response to glucose depletion occurs via 14-3-3-binding to transcriptional *co*-factor Adr1 which in turn prevents RNA polymerase II preinitiation complex formation, unless the co-regulatory transcriptional factors, either Cat8 or Oaf1/Pip2, is present (Parua et al., 2014). However, the participation of this mechanism in *Giardia* still needs to be proved.

It has been suggested that 14-3-3 proteins can play several roles in regulating P-bodies assembly, maintenance, and/or disassembly. Processing bodies (P-bodies) are dynamic cytoplasmic foci hallmarked for the storage of untranslated mRNA and for mRNA degradation. P-bodies contains factors involved in the mRNA degradative pathway (i.e. mRNA deadenylase, to short the 3′ poly (A) tail, mRNAs decapping enzymes, that remove the 5′ cap, as well as exosome for 3′–5′ degradation 5′–3′ exonuclease), but also components of the AU-rich element- and nonsense-mediated mRNA decay and RNA-mediated silencing pathways (Courchet et al., 2008). The presence of 14-3-3 proteins in P-bodies, as well as interaction of these proteins with components of RNA interference machinery such as DDX6 (Zheng et al., 2011) and Argonaute (Stoica et al., 2006), have been reported. Moreover, binding of 14-3-3 proteins to the enhancer of mRNA decapping complex EDC3 affects its interaction with other protein and results in miRNA-mediated gene silencing inhibition and in altered P-body morphology (Larance et al., 2010). Proteins belonging to the *Giardia* deadenylation machinery (GL50803_96732), the decapping machinery (GL50803_2098) and the nonsense-mediated decay pathway (UPF1-like, GL50803_13452) (Williams and Elmendorf, 2011) were found in the g14-3-3 interactome, together with several proteins ascribable to DEAD/DExH-box RNA helicases (Lalle et al., 2012). RNA helicases catalyse the ATP-dependent separation of double-stranded RNA molecules or displace bound proteins to remodel RNA-protein complexes. The DEAD/DExH-box families of RNA helicases, named based on the four amino acids Asp-Glu-Ala-Asp (DEAD) or Asp-Glu-x-His (DExH) in motif II, have been well studied in several organisms and 32 putative members were detected in *Giardia* (Marchat et al., 2015). Two of the identified RNA helicases in the g14-3-3 trophozoite interactome, namely, GL50803_15048 and GL50803_2098 (Lalle et al., 2012), show homology with *D. melanogaster*

Belle (Bel) DEAD-box RNA helicase and human DDX6 helicase (p54), respectively. It is suggested that these molecules are components of the RNA interference mechanism governing antigenic variation by post-transcriptional silencing in *Giardia* (Gargantini et al., 2012). Binding of the g14-3-3 to these enzymes would likely contribute to regulate antigenic variation, as well as other transcripts. Noteworthy, the *Giardia* upstream frameshift 1 (UPF1) homolog (GL50803_13452) was identified in the g14-3-3 interactome only in encysting parasites (Lalle et al., 2012), suggesting either a stage dependent interaction or the formation of a more stable complex only during encystation. Despite UFP1 is transcribed at trophozoite stage (Einarsson et al., 2016), conflicting results have been reported on the protein expression in trophozoites and encysting parasites (Chen et al., 2008b; Faso et al., 2013). The DEAD-box RNA helicase UPF1 is the central factor in eukaryotic nonsense-mediated mRNA decay (NMD) surveillance pathway. NMD ensures rapid degradation of mRNAs that have acquired premature termination codons, promote translation termination fidelity, and contribute in regulating the abundance of some naturally occurring mRNAs. In *Giardia*, UPF1 has been implicated in regulation of mRNA levels and stability of some naturally occurring mRNAs including encystation-induced genes, *cwp1–3*, and *myb2* (Chen et al., 2008b). Overexpression of UPF1 indeed decreases mRNA level of *cwp1–3* and *myb2*, leading to reduced CWP1 protein level and hampering cyst formation (Chen et al., 2008b). In human cells and in *Caenorhabditis elegans*, phosphorylated UPF1 interacts with SMG5, SMG6, and SMG7, three proteins with an N-terminal 14-3-3-like binding domain. SMG5-SMG7 bind to UPF1 as heterodimers whereas SMG6 bind as monomer. SMG5-SMG7 or SMG6 interaction recruits both protein phosphatase 2A, favouring UPF1 dephosphorylation and NMD activity, and decay factors, such as the CCR4-NOT deadenylase complex (Loh et al., 2013), thus promoting target mRNA degradation (Jonas et al., 2013). Interaction with SMG5/SMG7 and SMG6 homologs has been shown also in yeast, although, Nam7p (the yeast homolog of UFP1) have been identified in a large-scale proteomic analysis of *S. cerevisiae* 14-3-3 interactions (Dehecq et al., 2018). Despite NMD is functional in *Giardia*, no homolog of SMG5, SMG6, and SMG7 has been detected (Williams and Elmendorf, 2011), suggesting that the g14-3-3 could replace their functions in a simplified organism. Indeed, subunits of the protein phosphatase 2A and a putative subunit of the CCR4-NOT deadenylase complex also co-purified with the g14-3-3 (Lalle et al., 2012). If g14-3-3-binding to UPF1 enhances the NMD activity, it is reasonable that the occurrence of g14-3-3/UPF1 interaction during encystation would likely reflect the prerequisite to carefully control the quality and quantity of hiper-transcribed encystation-related genes (i.e. *cwp1–3*).

4.3 The g14-3-3 in cell cycle regulation

Eukaryotic cell cycle has four phases: G1 phase (in which the cell grows, copies organelles and accumulates nutrients needed for next phases), S phase (in which the cell synthesizes a complete copy of nuclear DNA in its nucleus); G2 phase (in which the cell further grows and accumulates proteins needed for cell division); M phase (the mitotic phase, during which the cell divides into two daughter cells). The 14-3-3 proteins play a pivotal role in cell cycle progression and regulation being part of integral components of several checkpoints. In particular, 14-3-3 proteins function in G1/S- and G2/M-transition checkpoints by binding to and modulating the function of several regulatory proteins (Gardino and Yaffe, 2011).

In *Giardia* trophozoites as well as in encysting parasites, the g14-3-3 co-precipitates with gCDC7 (GL50803_112076) and with a highly divergent gDBF4 (GL50803_94117), a Cdc7-regulatory subunit, forming a highly stable ternary complex, thus confirming the occurrence also in *Giardia* of the CDC7-DBF4 kinase complex (Dbf4-Dependent Kinase, DDK) (Lalle et al., 2012). In eukaryotes, DDK regulates the G1/S-transition, in addition to cyclin-dependent kinase, and it is essential for cell cycle progression and in response to DNA damage or replication fork stalling. DDK phosphorylates and activates the Mini-chromosome maintenance protein complex (Mcm2–7 helicases) thus promoting the assembly of the replication forks and their firing controlling DNA replication, chromatin structure and chromosome segregation during mitosis (Labib, 2010). A similar function is expected to occur also in *Giardia*, and indeed, the giardial Mcm3 homolog (GL50803_16210) was detected in the g14-3-3 interactome (Lalle et al., 2012). In eukaryotic cells, the expression level of Cdc7 remains constant throughout the cell cycle whereas the DDK activity increases during S phase following the increase in Dbf4 protein level. In turn Dbf4 protein level is low in G1, increases at the G1/S-transition, and persists at high levels during S phase and then it declines during G2/M (Gómez-Escoda and Wu, 2017). In contrast, both gCDC7 (Lalle et al., 2012) and gDBF4 (https://giardiadb.org/) are constitutively expressed at almost constant level in *Giardia*. Affinity purified gDDK displays both protein kinase and auto-phosphorylation activities *in vitro*, with phosphorylation being reduced in presence of a phosphopeptide that reproduces a mode-1 consensus 14-3-3-binding motif, thus suggesting that protein kinase activity could be regulated via g14-3-3-binding (Marco Lalle et al., unpublished). The interaction with the g14-3-3 likely affects also gDDK intracellular localization. Several potential 14-3-3 binding motifs, mostly outside of the kinase domain, were detected and one of them was located inside a putative nuclear localization signal (NLS) (Lalle et al., 2012). In trophozoites, the gDDK signal is cytosolic and prominently associated to axonemal exit points, or flagellar pores, as supported also by the co-precipitation of gDDK with axonemal proteins (Lalle et al., 2012). Since intracellular localization was detected in asynchronous culture at stationary phase (largely in post-replicative G2 stage) localization of gDDK in nuclei of trophozoites has not been reported (Lalle et al., 2012). On the contrary, re-localization of gDDK from flagellar pores to nuclei was observed in 12h encysting parasites (Lalle et al., 2012), likely because parasite triggered to encystation exits the cell cycle in G2 and replicates again DNA later during the differentiation process, but without a cell division event (endoreplication) (Reiner et al., 2008). The re-localization of gDDK in encysting nuclei is compatible with its function in both DNA replication and chromosome segregation. In budding yeast, preparation of chromosomes for reductional segregation during meiosis I is controlled by DDK (Matos et al., 2008). The nuclear localization of the g14-3-3 following the shortening of polyglycine chain could allow the g14-3-3/gDDK complex to shuttle into the nuclei during encystation. However, g14-3-3-independent nuclear localization of gDDK could not be excluded. The g14-3-3-binding could also mediate assemblage of gDDK into the pre-Replication Complex (pre-RC) promoting the firing of DNA replication origin by activating the replicative MCM helicases. The yeast 14-3-3 isoform Bmh2 binds to Mcm2 and Orc2, two members of the pre-RC and, together with the ORC (Origin Replication Complex) and promotes the MCM proteins binding to replication origins at G1 phase (Yahyaoui and Zannis-Hadjopoulos, 2009). In several proteomic studies, 14-3-3 proteins were also found to interact directly with replication-initiation proteins, including mammalian Mcm3, Mcm5 and Mcm10 (Pozuelo Rubio et al., 2004). A recently developed method to obtain synchronized *Giardia* trophozoites without the use of cell cycle blocking drugs (Horlock-Roberts et al., 2017) might help in defining the dynamics and exact significance of g14-3-3/gDDK complex in different cell cycle steps.

An indication of a role of the g14-3-3 in the regulation of the G2/M checkpoint in *Giardia* is supported by the identification of homologs of the dual specificity protein phosphatase CDC14A (GL50803_9270), the G2/M-specific cyclin B (GL50803_3977) and a CDK2 (cdc28/cdc2) protein kinase (GL50803_16802). The G2/M-transition is generally regulated by 14-3-3 proteins via binding to phosphorylated and inactive phosphatase CDC25C and sequestration of the complex in the cytoplasm. This results in an increased Cdk1(cdc2) phosphorylation that reduces protein kinase activity and inhibits mitotic entry (Gardino and Yaffe, 2011). Additionally, 14-3-3 proteins also bind and stimulate the activity of Wee1 kinase that in turn inactivates the cdc2-cyclin B1 complex by tyrosine phosphorylation (Gardino and Yaffe, 2011). A third mechanism has been associated only to mammalian 14-3-3σ. This isoform prevents cells from entering mitosis by sequestering the cyclin-dependent kinase cdc2/cyclin B1 complex in cytoplasm (Laronga et al., 2000). Noteworthy, *Giardia* CDK2 localizes in trophozoites at plasma membrane, basal bodies and cytoplasmic axonemes, supporting a g14-3-3-mediated CDK2 compartmentalization. It has been also observed that in *Giardia*, in the absence of an anaphase-promoting complex (APC), degradation of cyclin B at the metaphase-anaphase transition and progression through mitosis, is mediated by direct phosphorylation of cyclin B or cyclin interacting proteins (Gourguechon et al., 2013). However, it cannot be ruled out that g14-3-3-mediated degradation of cyclin B may occur in *Giardia*.

Further, regulation of mitosis could be achieved in *Giardia* by g14-3-3/CDC14 interaction. In the yeast *S. pombe*, the 14-3-3 isoform Rad24 promotes mitotic exit and cytokinesis in late mitosis through the binding and the cytosolic retention of Clp1, a member of the Cdc14-family phosphatases that dephosphorylates substrates of cyclin-dependent kinase (Chen et al., 2008a,b). The absence of canonical cell cycle regulators among the g14-3-3 interactors suggests either the existence of divergent checkpoints or a less stringent control of the cell cycle in *Giardia*. The occurrence of defective cell cycle checkpoint in *Giardia*, or the existence of mechanism able to overcome checkpoints, is supported by the observation that the arrest of DNA synthesis does not impair cell growth and defective spindles and double-stranded DNA breaks do not prevent enter in mitosis (Horlock-Roberts et al., 2017).

4.4 The g14-3-3 in protein trafficking and vesicular transport

The participation of the g14-3-3 in protein trafficking and vesicular transport in *Giardia* trophozoites is strongly supported by co-precipitation with multiple proteins involved in nucleo-cytoplasmic shuttling, membrane fusion and vesicle transport (Lalle et al., 2012). In particular, subunits of the coatomer complexes COPI and COPII, functioning in higher eukaryotes in ER-to-Golgi transport, the adaptor protein complex AP2, involved in endocytosis, RABs, such as Rab11, belonging to the Ras superfamily of small GTP-binding proteins, and guanine-nucleotide exchange factors (GEFs), and components of the endosomal sorting complex required for transport II (ESCRT-II). Despite a number of high throughput 14-3-3 interactome studies that recognize many different components of the vesicular transport machinery, including coat components and motor proteins, GEFs and GTPase-activating proteins (GAPs) associated to Arf and Rab GTPases, the direct protein binding to 14-3-3 and the functional role of the interaction remain elusive (Mrowiec and Schwappach, 2006). The binding of 14-3-3 proteins to cargo proteins mediates transport of a number of multimeric membrane proteins from ER-to-Golgi. The correct assembly of multimers is sensed by 14-3-3 proteins, that in turn prevent COPI binding to the cargo protein for anterograde transport and lead to proper export to the plasma membrane (Smith et al., 2011). Despite the lack of a proper Golgi apparatus, *Giardia* possesses a complex system for protein and vesicles trafficking cantered on the ER network (Faso and Hehl, 2011), as well as a complex microtubule (MT) cytoskeleton that is of critical importance and deeply involved in intracellular protein trafficking. In *Giardia* trophozoites the synthesis and export to plasma membrane (PM) of transmembrane-anchored variant surface antigens (VSPs) and cysteine-rich, non-variable protein, constitute a major part of the secretory activity, whereas export of CWPs to membrane is predominant during encystation. Intriguingly, without a Golgi complex, ER exit sites (ERES) have been identified as the sites in which protein sorting occurs and the Sec23, a component of the COPII complex, localize in the ERES (Touz and Zamponi, 2017). Since Sec23 is included in the g14-3-3 interactome, this result strengthens the involvement of the g14-3-3 in the early event of protein sorting. In mammalian cells has been proven that 14-3-3 serves as an adaptor protein for export from the ER of SAC1, and possibly other client proteins, simultaneously interacting with the COPII sorting subunit, Sec24, and the cargo protein (Bajaj Pahuja et al., 2015).

In *Giardia*, Rab GTPases are essentially involved in the vesicle trafficking machinery. Rab2 localizes in the ER, in the PVs and at the membrane level of the ESVs during encystation, whereas Rab11 participate in ESVs transport in accordance with its co-localization with ESVs and actin microfilaments during encystation. Remarkably, depletion of 14-3-3 proteins in *Trypanosoma brucei* reduces the size of the Rab11-positive recycling endosome compartment negatively affecting the return rate of recycling Variant Surface Glycoprotein to the plasma membrane surface (Benz et al., 2010). In *C. elegans*, the 14-3-3 isoform Par5 is necessary to maintain the apical polarity of Rab11-positive recycling endosomes by acting as regulatory for a cell polarity-protein network including F-actin. Such interactions are critical to maintain the low net levels of F-actin and other apical domain components at the basolateral cortex (Winter et al., 2012).

ESCRT is a membrane remodelling machinery made of multiprotein complexes (ESCRT-0–III and Vps4 complex) sequentially recruited to plasma membrane to induce the negative curvature of the membrane, promote membrane evagination and then its removal. Among the several functions, they are required for transmembrane proteins sorting into vacuole lumen, autophagy, and biogenesis of MVB, exosomes and ectosomes. *Giardia* encodes one of the simplest but functional ESCRT machinery that compared with other eukaryotes is composed of fewer subunits and lacks ESCRT-0 and I (Saha et al., 2018). In a protein-protein interaction assay using high-density protein microarray, Vps22 of ESCRT-II directly interacted with h14-3-3ε protein, although the functional role of this remains unclear (Satoh et al., 2006).

4.5 The g14-3-3 in cytoskeleton dynamic

In addition to proteins involved in trafficking, components of the *Giardia* cytoskeleton, tubulins, actin, plus-end and minus-end motor proteins (kinesin, dynein) and intraflagellar transport machinery (IFT complexes) have been detected in the g14-3-3 interactome (Lalle et al., 2012). This provide evidence that the g14-3-3 could orchestrate a coordinated bidirectional motility of cargo proteins and coated vesicle along the cellular microtubules. Indeed, the g14-3-3 knockdown induce polarity and cytokinesis defects, confirming that the g14-3-3 has a pivotal roles in regulating both actin and tubulin cytoskeletal organization (Krtková et al., 2017). Tubulins complexes with 14-3-3 proteins have been widely reported (Paul et al., 2009; Pozuelo Rubio et al., 2004). It has been suggested that the binding of 14-3-3 to microtubule associated proteins (MAPs) and several microtubule associated proteins kinases (MARKs) affect the rate of microtubule assembly.

It has been reported that 14-3-3 protein bind and regulate kinesins in different way. In mammals, kinesin KIF1C involved in the retrograde vesicle transport from the Golgi- to the ER and binds to 14-3-3 proteins in a phosphorylation-dependent fashion (Dorner et al., 1999). Meiosis in *Drosophila* oocyte is partially and spatially regulated via 14-3-3-binding to the kinesin-14 like Ncd to prevent its association with microtubules far from the meiotic spindle. In proximity of the meiotic spindle 14-3-3-binding is abrogate by Ncd hyper-phosphorylation, thus directing Ncd to bind specifically to spindle microtubules (Beaven et al., 2017). More direct evidences on the nature of 14-3-3-actin interaction (Krtková et al., 2017) show that actin was identified in different proteomic studies as 14-3-3 interactor (Paul et al., 2009) and interaction between the g14-3-3 and actin in *Giardia* has been reported in two independent proteomic studies (Lalle et al., 2012; Paredez et al., 2014). In mammals, 14-3-3 proteins regulate actin through the phosphorylation-dependent sequestration of the actin-depolymerizing protein cofilin (Gohla and Bokoch, 2002). 14-3-3 isoforms participate in the remodelling of the actin cytoskeleton in the priming phase of exocytosis (Chamberlain et al., 1995). In breast cancer cells, upregulated 14-3-3σ isoform forms a complex with actin and intermediate filament proteins that sequesters soluble actin in a bioavailable form that is used for directional assembly of the cytoskeleton during cell migration (Boudreau et al., 2013). In *Giardia*, actin assembly to specific subcellular regions is regulated by the g14-3-3, as g14-3-3 knockdown results in short actin filaments dispersed throughout the cell with loss of the typical actin organization. Increased actin phosphorylation, following phosphatase inhibitor treatment, destabilizes the actin network and promotes complex formation with the g14-3-3. Conversely, low phosphorylation stabilizes actin filaments and decreases g14-3-3-association (Krtková et al., 2017). Noteworthy, Rho GTPase signalling by the sole *Giardia* Rac modulates the g14-3-3-actin complex formation. Induction of a constitutive active gRac results in reduced association of the g14-3-3 and actin, and to actin filament stabilization (Krtková et al., 2017). Despite of the fact that several 14-3-3-binding consensus motifs centred on pSer have been detected in *Giardia* actin, mutation of single or multiple of them only partially affects 14-3-3 complex formation. Furthermore, overlay assays and native gels do not provide evidence for a direct interaction between g14-3-3 and actin (Krtková et al., 2017). In the absence of canonical actin-binding proteins such as cofilin, regulation of actin by the g14-3-3 in *Giardia* is likely involves intermediate proteins, not yet identified, to support a phosphorylation-dependent 14-3-3/actin complex formation (Krtková et al., 2017). Actin-associated protein, such as TCP-1, TIP49, SMC domain protein and dynein heavy-chain, could mediate actin/g14-3-3 complex formation. Overall, g14-3-3 regulates monomeric vs filamentous actin homeostasis, as well as partitioning of actin in different complexes for sub functionalization (Krtková et al., 2017).

4.6 The g14-3-3 in metabolism

From yeast to humans, 14-3-3 proteins have been shown to be heavily involved in multiple signalling pathways that modulate cellular energy and nutrient homeostasis. In accordance with this, key enzymes of the glycolytic/gluconogenetic pathway and of the pyruvate metabolism have been identified in the g14-3-3 interactome, thus highlighting a role of the g14-3-3 in energy metabolism (Lalle et al., 2012). *Giardia* relies on both fermentative metabolism and arginine catabolism via arginine dehydrolase as source of energy, as no functional mitochondria are present (Adam, 2001). Carbohydrates, including glucose, are the main carbon sources and, depending on oxygen concentration, are incompletely catabolized to acetate, ethanol, alanine, and CO_2 (Adam, 2001). Three enzymes of the metabolism of glucose to phosphoenolpyruvate, namely, glucokinase (GL50803_8826), fructose-bisphosphate aldolase (GL50803_11043), glyceraldehyde 3-phosphate dehydrogenase (GL50803_6687) co-purify with the g14-3-3, with fructose-bisphosphate aldolase being confirmed also by reverse co-immunoprecipitation (Lalle et al., 2012). Direct modulation of metabolic enzymes function by 14-3-3 proteins has been reported. A general role of 14-3-3 proteins in down-regulation of carbohydrate metabolism has been observed in plants and in yeast *S. cerevisiae* (Bruckmann et al., 2007; Zuk et al., 2005). If a similar negative regulation of carbohydrates metabolism by the g14-3-3 also occurs in *Giardia* cannot yet be ruled out. Conversely, g14-3-3-interaction with enzyme working almost sequentially could promote the formation of a multiproteins complex thus favouring glycolysis. Enzymes involved in the glycogen synthesis are also present in the g14-3-3 interactome, the glycogen synthase (GL50803_104031) and the homolog of glycogen synthase kinase 3 (GL50803_17625) in encysting parasites and trophozoites interactome, respectively, and the UTP-glucose-1-phosphate uridylyltransferase (GL50803_29307) in both interactomes (Lalle et al., 2012). In mammals, insulin stimulates glucose uptake and its storage as glycogen by the protein kinase AKT pathways. In turn, AKT mediates phosphorylation-dependent inactivation of glycogen synthase kinase 3 (GSK3), which is a suppressor of the glycogen synthesis. Ser9 phosphorylation of GSK3b is a docking site for 14-3-3 proteins (Kleppe et al., 2011). *Giardia* synthesizes and stores glycogen during logarithmic phases of growth and uses it in late growth phase, and glycogen synthesis increases in early encystation and then diminishes throughout the transition to the cyst form (Pradhan et al., 2012). This could be in agreement with a g14-3-3-mediated inhibition of GSK3 in growing *Giardia* trophozoites. On the contrary in human cells, dephosphorylation of glycogen synthase by protein phosphatase 1 (PP1) stimulates glycogen synthesis and it is mediated by 14-3-3-binding to PPI subunits (Rubio-Villena et al., 2015).

In *Giardia* the synthesis of phosphoenolpyruvate and pyruvate, the intermediate products of carbohydrate metabolism, occupy a central node at the crossroads of several metabolic pathways. Noteworthy, the acetyl-coenzyme A (CoA) synthase (ADP forming) (gACD, GL50803_13608) interacts with g14-3-3, as supported by reverse co-precipitation experiments (Lalle et al., 2012). In *Giardia*, gACD can provide ATP via substrate-level phosphorylation thus forming acetate and function in CoA recycling but it can also function in the reverse direction for acetate utilization (acetyl-CoA + ADP + Pi $\rightleftharpoons$ acetate + ATP + CoA) (Sánchez et al., 2000). Alanine aminotransferase (GL50803_16363) catalyses the conversion of pyruvate in alanine as the end product under strictly anaerobic condition (Adam, 2001). Since the balance of end product formation in *Giardia* is sensitive to both O_2 tension and glucose concentration in the medium, it is reasonably advantageous to post-translationally regulate two of the terminal enzymes by g14-3-3-interaction, to quickly respond to environmental changes, as those occurring in the host gut. A further way in which the g14-3-3 could affect glucose metabolism during encystation is suggested by the identification in the interactome of encystating parasites of phosphoacetylglucosamine mutase (GL50803_16069) (Lalle et al., 2012). Phosphoacetylglucosamine mutase is one of the enzymes in the pathway for the synthesis of N-acetylgalactosamine, the major carbohydrate portion of the cyst wall. Despite the protein expression of all the enzymes that make up the N-acetylgalactosamine pathway, as well as those for the CWPs, is up-regulated during encystation, phosphoacetylglucosamine mutase was the only one identified and confirmed by immunoblot experiments (Lalle et al., 2012).

Giardia lacks pyrimidine synthetic pathways and depends on salvage pathways for obtaining both purine and pyrimidine nucleosides (Adam, 2001). Also enzymes of the pyrimidine salvage pathways are potentially targeted and regulated by the g14-3-3 (Lalle et al., 2012)

Giardia actively imports phosphatidylcholine (PC) and lyso-phosphatidylcholine (PC) from the external environment and can efficiently convert these molecules into various downstream lipids (Yichoy et al., 2011). Evidence are also emerging that the g14-3-3 can participate in lipid metabolism in *Giardia* (Lalle et al., 2012). In particular, the association of the g14-3-3 and the unusual FAD-dependent glycerol-3-phosphate dehydrogenase (gG3PD, GL50803_16125) have been partially characterized (Lalle et al., 2015). The gG3PD catalyses the (inter) convertion of glycerol-3-phosphate (g3p) to dihydroxyacetone phosphate (DHAP) with the simultaneous reduction of FAD to FADH2 and with the electron transfer to an unknown final acceptor protein. In *Giardia* trophozoites, the gG3PD localizes to the ventral plasma membrane where, similarly to bacteria, is part of a putative functional glycerol biosynthetic pathway able to sustain energy metabolism providing an extra source of DHAP for glycolysis and reducing equivalents to putative electron transfer chain (Lalle et al., 2015). The source of g3p, the substrate of gG3PD could derive from PC catabolism by combined activity of *Giardia* encoded phospholipase PLB and a putative GPC-PDE (Morrison et al., 2007). Complex formation with the g14-3-3 mainly occurs at the trophozoite stage and has been linked to gG3PD localization to plasma membrane (Lalle et al., 2015). Despite several gG3PD mutants in putative g14-3-3-binding motif have been produced, the interaction mechanism has not been clarified, thus leaving still open the possibility that both proteins are present in a multiprotein complex (Lalle et al., 2015). However, a relationship between the g14-3-3 and gG3PD localization and, likely, its enzymatic activity, have been suggested by the reduced gG3PD enzymatic activity associate with a reduced co-precipitation with the g14-3-3 and the partial re-localization of gG3PD to mitosomes during encystation.

In *Giardia*, it is reasonable to propose that energy metabolism can be regulated in a coordinate manner in response to glucose (and other nutrients), ATP and oxygen level and this is orchestrated by the g14-3-3. Identification in the g14-3-3 interactome of homologs of α, β and γ subunits of the V-ATPase further supports this scenario. Biosynthetic pathways can be heavy users of ATP and, in a number of organisms, mitochondrial and chloroplastic ATP synthases have been reported to bound to and be regulated by 14-3-3 that can indeed act as a molecular switcher from ATP synthesis to ATP hydrolysis (Bunney et al., 2001). Protein classified as AMPK homolog subunits (α subunit, GL50803_16034 and γ subunit, GL50803_3414) and CaMKK are present in the g14-3-3 interactome, suggesting an additional level of the 14-3-3 protein in integrate and control the energy metabolism in *Giardia* (Lalle et al., 2012). The heterotrimeric AMPKs (α, β, γ subunits) are energy sensor that detect cellular AMP/ATP ratio and are activated by AMP binding to γ subunits and phosphorylation by an upstream AMPK Kinase. AMPKs ensure the maintenance of ATP balance during energy metabolism inhibiting glycogen, fatty acid, and protein synthesis and enhancing glucose/fatty uptake, mitochondrial metabolism, and cellular autophagy (Ke et al., 2018). The calcium/calmodulin-dependent protein kinase kinases family, CaMKKs, are involved in glucose homeostasis and are, among others, upstream activator of AMPKs. Protein kinase activity of both AMPKs and CaMKKs can be modulated upon 14-3-3-binding as proven in *D. melanogaster* and in mammals (Benton et al., 2002; Psenakova et al., 2018)

5. The g14-3-3 druggability (g14-3-3 as a potential target for antigiardial drugs)

Protein-protein interactions (PPIs) have long been regarded as "no drug targets" because the surfaces involved in PPIs are generally wide and lack cavities. However, the presence of "hot spots" in most PPI interfaces, i. e., residues that make a major contribution to the binding energy, implies the presence of restricted sites that are critical for the interaction, supporting the feasibility of targeting PPIs. Therefore, in the last years, the modulation of PPIs has emerged as a new and promising resource in drug development (Mullard, 2012; Stevers et al., 2018). Expanding the knowledge in the field of 14-3-3 proteins as well as in 14-3-3/ligand interactions is emerging as an important starting point in drug discovery process to develop new anti-parasitic therapeutic approaches (Stevers et al., 2018).

The first inhibitor described for 14-3-3 PPIs was the peptide R18, identified by phage display experiments, with a high affinity for virtually all 14-3-3 isoforms and the ability to abolish 14-3-3 interaction with Raf-1 protein kinase (Petosa et al., 1998). The R18 core sequence, WLDLE, fulfil the amphipathic character of the binding groove by establishing both salt bridges and extensive hydrophobic interactions. The longer peptide difopein, containing two tandem repeats of R18, is indeed capable, once overexpressed in transfected cancer cell to induce pro-apoptotic activity (Masters and Fu, 2001). However, the limit of these molecules resides in their inability to penetrate the cell membranes. Regarding the use of stabilizers of 14-3-3 interactions, initial studies were done with fusicoccin A (FC-A), a diterpenoid glycoside produced by the phytopathogenic fungus

Phomopsis amygdali. The toxin strongly stabilizes the binary complex between 14-3-3 proteins and the regulatory domain of the plasma membrane H+-ATPase (PMA), causing the irreversible opening of stomata and plant wilting (Oecking et al., 1994). The stabilizing effect of FC-A is although limited to 14-3-3 interaction with mode-3 binding motif as the short C-terminal phosphomotif occupies only part of the 14-3-3 binding groove, thus leaving a cavity filled by PC-A (Würtele et al., 2003). Further studies have shown that many natural and semisynthetic active fusicoccanes can be active even on human 14-3-3 proteins (Andrei et al., 2018). Intriguingly, cotylenin A, a molecule closely related to FC-A, possess a broader stabilizing effect on 14-3-3 interaction with all consensus motifs, thus exerting an anti-cancer activity (Ottmann et al., 2009). These remarkable results opened the way to the discovery of 14-3-3 PPI modulators through various approaches, such as *in vitro* or in silico screening of chemical libraries and rational design of peptides and peptidomimetics derived from natural binding motifs (for extensive review see Stevers et al., 2018). As a result, several small molecules, natural products, peptides and peptidomimetics able to both inhibit and stabilize specific 14-3-3 protein complexes have been developed (Fig. 8).

In the case of anti-parasitic drugs, a promising target must be critical for parasite growth or survival and sufficiently different from host homologue in order to allow specific activity of the drug and minimize its side effects. *Giardia* 14-3-3 potentially fulfils all these requirements: the protein has been shown to be critical for parasite survival (Krtková et al., 2017; Lalle et al., 2010) and its structure, extensively characterized and described above (Cau et al., 2015; Fiorillo et al., 2014). Druggability of the g14-3-3 is supported by the positive results obtained in define human 14-3-3 PPI modulator. On the other hand, the similarity between the target (parasite protein) and the off-targets (host homologues) can be a disadvantage in the case of anti-infective drugs, making difficult the identification of highly selective drugs and increasing the probability of unwanted secondary effects. Structure-based drug discovery is one of the most diffused approaches to overcome such limitation although it strongly relies on a deep characterization of target 3-D structure, followed by the selection and validation of lead compounds through *in vitro* or in silico techniques. The structural analysis performed on the g14-3-3 protein highlighted some peculiarities that provide a concrete possibility to target specifically this protein. Structural characterization, described above, shows that client binding of 14-3-3 proteins relies on a "primary interaction" due to a core of highly conserved residues

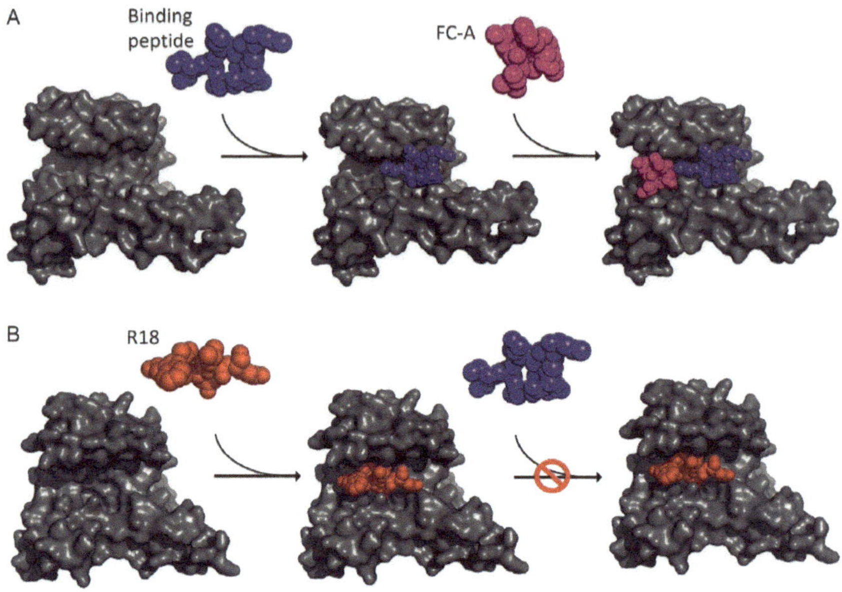

Fig. 8 Modulation of 14-3-3s interaction. (A) fusicoccin (FC-s) stabilizes interaction between 14-3-3 and target proteins containing mode-3 binding motif (e.g. potassium channel subfamily K or plant plasma membrane H^+-ATPase) since it is able to bind a hydrophobic pocket that arises upon mode-3 peptides binding. (B) R18 inhibits partners binding by occupying the middle of the binding cleft and competing with 14-3-3 binding to protein targets. The scheme is based on the structures of human 14-3-3σ in complex with TASK-3 (potassium channel subfamily K) peptide and FC-A (pdb 3p1q, (A)) and human 14-3-3ζ in complex with R18 peptide (pdb 1A38, (B)).

directly interacting with the phosphopeptide followed by rearrangements involving more plastic regions that contribute to the formation of specific contacts. Subtle differences in these "secondary interactions" among human and *Giardia* 14-3-3 could be decisive in developing selective modulators.

Many observations point to a critical role of the α8-α9 loop, in partners binding and recognition (Obsil et al., 2001; Yang et al., 2006). In the case of the g14-3-3, constitutive phosphorylation occurs just on α8-α9 loop and the phosphomimetic mutation Thr214Glu has been shown to affect *in vitro* the binding affinity towards a subset of synthetic phosphopeptides, reproducing known 14-3-3 binding sequences of human and *Drosophila* proteins (Lalle et al., 2010). Computational studies aimed at modelling the interaction of selected peptides with g14-3-3 also support a critical role for α8-α9 loop phosphorylation in partner binding (Cau et al., 2015). In fact, phosphopeptides endowed with balanced hydrophobic/hydrophilic character have shown, at least in silico, a high electrostatic complementarity with the "closed" conformation of g14-3-3, thus highlighting the key structural role of Thr214 phosphorylation as well as its phosphomimetic mutation in binding. Moreover, in the case of peptide CDC25C$_{S216}$, a direct interaction occurs between the phosphate group of Thr214 and a residue with a positive net charge in the target peptide, such as the arginine at position +7 (Fig. 9). This "hot-spot" in PPI interface of g14-3-3 could represent a specific feature relevant to the design of small molecules selectively acting on g14-3-3, opening up to the concrete possibility to design innovative antigiardial drugs.

An intriguing possibility would be to target the phosphorylated Thr214 residue thus introducing a steric hindrance that would hamper the target binding. Indeed, molecular tweezer (a synthetic U-shaped receptors molecule with aromatic side walls) has been design to bind human 14-3-3σ at Lys 214, located at the beginning of the helix α9 and facing the central binding channel, proving inhibitory effect on 14-3-3 binding to two clients (Bier et al., 2013). However, molecular tweezers to target selectively negative charged residues have not yet been designed.

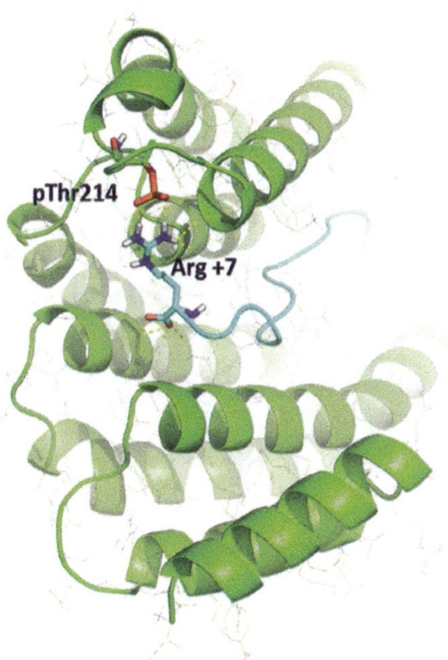

Fig. 9 Interaction of phosphorylated g14-3-3 with the peptide CDC25C-S216. Arginine residue directly interacting with pThr214 is shown. *Reprinted and adapted with permission from Cau, Y., Fiorillo, A., Mori, M., Ilari, A., Botta, M., Lalle, M. 2015. Molecular dynamics simulations and structural analysis of* Giardia duodenalis *14-3-3 protein-protein interactions. J. Chem. Inf. Model 55, 2611–2622. Copyright 2015 American Chemical Society.*

To date, a selective molecule targeting g14-3-3 is still far to be identified. Once 14-3-3 consensus binding sequences will be experimentally defined in naturally occurring g14-3-3 client proteins, a depth characterization, at structural and biochemical level, of g14-3-3 in complexes with corresponding phosphopeptides (or eventually with larger portion of the client proteins) will provide further outcomes elements for approaching the structure-guided design of g14-3-3 targeting modulators.

6. Concluding remarks

After decades of intense research, the definition of the complexity and the biological meaning, both in physiological and in pathological conditions, of the interaction networks established by the 14-3-3 proteins in human and in model organisms has just started. However, the knowledge of the single 14-3-3 protein in the deep-branching protozoan parasite *Giardia* is still limited. Nevertheless, more and more evidences are accumulating on the central role of giardial 14-3-3 as a master regulator in multiple processes. However, future studies are needed to define, at mechanistic and functional levels, the interactions of the g14-3-3 with other proteins, as well as to evaluate the impact of multiple stimuli, other than encystation, on the g14-3-3 interactome. Furthermore, according to the "guilty by association" principle, identification of the different g14-3-3-containing complexes can help to predict the function of the wide amount of proteins of *Giardia* yet classified as "unknown protein function." Even more relevant is to assess the role of the g14-3-3 in the pathogenesis of giardiasis taking advantage of new available tools to manipulate genetically the parasite and of *in vitro* and *in vivo* models of *Giardia*-host-parasite interaction. Finally, the unique structural features of the g14-3-3 together with the existence of *Giardia*-specific 14-3-3 PPIs offer the basis for the discovery of compounds able to modulate selectively such interaction, thus these can be considered as new targets for new antigiardial drugs.

Acknowledgements

We are sincerely grateful to all the colleagues (particularly to Serena Cecchetti and Serena Camerini, from Istituto Superiore di Sanità, Italy, and Anna Maria Salzano and Andrea Ilari, from National Research Council of Italy) and to the students that with their work, expertise, enthusiasm and perseverance have provided substantial contribution to collate, during the years, the knowledge presented herein.

References

Adam, R.D., 2001. Biology of *Giardia lamblia*. Clin. Microbiol. Rev. 14, 447–475.

Aitken, A., 2006. 14-3-3 proteins: a historic overview. Semin. Cancer Biol. 16, 162–172.

Aitken, A., 2011. Post-translational modification of 14-3-3 isoforms and regulation of cellular function. Semin. Cell Dev. Biol. 22, 673–680.

Alblova, M., Smidova, A., Docekal, V., Vesely, J., Herman, P., Obsilova, V., Obsil, T., 2017. Molecular basis of the 14-3-3 protein-dependent activation of yeast neutral trehalase Nth1. Proc. Natl. Acad. Sci. U. S. A. 114, E9811–E9820.

Allain, T., Amat, C.B., Motta, J.P., Manko, A., Buret, A.G., 2017. Interactions of Giardia sp. with the intestinal barrier: epithelium, mucus, and microbiota. Tissue Barriers 5, e1274354.

Alvarado, M.E., Wasserman, M., 2010. Analysis of phosphorylated proteins and inhibition of kinase activity during Giardia intestinalis excystation. Parasitol Int. 59 (1), 54–61.

Andrei, S.A., de Vink, P., Sijbesma, E., Han, L., Brunsveld, L., Kato, N., Ottmann, C., Higuchi, Y., 2018. Rationally designed semisynthetic natural product analogues for stabilization of 14-3-3 protein-protein interactions. Angew. Chem. Int. Ed. Engl. 57, 13470–13474.

Ankarklev, J., Jerlström-Hultqvist, J., Ringqvist, E., Troell, K., Svärd, S.G., 2010. Behind the smile: cell biology and disease mechanisms of Giardia species. Nat. Rev. Microbiol. 8, 413–422.

Argüelles, S., Camandola, S., Hutchison, E.R., Cutler, R.G., Ayala, A., Mattson, M.P., 2013. Molecular control of the amount, subcellular location, and activity state of translation elongation factor 2 in neurons experiencing stress. Free Radic. Biol. Med. 61, 61–71.

Argüello-Garciá, R., Bazán-Tejeda, M.L., Ortega-Pierres, G., 2009. Encystation commitment in *Giardia duodenalis*: a long and winding road. Parasite 16, 247–258.

Bagchi, S., Oniku, A.E., Topping, K., Mamhoud, Z.N., Paget, T.A., 2012. Programmed cell death in Giardia. Parasitology 139, 894–903.

Bajaj Pahuja, K., Wang, J., Blagoveshchenskaya, A., Lim, L., Madhusudhan, M.S., Mayinger, P., Schekman, R., 2015. Phosphoregulatory protein 14-3-3 facilitates SAC1 transport from the endoplasmic reticulum. Proc. Natl. Acad. Sci. U. S. A. 112, E3199–E3206.

Beaven, R., Bastos, R.N., Spanos, C., Romé, P., Cullen, C.F., Rappsilber, J., Giet, R., Goshima, G., Ohkura, H., 2017. 14-3-3 regulation of Ncd reveals a new mechanism for targeting proteins to the spindle in oocytes. J. Cell Biol. 216, 3029–3039.

Benton, R., Palacios, I.M., St Johnston, D., 2002. Drosophila 14-3-3/PAR-5 is an essential mediator of PAR-1 function in axis formation. Dev. Cell 3, 659–671.

Benz, C., Engstler, M., Hillmer, S., Clayton, C., 2010. Depletion of **14-3-3 proteins** in bloodstream-form Trypanosoma brucei inhibits variant surface glycoprotein recycling. Int. J. Parasitol. 40 (5), 629–634.

Bier, D., Rose, R., Bravo-Rodriguez, K., Bartel, M., Ramirez-Anguita, J.M., Dutt, S., Wilch, C., Klarner, F.G., Sanchez-Garcia, E., Schrader, T., Ottmann, C., 2013. Molecular tweezers modulate 14-3-3 protein-protein interactions. Nat. Chem. 5, 234–239.

Boudreau, A., Tanner, K., Wang, D., Geyer, F.C., Reis-Filho, J.S., Bissell, M.J., 2013. 14-3-3 sigma stabilizes a complex of soluble actin and intermediate filament to enable breast tumor invasion. Proc. Natl. Acad. Sci. U. S. A. 110, E3937–E3944.

Brennand, A., Gualdrón-López, M., Coppens, I., Rigden, D.J., Ginger, M.L., Michels, P.A., 2011. Autophagy in parasitic protists: unique features and drug targets. Mol. Biochem. Parasitol. 177, 83–99.

Bridges, D., Moorhead, G.B., 2005. 14-3-3 proteins: a number of functions for a numbered protein. Sci. STKE 2005 (296), re10.

Brock, T.G., 2008. Arachidonic acid binds 14-3-3zeta, releases 14-3-3zeta from phosphorylated BAD and induces aggregation of 14-3-3zeta. Neurochem. Res. 33, 801–807.

Bruckmann, A., Hensbergen, P.J., Balog, C.I., Deelder, A.M., de Steensma, H.Y., van Heusden, G.P., 2007. Post-transcriptional control of the *Saccharomyces cerevisiae* proteome by 14-3-3 proteins. J. Proteome Res. 6, 1689–1699.

Bunney, T.D., van Walraven, H.S., de Boer, A.H., 2001. 14-**3-3** protein is a regulator of the mitochondrial and chloroplast ATP synthase. Proc. Natl. Acad. Sci. U S A 98 (7), 4249–4254.

Bustos, D.M., 2012. The role of protein disorder in the 14-3-3 interaction network. Mol. Biosyst. 8, 178–184.

Cacciò, S.M., Lalle, M., Svärd, S.G., 2018. Host specificity in the *Giardia duodenalis* species complex. Infect. Genet. Evol. 66, 335–345.

Cau, Y., Fiorillo, A., Mori, M., Ilari, A., Botta, M., Lalle, M., 2015. Molecular dynamics simulations and structural analysis of *Giardia duodenalis* 14-3-3 protein-protein interactions. J. Chem. Inf. Model. 55, 2611–2622.

Chalupska, D., Różycki, B., Humpolickova, J., Faltova, L., Klima, M., Boura, E., 2019. Phosphatidylinositol 4-kinase IIIβ (PI4KB) forms highly flexible heterocomplexes that include ACBD3, 14-3-3, and Rab11 proteins. Sci. Rep. 9, 567.

Chamberlain, L.H., Roth, D., Morgan, A., Burgoyne, R.D., 1995. Distinct effects of alpha-SNAP, 14-3-3 proteins, and calmodulin on priming and triggering of regulated exocytosis. J. Cell Biol. 130, 1063–1070.

Chatterjee, D., Zhiping, L.L., Tan, S.M., Bhattacharjya, S., 2016. Interaction analyses of the integrin beta2 cytoplasmic tail with the F3 FERM domain of talin and 14-3-3zeta reveal a ternary complex with phosphorylated tail. J. Mol. Biol. 428, 4129–4142.

Chaudhri, M., Scarabel, M., Aitken, A., 2003. Mammalian and yeast 14-3-3 isoforms form distinct patterns of dimers in vivo. Biochem. Biophys. Res. Commun. 300, 679–685.

Chen, C.T., Feoktistova, A., Chen, J.S., Shim, Y.S., Clifford, D.M., Gould, K.L., McCollum, D., 2008a. The SIN kinase Sid2 regulates cytoplasmic retention of the *S. pombe* Cdc14-like phosphatase Clp1. Curr. Biol. 18, 1594–1599.

Chen, Y.H., Su, L.H., Huang, Y.C., Wang, Y.T., Kao, Y.Y., Sun, C.H., 2008b. UPF1, a conserved nonsense-mediated mRNA decay factor, regulates cyst wall protein transcripts in *Giardia lamblia*. PLoS One 3, e3609.

Coblitz, B., Wu, M., Shikano, S., Li, M., 2006. C-terminal binding: an expanded repertoire and function of 14-3-3 proteins. FEBS Lett. 580, 1531–1535.

Courchet, J., Buchet-Poyau, K., Potemski, A., Brès, A., Jariel-Encontre, I., Billaud, M., 2008. Interaction with 14-3-3 adaptors regulates the sorting of hMex-3B RNA-binding protein to distinct classes of RNA granules. J. Biol. Chem. 283, 32131–32142.

de Boer, A.H., van Kleeff, P.J., Gao, J., 2013. Plant 14-3-3 proteins as spiders in a web of phosphorylation. Protoplasma 250, 425–440.

Dehecq, M., Decourty, L., Namane, A., Proux, C., Kanaan, J., Le Hir, H., Jacquier, A., Saveanu, C., 2018. Nonsense-mediated mRNA decay involves two distinct Upf1-bound complexes. EMBO J. 37, e99278.

Denison, F.C., Gokirmak, T., Ferl, R.J., 2014. Phosphorylation-related modification at the dimer interface of 14-3-3omega dramatically alters monomer interaction dynamics. Arch. Biochem. Biophys. 541, 1–12.

Dorner, C., Ullrich, A., Häring, H.U., Lammers, R., 1999. The kinesin-like motor protein KIF1C occurs in intact cells as a dimer and associates with proteins of the 14-3-3 family. J. Biol. Chem. 274 (47), 33654–33660.

Einarsson, E., Troell, K., Hoeppner, M.P., Grabherr, M., Ribacke, U., Svärd, S.G., 2016. Coordinated changes in gene expression throughout encystation of *Giardia intestinalis*. PLoS Negl. Trop. Dis. 10, e0004571.

Emery, S.J., Mirzaei, M., Vuong, D., Pascovici, D., Chick, J.M., Lacey, E., Haynes, P.A., 2016. Induction of virulence factors in *Giardia duodenalis* independent of host attachment. Sci. Rep. 6, 20765.

Emery, S.J., Baker, L., Ansell, B.R.E., Mirzaei, M., Haynes, P.A., McConville, M.J., Svärd, S.G., Jex, A.R., 2018. Differential protein expression and post-translational modifications in metronidazole-resistant *Giardia duodenalis*. Gigascience 7.

Evans-Osses, I., Mojoli, A., Monguió-Tortajada, M., Marcilla, A., Aran, V., Amorim, M., Inal, J., Borràs, F.E., Ramirez, M.I., 2017. Microvesicles released from *Giardia intestinalis* disturb host-pathogen response in vitro. Eur. J. Cell Biol. 96, 131–142.

Faso, C., Hehl, A.B., 2011. Membrane trafficking and organelle biogenesis in *Giardia lamblia*: use it or lose it. Int. J. Parasitol. 41, 471–480.

Faso, C., Bischof, S., Hehl, A.B., 2013. The proteome landscape of *Giardia lamblia* encystation. PLoS One 8 e83207.

Fiorillo, A., di Marino, D., Bertuccini, L., Via, A., Pozio, E., Camerini, S., Ilari, A., Lalle, M., 2014. The crystal structure of *Giardia duodenalis* 14-3-3 in the apo form: when protein post-translational modifications make the difference. PLoS One 9, e92902.

Furukawa, Y., Ikuta, N., Omata, S., Yamauchi, T., Isobe, T., Ichimura, T., 1993. Demonstration of the phosphorylation-dependent interaction of tryptophan hydroxylase with the 14-3-3 protein. Biochem. Biophys. Res. Commun. 194, 144–149.

Gardino, A.K., Yaffe, M.B., 2011. 14-3-3 proteins as signaling integration points for cell cycle control and apoptosis. Semin. Cell Dev. Biol. 22, 688–695.

Gardino, A.K., Smerdon, S.J., Yaffe, M.B., 2006. Structural determinants of 14-3-3 binding specificities and regulation of subcellular localization of 14-3-3-ligand complexes: a comparison of the X-ray crystal structures of all human 14-3-3 isoforms. Semin. Cancer Biol. 16, 173–182.

Gargantini, P.R., Serradell, M.C., Torri, A., Lujan, H.D., 2012. Putative SF2 helicases of the early-branching eukaryote *Giardia lamblia* are involved in antigenic variation and parasite differentiation into cysts. BMC Microbiol. 12, 284.

Gohla, A., Bokoch, G.M., 2002. 14-3-3 regulates actin dynamics by stabilizing phosphorylated cofilin. Curr. Biol. 12, 1704–1710.

Gómez-Escoda, B., Wu, P.J., 2017. Roles of CDK and DDK in genome duplication and maintenance: meiotic singularities. Genes (Basel) 8, E105.

Gourguechon, S., Holt, L.J., Cande, W.Z., 2013. The Giardia cell cycle progresses independently of the anaphase-promoting complex. J. Cell Sci. 26, 2246–2255.

Henriksson, M.L., Francis, M.S., Peden, A., Aili, M., Stefansson, K., Palmer, R., Aitken, A., Hallberg, B., 2002. A nonphosphorylated 14-3-3 binding motif on exoenzyme S that is functional in vivo. Eur. J. Biochem. 269, 4921–4929.

Hirt, R.P., de Miguel, N., Nakjang, S., Dessi, D., Liu, Y.C., Diaz, N., Rappelli, P., Acosta-Serrano, A., Fiori, P.L., Mottram, J.C., 2011. *Trichomonas vaginalis* pathobiology new insights from the genome sequence. Adv. Parasitol. 77, 87–140.

Horlock-Roberts, K., Reaume, C., Dayer, G., Ouellet, C., Cook, N., Yee, J., 2017. Drug-free approach to study the unusual cell cycle of *Giardia intestinalis*. mSphere 2, e00384-16.

Ichimura, T., Isobe, T., Okuyama, T., Yamauchi, T., Fujisawa, H., 1987. Brain 14-3-3 protein that activates tryptophan 5-mono-oxygenase and tyrosine 3-mono-oxygenase in the presence of Ca2+, calmodulindependent protein kinase II. FEBS Lett. 219, 79–82.

Jedelský, P.L., Doležal, P., Rada, P., Pyrih, J., Smíd, O., Hrdý, I., Sedinová, M., Marcinčiková, M., Voleman, L., Perry, A.J., Beltrán, N.C., Lithgow, T., Tachezy, J., 2011. The minimal proteome in the reduced mitochondrion of the parasitic protist *Giardia intestinalis*. PLoS One 6, e17285.

Jia, H., Liang, Z., Zhang, X., Wang, J., Xu, W., Qian, H., 2017. 14-3-3 proteins: an important regulator of autophagy in diseases. Am. J. Transl. Res. 9, 4738–4746.

Jin, J., Pawson, T., 2012. Modular evolution of phosphorylation-based signalling systems. Philos. Trans. R. Soc. Lond. B Biol. Sci. 367, 2540–2555.

Jin, J., Smith, F.D., Stark, C., Wells, C.D., Fawcett, J.P., Kulkarni, S., Metalnikov, P., O'Donnell, P., Taylor, P., Taylor, L., Zougman, A., Woodgett, J.R., Langeberg, L.K., Scott, J.D., Pawson, T., 2004. Proteomic, functional, and domain-based analysis of in vivo 14-3-3 binding proteins involved in cytoskeletal regulation and cellular organization. Curr. Biol. 14, 1436–1450.

Johnson, C., Crowther, S., Stafford, M.J., Campbell, D.G., Toth, R., MacKintosh, C., 2010. Bioinformatic and experimental survey of 14-3-3-binding sites. Biochem. J. 427, 69–78.

Jonas, S., Weichenrieder, O., Izaurralde, E., 2013. An unusual arrangement of two 14-3-3-like domains in the SMG5-SMG7 heterodimer is required for efficient nonsense-mediated mRNA decay. Genes Dev. 27, 211–225.

Kaplan, A., Bueno, M., Fournier, A.E., 2017. Extracellular functions of 14-3-3 adaptor proteins. Cell. Signal. 31, 26–30.

Ke, R., Xu, Q., Li, C., Luo, L., Huang, D., 2018. Mechanisms of AMPK in the maintenance of ATP balance during energy metabolism. Cell Biol. Int. 42, 384–392.

Kjarland, E., Keen, T.J., Kleppe, R., 2006. Does isoform diversity explain functional differences in the 14-3-3 protein family? Curr. Pharm. Biotechnol. 7, 217–223.

Kleppe, R., Martinez, A., Døskeland, S.O., Haavik, J., 2011. The 14-3-3 proteins in regulation of cellular metabolism. Semin. Cell Dev. Biol. 22, 713–719.

Krtková, J., Xu, J., Lalle, M., Steele-Ogus, M., Alas, G.C.M., Sept, D., Paredez, A.R., 2017. 14-3-3 regulates actin filament formation in the deep-branching eukaryote *Giardia lamblia*. mSphere 2, e00248-17.

Labib, K., 2010. How do Cdc7 and cyclin-dependent kinases trigger the initiation of chromosome replication in eukaryotic cells? Genes Dev. 24, 1208–1219.

Lalle, M., Hanevik, K., 2018. Treatment-refractory giardiasis: challenges and solutions. Infect. Drug Resist. 11, 1921–1933.

Lalle, M., Salzano, A.M., Crescenzi, M., Pozio, E., 2006. The *Giardia duodenalis* 14-3-3 protein is post-translationally modified by phosphorylation and polyglycylation of the C-terminal tail. J. Biol. Chem. 281, 5137–5148.

Lalle, M., Bavassano, C., Fratini, F., Cecchetti, S., Boisguerin, P., Crescenzi, M., Pozio, E., 2010. Involvement of 14-3-3 protein post-translational modifications in *Giardia duodenalis* encystation. Int. J. Parasitol. 40, 201–213.

Lalle, M., Camerini, S., Cecchetti, S., Blasetti Fantauzzi, C., Crescenzi, M., Pozio, E., 2011. *Giardia duodenalis* 14-3-3 protein is polyglycylated by a tubulin tyrosine ligase-like member and deglycylated by two metallocarboxypeptidases. J. Biol. Chem. 286, 4471–4484.

Lalle, M., Camerini, S., Cecchetti, S., Sayadi, A., Crescenzi, M., Pozio, E., 2012. Interaction network of the 14-3-3 protein in the ancient protozoan parasite *Giardia duodenalis*. J. Proteome Res. 11, 2666–2683.

Lalle, M., Leptourgidou, F., Camerini, S., Pozio, E., Skoulakis, E.M.C., 2013. Interkingdom complementation reveals structural conservation and functional divergence of 14-3-3 proteins. PLoS One 8, e78090.

Lalle, M., Camerini, S., Cecchetti, S., Finelli, R., Sferra, G., Müller, J., Ricci, G., Pozio, E., 2015. The FAD-dependent glycerol-3-phosphate dehydrogenase of *Giardia duodenalis*: an unconventional enzyme that interacts with the g14-3-3 and it is a target of the antitumoral compound NBDHEX. Front. Microbiol. 6, 544.

Larance, M., Rowland, A.F., Hoehn, K., Humphreys, D.T., Preiss, T., Guilhaus, M., James, D.E., 2010. Global phosphoproteomics identifies a major role for akt and 14-3-3 in regulating Edc3. Mol. Cell. Proteomics 9, 682–694.

Laronga, C., Yang, H.Y., Neal, C., Lee, M.H., 2000. Association of the cyclin-dependent kinases and 14-3-3 sigma negatively regulates cell cycle progression. J. Biol Chem. 275 (30), 23106–23112.

Lauwaet, T., Davids, B.J., Reiner, D.S., Gillin, F.D., 2007. Encystation of *Giardia lamblia*: a model for other parasites. Curr. Opin. Microbiol. 10, 554–559.
Lauwaet, T., Smith, A.J., Reiner, D.S., Romijn, E.P., Wong, C.C., Davids, B.J., Shah, S.A., Yates 3rd, J.R., Gillin, F.D., 2011. Mining the Giardia genome and proteome for conserved and unique basal body proteins. Int. J. Parasitol. 41, 1079–1092.
Lingdan, L., Pengtao, G., Wenchao, L., Jianhua, L., Ju, Y., Chengwu, L., He, L., Guocai, Z., Wenzhi, R., Yujiang, C., Xichen, Z., 2012. Differential dissolved protein expression throughout the life cycle of *Giardia lamblia*. Exp. Parasitol. 132, 465–469.
Liu, D., Bienkowska, J., Petosa, C., Collier, R.J., Fu, H., Liddington, R., 1995. Crystal structure of the zeta isoform of the 14-3-3 protein. Nature 376, 191–194.
Liu, P., Gan, W., Guo, C., Xie, A., Gao, D., Guo, J., Zhang, J., Willis, N., Su, A., Asara, J.M., Scully, R., Wei, W., 2015. Akt-mediated phosphorylation of XLF impairs non-homologous end-joining DNA repair. Mol. Cell 57, 648–661.
Loh, B., Jonas, S., Izaurralde, E., 2013. The SMG5-SMG7 heterodimer directly recruits the CCR4-NOT deadenylase complex to mRNAs containing nonsense codons via interaction with POP2. Genes Dev. 27, 2125–2138.
Lozano-Durán, R., Robatzek, S., 2015. 14-3-3 proteins in plant-pathogen interactions. Mol. Plant Microbe Interact. 28, 511–518.
Ma'ayeh, S.Y., Brook-Carter, P.T., 2012. Representational difference analysis identifies specific genes in the interaction of *Giardia duodenalis* with the murine intestinal epithelial cell line, IEC-6. Int. J. Parasitol. 42, 501–509.
Maia, C., Attias, M., Urbina, J., Gilbert, I., Magaraci, F., de Souza, W., 2007. Azasterols impair *Giardia lamblia* proliferation and induces encystation. Biochem. Biophys. Res. Commun. 363, 310–316.
Manning, G., Reiner, D.S., Lauwaet, T., Dacre, M., Smith, A., Zhai, Y., Svard, S., Gillin, F.D., 2011. The minimal kinome of *Giardia lamblia* illuminates early kinase evolution and unique parasite biology. Genome Biol. 12, R66.
Marchat, L.A., Arzola-Rodríguez, S.I., Hernandez- de la Cruz, O., Lopez-Rosas, I., Lopez-Camarillo, C., 2015. DEAD/DExH-box RNA helicases in selected human parasites. Korean J. Parasitol. 53, 583–595.
Masters, S.C., Fu, H., 2001. 14-3-3 proteins mediate an essential anti-apoptotic signal. Biol. Chem. 276, 45193–45200.
Matos, J., Lipp, J.J., Bogdanova, A., Guillot, S., Okaz, E., Junqueira, M., Shevchenko, A., Zachariae, W., 2008. Dbf4-dependent CDC7 kinase links DNA replication to the segregation of homologous chromosomes in meiosis I. Cell 135, 662–678.
McGowan, J.E., Kratch, J., Chattopadhyay, S., Joe, B., Conti, H.R., Chakravarti, R., 2017. Bioinformatic analysis reveals new determinants of antigenic 14-3-3 proteins and a novel antifungal strategy. PLoS One 12, e0189503.
Mizuno, E., Kitamura, N., Komada, M., 2007. 14-3-3-dependent inhibition of the deubiquitinating activity of UBPY and its cancellation in the M phase. Exp. Cell Res. 313, 3624–3634.
Moore, B.W., Perez, V.J., 1968. Specific acid proteins in the nervous system. In: Carlson, F.D. (Ed.), Physiological and Biochemical Aspects of Nervous Integration. Prentice Hall, New Jersey, U.S.A, pp. 343–359.
Morf, L., Spycher, C., Rehrauer, H., Fournier, C.A., Morrison, H.G., Hehl, A.B., 2010. The transcriptional response to encystation stimuli in *Giardia lamblia* is restricted to a small set of genes. Eukaryot. Cell 9, 1566–1576.
Morrison, H.G., McArthur, A.G., Gillin, F.D., Aley, S.B., Adam, R.D., Olsen, G.J., Best, A.A., Cande, W.Z., Chen, F., Cipriano, M.J., Davids, B.J., Dawson, S.C., Elmendorf, H.G., Hehl, A.B., Holder, M.E., Huse, S.M., Kim, U.U., Lasek-Nesselquist, E., Manning, G., Nigam, A., Nixon, J.E., Palm, D., Passamaneck, N.E., Prabhu, A., Reich, C.I., Reiner, D.S., Samuelson, J., Svard, S.G., Sogin, M.L., 2007.

Genomic minimalism in the early diverging intestinal parasite *Giardia lamblia*. Science 317, 1921–1926.

Mrowiec, T., Schwappach, B., 2006. 14-3-3 proteins in membrane protein transport. Biol. Chem. 387, 1227–1236.

Mullard, A., 2012. Protein–protein interaction inhibitors get into the groove. Nat. Rev. Drug Discov. 11, 173–175.

Muslin, A.J., Tanner, J.W., Allen, P.M., Shaw, A.S., 1996. Interaction of 14-3-3 with signaling proteins is mediated by the recognition of phosphoserine. Cell 84, 889–897.

Nagy, G., Oostenbrink, C., Hritz, J., 2017. Exploring the binding pathways of the 14-3-3ζ protein: structural and free-energy profiles revealed by Hamiltonian replica exchange molecular dynamics with distancefield distance restraints. PLoS One 12, e0180633.

Niño, C.A., Chaparro, J., Soffientini, P., Polo, S., Wasserman, M., 2013. Ubiquitination dynamics in the early-branching eukaryote *Giardia intestinalis*. Microbiologyopen 2, 525–539.

Obsil, T., Obsilova, V., 2011. Structural basis of 14-3-3 protein functions. Semin. Cell Dev. Biol. 22, 663–672.

Obsil, T., Ghirlando, R., Klein, D.C., Ganguly, S., Dyda, F., 2001. Crystal structure of the 14-3-3zeta:serotonin N-acetyltransferase complex. A role for scaffolding in enzyme regulation. Cell 105, 257–267.

Oecking, C., Eckerskorn, C., Weiler, E.W., 1994. The fusicoccin receptor of plants is a member of the 14-3-3 superfamily of eukaryotic regulatory proteins. FEBS Lett. 352, 163–166.

Ohtake, F., Tsuchiya, H., 2017. The emerging complexity of ubiquitin architecture. J. Biochem. 161, 125–133.

Ottmann, C., Weyand, M., Sassa, T., Inoue, T., Kato, N., Wittinghofer, A., Oecking, C., 2009. A structural rationale for selective stabilization of anti-tumor interactions of 14-3-3 proteins by cotylenin A. J. Mol. Biol. 386, 913–919.

Paredez, A.R., Nayeri, A., Xu, J.W., Krtková, J., Cande, W.Z., 2014. Identification of obscure yet conserved actin-associated proteins in *Giardia lamblia*. Eukaryot. Cell 13, 776–784.

Parua, P.K., Dombek, K.M., Young, E.T., 2014. Yeast 14-3-3 protein functions as a comodulator of transcription by inhibiting coactivator functions. J. Biol. Chem. 289, 35542–35560.

Paul, A.L., Liu, L., McClung, S., Laughner, B., Chen, S., Ferl, R.J., 2009. Comparative interactomics: analysis of arabidopsis 14-3-3 complexes reveals highly conserved 14-3-3 interactions between humans and plants. J. Proteome Res. 8, 1913–1924.

Pennington, K.L., Chan, T.Y., Torres, M.P., Andersen, J.L., 2018. The dynamic and stress-adaptive signaling hub of 14-3-3: emerging mechanisms of regulation and context-dependent protein-protein interactions. Oncogene 37, 5587–5604.

Petosa, C., Masters, S.C., Bankston, L.A., Pohl, J., Wang, B., Fu, H., Liddington, R.C., 1998. 14-3-3zeta binds a phosphorylated Raf peptide and an unphosphorylated peptide via its conserved amphipathic groove. J. Biol. Chem. 273, 16305–16310.

Pham, J.K., Nosala, C., Scott, E.Y., Nguyen, K.F., Hagen, K.D., Starcevich, H.N., Dawson, S.C., 2017. Transcriptomic profiling of high-density Giardia foci encysting in the murine proximal intestine. Front. Cell. Infect. Microbiol. 7, 227.

Pozuelo Rubio, M., Geraghty, K.M., Wong, B.H., Wood, N.T., Campbell, D.G., Morrice, N., Mackintosh, C., 2004. 14-3-3-affinity purification of over 200 human phosphoproteins reveals new links to regulation of cellular metabolism, proliferation and trafficking. Biochem J. 379 (Pt 2), 395–408.

Pradhan, P., Lundgren, S.W., Wilson, W.A., Brittingham, A., 2012. Glycogen storage and degradation during in vitro growth and differentiation of *Giardia intestinalis*. J. Parasitol. 98, 442–444.

Psenakova, K., Petrvalska, O., Kylarova, S., Lentini Santo, D., Kalabova, D., Herman, P., Obsilova, V., Obsil, T., 2018. 14-3-3 protein directly interacts with the kinase domain of calcium/calmodulin-dependent protein kinase kinase (CaMKK2). Biochim. Biophys. Acta Gen. Subj. 1862, 1612–1625.
Reiner, D.S., Ankarklev, J., Troell, K., Palm, D., Bernander, R., Gillin, F.D., Andersson, J.O., Svärd, S.G., 2008. Synchronisation of *Giardia lamblia*: identification of cell cycle stage-specific genes and a differentiation restriction point. Int. J. Parasitol. 38, 935–944.
Rittinger, K., Budman, J., Xu, J., Volinia, S., Cantley, L.C., Smerdon, S.J., Gamblin, S.J., Yaffe, M.B., 1999. Structural analysis of 14-3-3 phosphopeptide complexes identifies a dual role for the nuclear export signal of 14-3-3 in ligand binding. Mol. Cell 4, 153–166.
Rogowski, K., Juge, F., van Dijk, J., Wloga, D., Strub, J.M., Levilliers, N., Thomas, D., Bre´, M.H., Van Dorsselaer, A., Gaertig, J., Janke, C., 2009. Evolutionary divergence of enzymatic mechanisms for posttranslational polyglycylation. Cell 137, 1076–1087.
Roque, A.C., Lowe, C.R., 2005. Lessons from nature: on the molecular recognition elements of the phosphoprotein binding-domains. Biotechnol. Bioeng. 91, 546–555.
Rosenquist, M., Sehnke, P., Ferl, R.J., Sommarin, M., Larsson, C., 2000. Evolution of the 14-3-3 protein family: does the large number of isoforms in multicellular organisms reflect functional specificity? J. Mol. Evol. 51, 446–458.
Rubio-Villena, C., Sanz, P., Garcia-Gimeno, M.A., 2015. Structure-function analysis of PPP1R3D, a protein phosphatase 1 targeting subunit, reveals a binding motif for 14-3-3 proteins which regulates its glycogenic properties. PLoS One 10, e0131476.
Saha, N., Dutta, S., Datta, S.P., Sarkar, S., 2018. The minimal ESCRT machinery of *Giardia lamblia* has altered inter-subunit interactions within the ESCRT-II and ESCRT-III complexes. Eur. J. Cell Biol. 97, 44–62.
Sánchez, L.B., Galperin, M.Y., Müller, M., 2000. Acetyl-CoA synthetase from the amitochondriate eukaryote *Giardia lamblia* belongs to the newly recognized superfamily of acyl-CoA synthetases (nucleoside diphosphate-forming). J. Biol. Chem. 275, 5794–5803.
Satoh, J., Nanri, Y., Yamamura, T., 2006. Rapid identification of 14-3-3-binding proteins by protein microarray analysis. J. Neurosci. Methods 152, 278–288.
Shen, W., Clark, A.C., Huber, S.C., 2003. The C-terminal tail of Arabidopsis 14-3-3omega functions as an autoinhibitor and may contain a tenth alpha-helix. Plant J. 34, 473–484.
Sluchanko, N.N., 2018. Association of multiple phosphorylated proteins with the 14-3-3 regulatory hubs: problems and perspectives. J. Mol. Biol. 430, 20–26.
Sluchanko, N.N., Beelen, S., Kulikova, A.A., Weeks, S.D., Antson, A.A., Gusev, N.B., Strelkov, S.V., 2017. Structural basis for the interaction of a human small heat shock protein with the 14-3-3 universal signaling regulator. Structure 25, 305–316.
Smith, A.J., Daut, J., Schwappach, B., 2011. Membrane proteins as 14-3-3 clients in functional regulation and intracellular transport. Physiology (Bethesda) 26, 181–191.
Sonda, S., Morf, L., Bottova, I., Baetschmann, H., Rehrauer, H., Caflisch, A., Hakimi, M.A., Hehl, A.B., 2010. Epigenetic mechanisms regulate stage differentiation in the minimized protozoan Giardia lamblia. Mol Microbiol. 76 (1), 48–67.
Stevers, L.M., Sijbesma, E., Botta, M., MacKintosh, C., Obsil, T., Landrieu, I., Cau, Y., Wilson, A.J., Karawajczyk, A., Eickhoff, J., Davis, J., Hann, M., O'Mahony, G., Doveston, R.G., Brunsveld, L., Ottmann, C., 2018. Modulators of 14-3-3 protein-protein interactions. J. Med. Chem. 10, 3755–3778.
Stoica, C., Carmichael, J.B., Parker, H., Pare, J., Hobman, T.C., 2006. Interactions between the RNA interference effector protein Ago1 and 14-3-3 proteins: consequences for cell cycle progression. J. Biol. Chem. 281, 37646–37651.

Su, C.H., Zhao, R., Velazquez-Torres, G., Chen, J., Gully, C., Yeung, S.C., Lee, M.H., 2010. Nuclear export regulation of COP1 by 14-3-3σ in response to DNA damage. Mol. Cancer 9, 243.

Taoka, K., Ohki, I., Tsuji, H., Furuita, K., Hayashi, K., Yanase, T., Yamaguchi, M., Nakashima, C., Purwestri, Y.A., Tamaki, S., Ogaki, Y., Shimada, C., Nakagawa, A., Kojima, C., Shimamoto, K., 2011. 14-3-3 proteins act as intracellular receptors for rice Hd3a florigen. Nature 476, 332–335.

Thompson, R.C., Monis, P., 2012. Giardia-from genome to proteome. Adv. Parasitol. 78, 57–95.

Tinti, M., Madeira, F., Murugesan, G., Hoxhaj, G., Toth, R., Mackintosh, C., 2014. ANIA: annotation and integrated analysis of the 14-3-3 interactome. Database (Oxford) 2014, bat085.

Touz, M.C., Zamponi, N., 2017. Sorting without a Golgi complex. Traffic 18, 637–645.

Truong, A.B., Masters, S.C., Yang, H., Fu, H., 2002. Role of the 14-3-3 C-terminal loop in ligand interaction. Proteins 49, 321–325.

Urano, T., Saito, T., Tsukui, T., Fujita, M., Hosoi, T., Muramatsu, M., Ouchi, Y., Inoue, S., 2002. Efp targets 14-3-3 sigma for proteolysis and promotes breast tumour growth. Nature 417, 871–875.

van Heusden, G.P., 2005. 14-3-3 proteins: regulators of numerous eukaryotic proteins. IUBMB Life 57, 623–629.

van Heusden, G.P., Griffiths, D.J., Ford, J.C., Chin-A-Woeng, T.F., Schrader, P.A., Carr, A.M., Steensma, H.Y., 1995. The 14-3-3 proteins encoded by the BMH1 and BMH2 genes are essential in the yeast *Saccharomyces cerevisiae* and can be replaced by a plant homologue. Eur. J. Biochem. 229, 45–53.

Wampfler, P.B., Tosevski, V., Nanni, P., Spycher, C., Hehl, A.B., 2014. Proteomics of secretory and endocytic organelles in *Giardia lamblia*. PLoS One 9, e94089.

Weber, K., Schneider, A., Westermann, S., Müller, N., Plessmann, U., 1997. Posttranslational modifications of alpha- and beta-tubulin in Giardia lamblia, an ancient eukaryote. FEBS Lett. 419 (1), 87–91.

Williams, C.W., Elmendorf, H.G., 2011. Identification and analysis of the RNA degrading complexes and machinery of *Giardia lamblia* using an in silico approach. BMC Genomics 12, 586.

Winter, J.F., Höpfner, S., Korn, K., Farnung, B.O., Bradshaw, C.R., Marsico, G., Volkmer, M., Habermann, B., Zerial, M., 2012. *Caenorhabditis elegans* screen reveals role of PAR-5 in RAB-11-recycling endosome positioning and apicobasal cell polarity. Nat. Cell Biol. 14, 666–676.

Würtele, M., Jelich-Ottmann, C., Wittinghofer, A., Oecking, C., 2003. Structural view of a fungal toxin acting on a 14-3-3 regulatory complex. EMBO J. 22, 987–994.

Xiao, B., Smerdon, S.J., Jones, D.H., Dodson, G.G., Soneji, Y., Aitken, A., Gamblin, S.J., 1995. Structure of a 14-3-3 protein and implications for coordination of multiple signalling pathways. Nature 376, 188–891.

Yaffe, M.B., 2002. How do 14-3-3 proteins work?—gatekeeper phosphorylation and the molecular anvil hypothesis. FEBS Lett. 513, 53–57.

Yahyaoui, W., Zannis-Hadjopoulos, M., 2009. 14-3-3 proteins function in the initiation and elongation steps of DNA replication in *Saccharomyces cerevisiae*. J. Cell Sci. 122, 4419–4426.

Yang, X., Lee, W.H., Sobott, F., Papagrigoriou, E., Robinson, C.V., Grossmann, J.G., Sundström, M., Doyle, D.A., Elkins, J.M., 2006. Structural basis for protein-protein interactions in the 14-3-3 protein family. Proc. Natl. Acad. Sci. U. S. A. 103, 17237–17242.

Yichoy, M., Duarte, T.T., De Chatterjee, A., Mendez, T.L., Aguilera, K.Y., Roy, D., Roychowdhury, S., Aley, S.B., Das, S., 2011. Lipid metabolism in Giardia: a post-genomic perspective. Parasitology 138, 267–278.

Yu, I., Garnham, C.P., Roll-Mecak, A., 2015. Writing and reading the tubulin code. J. Biol. Chem. 290, 17163–17172.
Zheng, D., Chen, C.Y., Shyu, A.B., 2011. Unraveling regulation and new components of human P-bodies through a protein interaction framework and experimental validation. RNA 17, 1619–1634.
Zuk, M., Weber, R., Szopa, J., 2005. 14-3-3 protein down-regulates key enzyme activities of nitrate and carbohydrate metabolism in potato plants. J. Agric. Food Chem. 53, 3454–3460.

Further reading

Aghazadeh, Y., Papadopoulos, V., 2016. The role of the 14-3-3 protein family in health, disease, and drug development. Drug Discov. Today 21, 278–287.
Al-Hakim, A.K., Göransson, O., Deak, M., Toth, R., Campbell, D.G., Morrice, N.A., Prescott, A.R., Alessi, D.R., 2005. 14-3-3 cooperates with LKB1 to regulate the activity and localization of QSK and SIK. J. Cell Sci. 118, 5661–5673.
Frearson, J.A., Wyatt, P.G., Gilbert, I.H., Fairlamb, A.H., 2007. Target assessment for antiparasitic drug discovery. Trends Parasitol. 23, 589–595.
Joo, Y., Schumacher, B., Landrieu, I., Bartel, M., Smet-Nocca, C., Jang, A., Choi, H.S., Jeon, N.L., Chang, K.A., Kim, H.S., Ottmann, C., Suh, Y.H., 2015. Involvement of 14-3-3 in tubulin instability and impaired axon development is mediated by Tau. FASEB J. 29, 4133–4144.
Kaplan, A., Fournier, A.E., 2017. Targeting 14-3-3 adaptor protein-protein interactions to stimulate central nervous system repair. Neural Regen. Res. 12, 1040–1043.
Paiardini, A., Aducci, P., Cervoni, L., Cutruzzolà, F., Di Lucente, C., Janson, G., Pascarella, S., Rinaldo, S., Visconti, S., Camoni, L., 2014. The phytotoxin fusicoccin differently regulates 14-3-3 proteins association to mode III targets. IUBMB Life 66, 52–62.
Parua, P.K., Young, E.T., 2014. Binding and transcriptional regulation by 14-3-3 (Bmh) proteins requires residues outside of the canonical motif. Eukaryot. Cell 13, 21–30.
Stadelmann, J.B., Birkestedt, S., Hellman, U., Svärd, S.G., 2012. Plasmid vectors for proteomic analyses in Giardia: purification of virulence factors and analysis of the proteasome. Eukaryot. Cell 11, 864–873.
Williams, D.M., Ecroyd, H., Goodwin, K.L., Dai, H., Fu, H., Woodcock, J.M., Zhang, L., Carver, J.A., 2011. NMR spectroscopy of 14-3-3ζ reveals a flexible C-terminal extension: differentiation of the chaperone and phosphoserine-binding activities of 14-3-3ζ. Biochem. J. 437, 493–503.

CHAPTER THREE

A cytonaut's guide to protein trafficking in *Giardia lamblia*

Carmen Faso, Adrian B. Hehl*
Laboratory of Molecular Parasitology, Institute of Parasitology, University of Zurich (ZH), Zürich, Switzerland
*Corresponding author: e-mail address: adrian.hehl@uzh.ch

Contents

Abstract

Over the past years, the subcellular organization of the *Excavata* member *Giardia lamblia* (syn. *duodenalis, intestinalis*) has been investigated in considerable detail. There are several reasons for this endeavour which go beyond this parasite's medical importance and are mostly concerned with its reduced subcellular complexity and debated evolutionary status. One may say that simplification has emerged as a paradigm for the evolution of *Giardia*'s subcellular architecture. However, a complete appreciation of the evolutionary and ecological significance of this phenomenon is far from complete.

In this chapter, we present and discuss the most recent data on the main trafficking pathways in *G. lamblia* which include *endo*- and *exo*-cytosis, organellar import and function. We provide perspectives on open questions concerning organelle replication and inheritance and include a technical outlook on methods and approaches to genetic manipulations in *G. lamblia*.

A better understanding of *G. lamblia* subcellular organization at the morphological and molecular level complements any effort aimed at elucidating this parasitic species' evolutionary status and could provide us with the basis for novel strategies to interfere with parasite transmission and/or pathogenesis.

Advances in Parasitology, Volume 106
ISSN 0065-308X
https://doi.org/10.1016/bs.apar.2019.08.001

1. Introduction

Diarrheal diseases are the top second and fifth causes of death in low and middle income countries (LMICs), respectively (WHO, 2013). *Giardia lamblia* (*syn. intestinalis, duodenalis*) is a ubiquitous and broad-spectrum Diplomonad parasitic protist responsible for the diarrheal disease known as giardiasis. Prevalence of giardiasis reaches and frequently surpasses 30% in LMICs (Furness et al., 2000). As a consequence, this communicable disease is mainly a scourge of populations already confronted with a heavy burden of illness, often including other parasitic infections.

The life cycle of *G. lamblia* consists of two main stages, the infectious and environmentally-resistant cyst form and the feeding but non-infectious trophozoite (Adam, 2001). Cysts are shed in faeces which, in conditions of poor sanitation, contaminate water. When ingested, a flagellated trophozoite precursor actively emerges from the cyst's confinement (excystation) setting the stage for colonization of the new host's small intestine. *In vivo* and *in vitro*, trophozoites can be induced to stage-differentiate and become environmentally resistant. Encysting trophozoites secrete large amounts of cyst wall material to build a cyst wall encapsulating the parasite within in a state of incomplete cell division (encystation), (Faso et al., 2013a,b) and thus preparing for transmission to a new host. *Giardia*'s simplified subcellular organization consisting of just four identifiable subcellular compartments, namely, nuclei, endoplasmic reticulum (ER), peripheral vesicles (PVs) and mitosomes (Faso and Hehl, 2011), a small and compact genome (*ca.* 12 Mb), and minimal molecular machinery (Morrison et al., 2007), highlight this parasitic species' peculiar form of evolution by secondary reduction (Ankarklev et al., 2010).

In this chapter, we will summarize and discuss the main recent advances in our understanding of *G. lamblia*'s subcellular organization, including intra- and extra-cellular protein trafficking routes and functional aspects of organelle maintenance. Citing the late Christian de Duve, one of the founding fathers of cell biology (Bowers, 1998), we will attempt to compile a critical 'cytonaut's guide' to the *Giardia* cell. Finally, we will introduce topics and techniques in *Giardia* molecular and evolutionary cell biology which are likely to hold centre-stage in future research efforts into the biology of this fascinating and deceivingly simple cell.

2. Protein trafficking routes in *Giardia lamblia*: The main highways

2.1 The way in: Peripheral vacuoles and endocytosis

2.1.1 PV structure and morphology

PVs are single-membrane bounded organelles primarily occupying the cortical and dorsal region of the *Giardia* cell, with a small ventral cluster between the two nuclei (Feely and Dyer, 1987). Based on electron microscopy reconstruction and segmentation data derived from FIB-SEM experiments (Zumthor et al., 2016), their average size is estimated to be between 100 and 200 nm, and they are situated *ca.* 50 nm away from the inner PM leaflet. They have highly heterogenous morphology and do not appear to constitute an extended network, although transient short-lived connections between individual PVs cannot be excluded. PVs are frequently directly connected to ER membranes; the significance of these membrane contact sites is still unclear, although they may play a role in PV membrane remodelling and/or cargo transport.

2.1.2 PV-mediated uptake and clathrin assemblies

Fluid-phase uptake in *G. lamblia* directly depends on PVs. These organelles are the only point of entry to the *Giardia* trophozoite, meaning that any nutrient or pharmaceutical must be retained in the PV luminal environment before being metabolized by the cell. PVs acidify presumably in connection with cargo loading (Abodeely et al., 2009) and to sort and retain useful molecules while releasing unused material (including experimental fluid phase markers) back in the environment. Thus, PVs constitute a formidable barrier at the host-parasite interface with the qualities of an *endo*-lysosomal compartment (Rivero et al., 2013).

The question of how PV lumina contact the extracellular environment was addressed recently to show that the dorsal side of Giardia trophozoites is pock-marked by PM-associated invaginations that come in close proximity to underlying PV organelles (Zumthor et al., 2016). This suggests that continuity and exchange of fluid-phase material is achieved through transient PM-PV membrane fusion events. Although consisting of conserved elements the molecular details of the machinery responsible for PM deformation in funnel-shaped structures and membrane fusion at the PM-PV interface remain unknown. In addition, reports on receptor-mediated endocytosis in *G. lamblia* point to PVs as sorting stations for receptors and their ligands (Rivero et al., 2010b, 2012, 2013), further underscoring their identity as endolysosomal compartments.

Given the nature of PVs, it is perhaps not surprising that *Giardia*'s single clathrin heavy chain protein (GlCHC) localizes in close proximity to these organelles, organized in static assemblies of unclear structure (Zumthor et al., 2016). By starting with GlCHC as an affinity handle for a series of co-immunoprecipitation experiments, an extended clathrin-centred interactome at PVs was defined (Rivero et al., 2010b; Touz et al., 2004; Zumthor et al., 2016). This included well-characterized and conserved clathrin interaction partners such as adaptor protein-2 complex (AP2) and giardial dynamin-related protein GlDRP, and what appears to be a highly-diverged clathrin light chain called Gl4259 (Zumthor et al., 2016). Several proteins of unknown function were also identified, including a family of lipid-binding proteins called PX domain-containing proteins (Jana et al., 2017; Touz et al., 2018) which may function as membrane adaptors for clathrin assemblies. Adaptor protein-1 complex (AP1) was also identified as a GlCHC interaction partner, as was the single giardial epsin-related (EpsinR) homologue known as Glepsin or GlENTHp. Epsin is a known clathrin interactor in organisms with well-characterized clathrin-coated vesicle (CCV) intermediates as carriers for endocytosed material. However, there exist conflicting reports on Glepsin's subcellular localization and physical interaction with GlCHC (Feliziani et al., 2015; Zumthor et al., 2016). Furthermore, there is currently no data to support the hypothesis that CCVs are present in *G. lamblia*. This is also mirrored in the absence of both clathrin coat disassembly factors and uncoating motifs in GlCHC (Zumthor et al., 2016).

2.2 Internal traffic: Mitosomes

2.2.1 Identification and evolutionary history

Giardia species were long believed to belong to one of several primitive eukaryotic microaerophilic or anaerobic amitochondriate lineages, including genera *Entamoeba* (supergroup *Amoebozoa*), *Trichomonas* (supergroup *Excavata*) and *Blastocystis* (supergroup *SAR*) (Cavalier-Smith, 1987). The absence of morphologically distinguishable mitochondria associated to a lack of any respiration-related protein machinery was one of the strongest reasons for this classification. However, this widely-held view was convincingly disproved with the discovery of mitochondria-related organelles (MROs), first in *E. histolytica* (Tovar et al., 1999) and then in *G. lamblia* (Fig. 1) (Regoes et al., 2005; Tovar et al., 2003). Of paramount importance was also the realization that hydrogenosomes, organelles present in other *Excavata* lineages such as *Parabasalia*, were in fact MROs where substrate-level phosphorylation ultimately leads to the production of molecular hydrogen (Boxma et al., 2005; Muller, 1993). These data set the stage for an appreciation of the variety of MROs which include *bona fide* mitochondria, mitosomes, and hydrogenosomes presenting a mutually exclusive distribution in individual genera

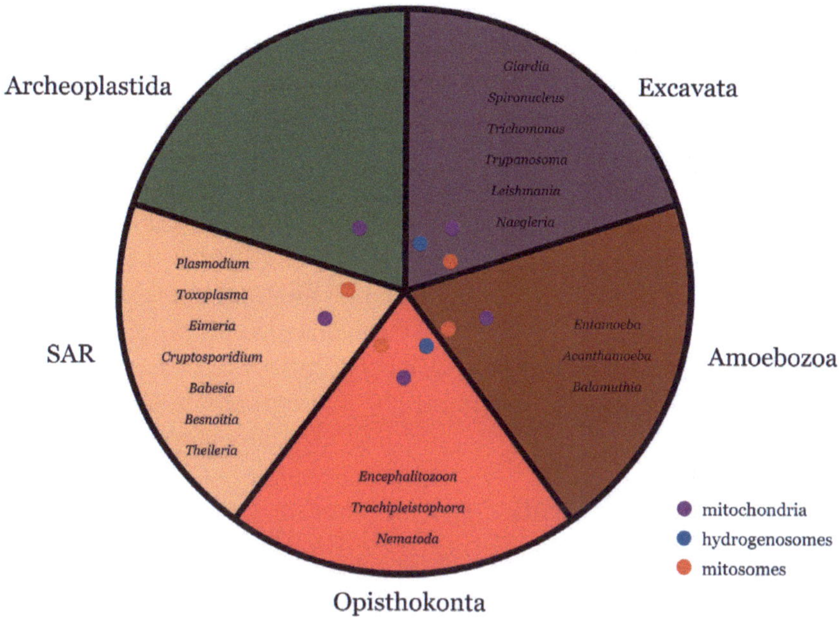

Fig. 1 The five main Eukaryotic supergroups and the distribution of MROs. The five most-characterized supergroups within the Eukaryotes are the *Excavata*, the *Amoebozoa*, the *Opisthokonta*, the *Stramenopile-Alevolates-Rhizaria* (SAR) and the *Archeoplastida*. The only supergroup that is not known to include animal parasites is the *Archeoplastida*. Representative parasitic genera for the other supergroups are indicated in each sector. The distribution of mitochondria and mitochondria-related organelles (MROs) is included at each sector's vertex. The presence of mitochondria is indicated by a violet dot. Blue and red dots indicate the presence of hydrogenosomes and mitosomes, respectively. *This scheme is a combined adaptation of data presented and discussed in Adl, S.M., Simpson, A.G., Lane, C.E., Lukes, J., Bass, D., Bowser, S.S., Brown, M.W., Burki, F., Dunthorn, M., Hampl, V., Heiss, A., Hoppenrath, M., Lara, E., Le Gall, L., Lynn, D.H., McManus, H., Mitchell, E.A., Mozley-Stanridge, S.E., Parfrey, L.W., Pawlowski, J., Rueckert, S., Shadwick, R.S., Schoch, C.L., Smirnov, A., Spiegel, F.W., 2012. The revised classification of eukaryotes. J. Eukaryot. Microbiol. 59 (5), 429–493 and Shiflett, A.M., Johnson, P.J., 2010. Mitochondrion-related organelles in eukaryotic protists. Annu. Rev. Microbiol. 64, 409–429.*

(Shiflett and Johnson, 2010), although all can be found within a single supergroup (Shiflett and Johnson, 2010). A more differentiated subcategorization of MROs (Muller et al., 2012) distinguishes five classes, based on the following criteria: oxygen as the only final electron acceptor (aerobic vs. anaerobic mitochondria, classes 1 and 2, respectively); use of alternative acceptors such as hydrogen in the presence of an electron transport chain (hydrogen-producing mitochondria vs. hydrogenosomes, classes 3 and 4, respectively) and absence of ATP production in the organelle (mitosomes, class 5). Previous studies indicate that *G. lamblia's* MROs are not involved in ATP synthesis which, as in genus *Entamoeba*, appears to be exclusively localized to the cytosol (Müller, 2003). Therefore, based on these criteria, *Giardia*'s MROs are defined as mitosomes. *G. lamblia*'s closest investigated relatives belonging to the *Spironucleus* genus all appear to carry hydrogenosomes (Millet et al., 2013). Importantly, this observation, supported by additional molecular phylogenetic data, has led to the recently-formulated hypothesis that, within Diplomonads, mitosomes evolved from hydrogenosomes and are not direct mitochondrial derivatives (Jerlstrom-Hultqvist et al., 2013; Martin, 2005). Interestingly, this hypothesis could also account for data on how *Giardia*'s ability to produce hydrogen (Lloyd et al., 2002) is linked to the presence of a cytosolic hydrogenase (Emelyanov and Goldberg, 2010) which was retargeted to the cytoplasm from the (presumably) hydrogenosome-like mitosome precursor.

2.2.2 Morphology, replication and metabolism

G. lamblia mitosomes are double membrane-bounded organelles which contain no detectable DNA. Based on confocal light and electron microscopy investigations, their numbers appear to be within the range of 20–50 units/cell (Regoes et al., 2005; Tovar et al., 2003). Their size is approximately 100 nm and their shape is mostly spherical, except for the central mitosome complex (CMC), which appears as a stable elongated cluster of 5–7 organelles embedded in the basal body—axoneme bundle between the two nuclei (Hehl et al., 2007). It is still unclear how these organelles replicate and whether the apparently stochastically-distributed peripheral mitosomes originate from the fixed CMC. However, recent reports point to a role for GlDRP (Fig. 2) in the regulation of mitosomal fission (Rout et al., 2016) and to the synchronization of mitosomal division with mitosis (Voleman et al., 2017).

Despite efforts towards obtaining a more comprehensive characterization of the organelles's proteome (Jedelsky et al., 2011), a full understanding of mitosomal metabolic networks remains elusive. To date, reliable information

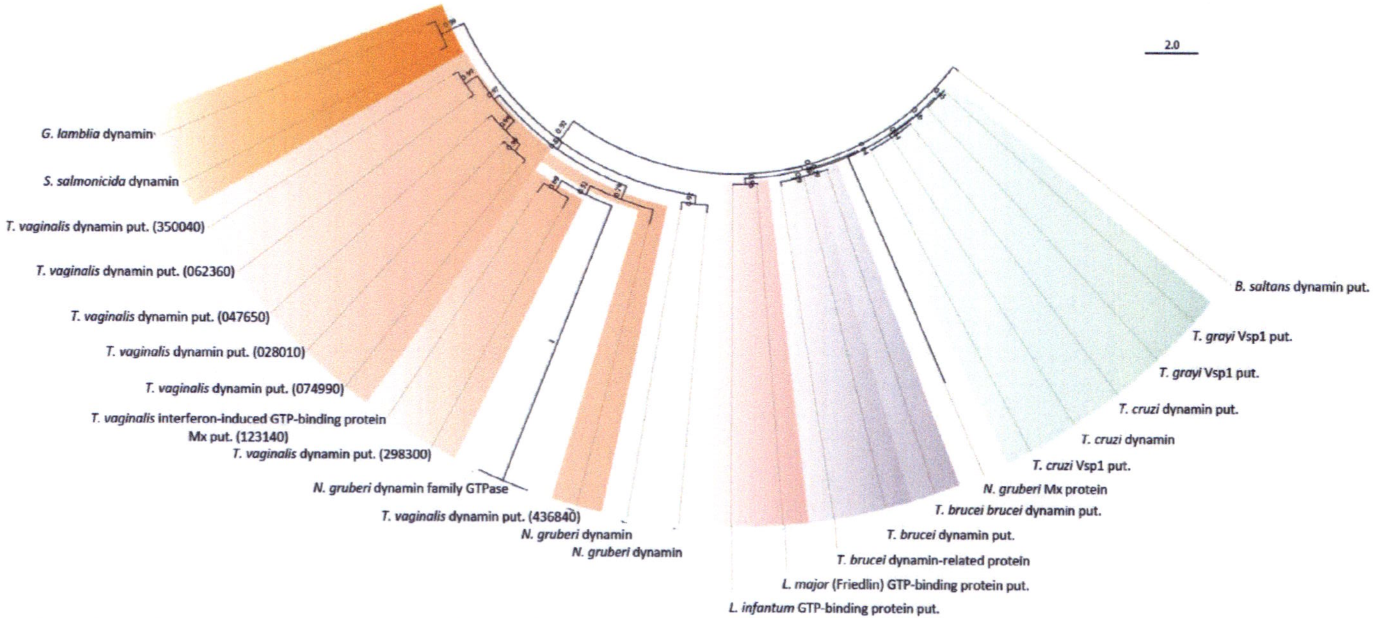

Fig. 2 A dynamin-centred phylogenetic tree for *Giardia* and other *Excavata* species. Dynamin sequences for 26 taxa were retrieved from public repositories, aligned using MUSCLE, trimmed using TRiMAL (STRICT setting) and subjected to a molecular phylogenetic analysis with PhyloBayes to construct a tree using a GTR-CAT substitution model. *G. lamblia* and *S. salmonicida* dynamins (orange) appear to be more closely related to the *T. vaginalis* family of dynamins (pink) than to *Kinetoplastida* proteins (fuchsia, violet and cyan). The bar on the right signifies branch length related to number of substitutions per residue analyzed.

on mitosome function in *G. lamblia* is limited to synthesis and maturation of iron-sulphur (Fe-S) clusters, an essential process which, with few exceptions, in Eukaryotes is limited to mitochondria and MROs (Lill, 2009; Lill and Kispal, 2000). This points to a possible explanation for the maintenance of mitosomes in otherwise highly reduced Protozoa such as *G. lamblia* and *E. histolytica* (Dellibovi-Ragheb et al., 2013). *Giardia*'s Fe-S cluster synthesis machinery includes the main components of this process, namely: cystein desulfurase (IscS), scaffold proteins IscA2, IscU and Nfu, glutaredoxin 5 (Grx5) and ferredoxin as electron transporters, and the chaperones Hsp70, Jac-1 and GrpE (Jedelsky et al., 2011; Muller et al., 2012). Notably, frataxin is missing, although this protein is present in other species harbouring mitosomes such as *C. parvum* (Abrahamsen et al., 2004) and *E. cuniculi* (Goldberg et al., 2008). Interestingly, although Fe-S cluster synthesis is known to require ATP, no giardial mitosomal ATP/ADP transporter has been identified so far (Hjort et al., 2010; Jedelsky et al., 2011), with no ATP synthesis occurring in the organelle. Therefore, the energy source for Fe-S cluster synthesis and chaperone function in giardial mitosomes remains unidentified.

2.2.3 Mitosomal protein targeting

The absence of a mitosomal genome requires that every component of this organelle's protein repertoire be imported from the cytosol across two membranes. This aspect of *Giardia* mitosomes places the spotlight on the machinery responsible for mediating protein trafficking into these organelles. This intracellular trafficking pathway has been well characterized in model organisms and it begins with the post-translational association of cytosolic chaperones to mitochondrial preproteins exhibiting targeting signals to the organelle (Pfanner et al., 1997). The interaction between preproteins and receptor components of the Translocon in the Outer Mitochondrial (TOM) complex leads to passage through Tom40, the outer membrane translocase (Pfanner et al., 1997). Tom40 homologues are beta-barrel proteins that function as the pore through which mitochondrial proteins cross the organelle's outer membrane. Proteins destined to the mitochondrial matrix are then transported through the Translocon in the Inner Mitochondrial membrane (TIM) complex (Pfanner et al., 1997).

The discovery of reduced mitochondrial remnants in *G. lamblia* inevitably raised the question whether mitosomal import machinery would be homologous to the one found in *bona fide* mitochondria. The first work that specifically addressed this (Dagley et al., 2009) reported on the identification *in silico* and localization of a putative Tom40 giardial homologue

(GlTom40; GL50803_17161). Tom40 homologues are part of the porin family of proteins, which includes both protein (Tom40-like) and metabolite (VDAC-like) translocases. Although an *in silico* analysis suggests that the giardial ORF is presumably more closely related to Tom40-like rather than to VDAC-like translocases (Dagley et al., 2009), definitive functional evidence for the protein translocase activity of GlTom40 is still lacking. However, given the absence of any other sequence closely related to GlTom40 in the predicted proteome, it is unlikely that *G. lamblia* possesses both Tom40 and VDAC. We could therefore speculate that transport across the outer mitosomal membrane occurs through a single porin family member. Alternatively, there may be an as-yet unidentified translocase which is either too diverged to be identified using conventional (e.g., BLAST tool suite) and sensitive (e.g., HMMER) homology-based search methods, or is entirely unrelated to members of the porin family. Interestingly, this is what was found in trypanosomes, fellow parasitic members of the *Excavata* supergroup. Although these organisms present *bona fide* class 1 mitochondria, protein translocation across the outer membrane is mediated by an atypical Tom40 homologue named ATOM, while a single VDAC-like porin family member is involved in metabolite transport (Pusnik et al., 2012).

Core components of the inner-membrane import and matrix machinery, such as Pam18, Pam16, mtHsp70 and the matrix-located processing peptidase (MPP), have been identified *in silico* and successfully localized to the *Giardia* mitosome (Dolezal et al., 2005; Regoes et al., 2005). Given the predicted location of PAM complex components at the inner membrane, this would suggest that an as-yet unidentified inner membrane translocation complex is indeed present in mitosomes. The possibility that a significant reduction in the mitosomal intermembrane space may obviate the need for a second inner translocon is appealing. However, there is currently no evidence for a direct physical association between giardial Pam18 or Pam16 homologs and GlTom40. Furthermore, although their exact subcellular location is unclear, highly diverged giardial TIM homologues have been recently identified using BirA-based *in vivo* enzymatic tagging techniques, coupled to protein co-immunoprecipitation and *in silico* searches using hidden Markov models (HMM) (Martincova et al., 2015; Pyrihova et al., 2018).

The first and only report on interaction partners for GlTom40 identified a single uncharacterized protein (Dagley et al., 2009). This left the question of the number of retained TOM complex components during the evolution of *Giardia* mitosomes, mostly unaddressed. Our own efforts over the past few years have led to a substantial increase in the size of the GlTom40 interactome (>40 protein partners), including the identification of a putative TOM complex receptor and novel matrix proteins of currently unknown function (Rout et al., 2016). Interestingly, specific GlTom40-associated SNARE proteins were found to localize both to the mitosomal surface and to the ER (Elias et al., 2008; Rout et al., 2016). SNARE proteins are almost invariably associated to vesicle trafficking where they mediate either vesicle-organelle or vesicle-vesicle fusion. Therefore, their association to mitosomes makes a compelling case for the presence of currently unknown trafficking routes involving this organelle. Alternatively, as found in other organisms and recently reported, these data also suggest the conservation of ER-mitochondria membrane contact sites (ERMES) that integrate mitosomes in a wider subcellular network (Rout et al., 2016; Voleman et al., 2017).

The acquisition of functional data by targeting the most promising GlTom40 interaction partners by means of mRNA or protein ablation approaches will be helpful to determine to what extent the metabolic reduction of the giardial mitosome is mirrored in the composition of its import machinery.

2.3 The way out: Exocytosis

2.3.1 Variant surface proteins and constitutive secretion

By far, the bulk of constitutive secretion cargo in *G. lamblia* cells is predicted to be composed of variant surface protein (VSP) which forms a dense protein coat covering the entire surface of every giardial cell (Adam, 2001). VSP is a large protein family whose members present some or all of the following features: an N-terminal signal sequence to direct secretion to the plasma membrane (PM), enrichment in Cys residues (usually in the Cys-X-X-Cys sequence configuration), a semi-conserved hydrophobic C-terminal sequence predicted to act as a transmembrane domain, and an invariable cytosolic tail consisting of residues Cys-Arg-Gly-Lys-Ala (CRGKA) that has been shown to play an important role in targeting to the PM (Marti et al., 2002). Based on the most comprehensive annotation efforts to date (Adam et al., 2010; Li et al., 2013; Morrison et al., 2007), the assemblage A WB strain presents up to 303 *vsp* genes, of which 228 are complete whereas the remaining 75 correspond to incomplete/partial open reading frames (ORF) (Adam et al., 2010). Previous reports (Adam et al., 2010) and our own unpublished investigations indicate that several incomplete or partial ORFs may need a manual re-annotation that would lengthen their sequences to include crucial missing elements such as *bona fide* N-terminal secretory leader sequences. This may in part explain recent data concerning the correct trafficking of VSPs which, in some cases, are predicted to be leader-less *in silico* (Li et al., 2013).

VSP trafficking has been investigated in some detail over the past years due to its role in antigenic switching. Every trophozoite is presumably covered by a single VSP species at any given time, with a switch to a new VSP type after 6 to 13 generations of division (Nash et al., 1990). The genomic organization of *vsp* genes is also peculiar, frequently presenting head-to-head or tail-to-tail configurations (Morrison et al., 2007). Factors affecting the frequency of VSP replacement have not yet been defined. Furthermore, this form of antigenic variation has been generally ascribed to a giardial immune evasion strategy, similarly to well-characterized antigenic variation mechanisms described in trypanosomes (Boothroyd, 1985).

Previous experiments have shown a correlation between surface antigen (VSP) coat variation and antibody-mediated responses (Gottstein and Nash, 1991). Furthermore, VSPs are the main antigens recognized by the host's immune system (Nash, 1997) and are surprisingly resistant to proteolysis (Muller and Gottstein, 1998). However, there is yet no 'smoking-gun' evidence that *Giardia* utilizes variations of its VSP coat to escape the host's immune response. In this context, it may be helpful to consider that antigenic variation *per se* is not aimed exclusively at host immune evasion. This phenomenon is present in free-living protozoa such as the ciliate genera *Paramecium* and *Tetrahymena* (Simon and Schmidt, 2007). Therefore, it is possible that antigenic variation in *Giardia* plays other as-yet unknown roles which may not be related to evasion of host immune responses.

Given that the Golgi organelle has not been detected in *Giardia* trophozoites, the question of how VSP secretion actually occurs in this organism is immediately raised. The large ER network which occupies most of the cell's volume clearly plays a fundamental role in sorting and directing secretory cargo to its final destination(s) (Zamponi et al., 2017). VSP secretion was shown to bypass any intermediate stations between the ER and the PM (Marti et al., 2002) and to associate to coatomer protein 1 and 2 (COP1 and COP2) complexes at ER exit sites (Marti et al., 2003a). There are conflicting reports on the structural requirements for correct VSP localization at the PM, with the C-terminal cytosolically-exposed tail CRGKA considered to be necessary and sufficient for correct VSP targeting (Marti et al., 2002) or more recently-identified motifs which would bring the number of potentially functional VSPs down to 73 from the reported 303 (Li et al., 2013). Although the exact role for antigenic variation in *Giardia* has not yet been determined, the mechanism by which a giardial cell expresses a single VSP on its surface has been partially elucidated. Work done mainly by the Lujan group on clonal populations which express a single VSP has shown that, although many different kinds of VSP transcript are produced, only 1 type accumulates and is translated to yield the VSP exposed on the parasite's surface (Prucca et al., 2008). Further investigations led to the conclusion that RNA interference (RNAi)-based mechanisms are at play in the regulation of VSP expression, supported by the presence of VSP-targeted small RNAs and three putative giardial homologues of the main components of the RNAi machinery, namely, RNA-dependent RNA polymerase, Dicer and Argonaute (Ago) (Prucca et al., 2011). Furthermore, two putative micro (mi)RNAs that co-immunoprecipitated with Ago are predicted to bind the 3′ end of over 200 VSP transcripts, further enriching the landscape of post-translational regulation of VSP expression (Li et al., 2012). Importantly, no mechanisms involving promoter activation or gene conversion (Boothroyd, 1985) have so far been implicated in *Giardia* antigenic variation. What still remains unknown is (a) how this mechanism is regulated in relation to the number of divisions required for antigenic switching, (b) why certain *vsp* genes are expressed and others not or only very rarely and, finally, (c) how VSP shedding and turnover at the surface is regulated on a molecular level. Importantly, VSPs are exemplary of how basic research on the molecular mechanisms underlying gene and protein expression can successfully steer biomedical applications such as vaccine development. Work done especially by the Lujan group in Argentina has uncovered the effectiveness of VSPs as vaccination antigens in companion animals. By de-regulating *vsp* gene expression, trophozoites exposing the full VSP panel on their surface were used in oral vaccination trials on gerbils (Rivero et al., 2010c). These animals were found to be largely protected from challenge infections by *Giardia* clones that express a unique VSP on their surface or by cysts obtained from infected individuals. Importantly, these data provide the strongest evidence yet that VSPs are indeed involved in immune-evasion. The same vaccine was tested on cats and dogs, showing high efficiency in preventing new infections and reducing chronic giardiasis in domestic animals both in experimental and natural infections (Serradell et al., 2016). A recent report on VSP 9B10A, highlights its proteolytic activity and damage to epithelial cells when expressed ectopically, suggesting novel roles for VSPs which await further investigation (Cabrera-Licona et al., 2017).

The investigation of constitutive secretion in *Giardia* trophozoites is still very much VSP-centred. However, recent reports on proteomic analyses of the *Giardia in vitro* secretome highlight the variety of secreted proteins found in conditioned media (Dubourg et al., 2018; Ma'ayeh et al., 2017), including the little-characterized family of secreted *Giardia* tenascins which have recently emerged as important virulence factors (Dubourg et al., 2018).

2.3.2 Cyst-wall proteins and regulated or inducible secretion

Cyst development requires a reorganization of cellular structures and building of an impermeable cyst wall (CW) during the process called encystation. During this process, flagellated binucleated trophozoites undergo significant morphological and biochemical cellular remodelling, culminating in the formation of oval quadrinucleated cysts presenting resorbed flagella, fragmented ventral disk cytoskeleton and surrounded by a sturdy CW. The CW is composed of a thick mesh of a unique GalNAc polymer complexed to cyst wall proteins (CWPs) (Samuelson and Robbins, 2011). Cysts are then shed through host faeces and were reported to remain viable for several months in water at temperatures below 10 °C and several weeks at room temperature (Bingham et al., 1979). The exact *in vivo* stimuli for encystation are not yet known. Recent studies on the dynamics of encystation in animal models point towards a link between high-density focal trophozoite populations in the proximal small intestine, and encystation (Barash et al., 2017). These data support the intriguing hypothesis that trophozoites can alter their local environment to generate conditions favourable to cyst differentiation.

CWPs are uniquely expressed during encystation by a promoter-based de-repression mechanism that is only partially elucidated (Morf et al., 2010; Sonda et al., 2010). In line with this, deposition of the CW is a tightly-regulated event that occurs exclusively in encysting trophozoites and requires neogenesis of specialized secretory organelles called encystation-specific vesicles (ESVs) (Konrad et al., 2010). ESVs traffic, sort and modify CWPs from their initial site of synthesis at the ER, to the parasite cell's surface. ESV and CW formation can be abolished by eliminating even a single CWP by complete gene disruption (Ebneter et al., 2016), demonstrating how CWPs, although similar in their sequence and overall predicted structure, are not functionally redundant. ESV neogenesis depends on active ER exit sites (Faso et al., 2013a) and is associated to coatomer and to COPII components Sec23 and Sec24 in the early stages of ESV development. ESVs were shown to partition and sort CWPs in two fractions, one more fluid and peripheral consisting mainly of CWP1 and one more condensed composed mainly of CWP3 with the fundamental contribution of a condensation-promoting short CWP2 fragment (Konrad et al., 2010). ESV sensitivity to brefeldin A (Marti et al., 2003b) and dependence on functional Sar1GTPase (Faso et al., 2013a; Stefanic et al., 2009) is clearly reminiscent of Golgi organelles. However, it is still unclear whether ESVs and Golgi are homologous or analogous to each other. Furthermore, the exact mechanism whereby ESV cargo is sequentially translocated across the PM to build the CW is still only partially understood (Konrad et al., 2010).

2.3.3 Atypical protein secretion

Symptoms of giardiasis are the result of trophozoite adhesion to host cells of the intestinal mucosa and proliferation in the small intestine. Over the past years, work done mainly by the Gillin and Svärd groups has probed the molecular aspects of *G. lamblia* trophozoite interaction with host cells *in vitro*. Their investigations showed that giardial enolase (ENO), ornithine carbamoyltransferase (OCT), translational elongation factor 1α (TEF1α) and arginine deiminase (ADI) are generally localized in the cytosol of trophozoites in axenic cultures. However, upon co-cultivation with intestinal cells, these proteins were found in the extracellular culture medium, suggesting they were secreted by the parasite as virulence factors in response to host cell-dependent cues (Eckmann et al., 2000; Ringqvist et al., 2008; Skarin et al., 2011; Touz et al., 2008). Strikingly, what ENO, ADI, OCT and TEF1α have in common is the absence of any *bona fide* predicted signal sequence (SS). Since protein secretion in Eukaryotes is almost universally dependent on SS interaction with the signal recognition particle to allow entry of the nascent secretory polypeptide into the ER lumen (Nyathi et al., 2013), the molecular mechanisms governing secretion of giardial ENO, ADI, OCT and TEF1α in response to host cells can be ascribed to unconventional or non-canonical secretion. Whether this occurs *via* extracellular vesicles such as in other protozoan parasites (Mantel et al., 2013; Twu et al., 2013) is currently unknown, although recent reports on the release of microvesicles upon exposure of host cells to *Giardia* trophozoites point in this direction (Evans-Osses et al., 2017).

The role for non-canonical secretion of ADI and OCT in *G. lamblia* host-pathogen interaction was specifically investigated in connection to arginine metabolism in the gut. The availability of arginine is one of the rate-limiting factors in host cell production of the pro-inflammatory signalling molecule nitric oxide (NO). Inducible NO synthesis from arginine by NO synthase (NOS) is important as a toxic defence molecule against infectious organisms (Wink et al., 1991). NO also regulates the functional activity, growth and death of many immune and inflammatory cell types including macrophages, T-lymphocytes, antigen-presenting cells, mast cells, neutrophils and natural killer cells (Kolios et al., 2004). Unlike NOS, giardial ADI and OCT degrade arginine to citrulline and ammonia, leading to a local depletion of arginine in the gut, thus negatively impacting host cell-dependent NO production (Banik et al., 2013; Stadelmann et al., 2012). Importantly, the inhibition of NO synthesis was shown to increase epithelial permeability *via* loosening of tight junctions and to reduce intestinal mucus secretion (Kochar et al., 2011; Kubes, 2000). Taken together, these data point towards giardial ADI and OCT non-canonical secretion as a strategy to promote parasite adhesion and invasion by lowering local NO concentration in the gut. In turn, this could inhibit inflammatory and toxic responses to parasite infection, thus allowing for the establishment of chronic *Giardia* infections.

3. Open questions and future directions

3.1 Organelle replication and partitioning in *G. lamblia*

Mitosomes are abundant organelles whose subcellular origin is still undetermined. The question of how new peripheral mitosomes arise still remains a puzzle. A hypothesis that has gained some traction postulates that the CMC is the source of new peripheral mitosomes (Regoes et al., 2005). However, there are currently no data to conclusively support or refute this hypothesis. While the central mitosome complex was shown to remain tightly associated and partition with the replicated basal body complexes into daughter cells early during cytokinesis, it is still unclear whether subcellular distribution of peripheral mitosomes and partitioning between daughter cells during cytokinesis is indeed random, as previously suggested (Regoes et al., 2005). Given that mitosomes were shown to constitutively interact with the ER (Voleman et al., 2017), this organelle may mediate both division and partitioning, as shown in other organisms (Friedman et al., 2011). Treatment with drugs that interfere with correct cytoskeletal structure was shown to disturb mitosome homeostasis, with cytochalasin-B causing an over-proliferation of organelles and nocodazole displacing the CMC at the cell's periphery (Regoes et al., 2005). This may be an indirect effect of impacting ER structure which is known to depend on the cytoskeleton for its correct configuration. However, the question of how mitosomes divide to give rise to a new set of organelles and whether dynamin-like proteins are involved in this process (Rout et al., 2016; Voleman et al., 2017), still needs to be addressed.

Similar to mitosomes, PVs are abundant organelles whose morphogenesis and replication during cell division are currently unknown. Although their role in endocytosis is well-established, PV division and partitioning among daughter cells remains mostly uncharacterized. It is unclear at what point of the cell cycle a new set of PVs is made and what the membrane source for this process is. Once again, the ER may play an important role, given that it is the largest organelle in the *Giardia* trophozoite and has been shown to contact PVs frequently (Abodeely et al., 2009; Zumthor et al., 2016). These membrane contacts were implicated in the translocation of selected cargo from PVs to the ER (Abodeely et al., 2009) but may also provide a membrane source for new PV organelles. GlDRP is implicated in PV homeostasis as shown by the enlarged PV phenotype resulting from expression of a predicted GTP-locked mutant GlDRP variant (Gaechter et al., 2008). However, GlDRP was also shown to be a component of the core clathrin heavy chain interactome and to localize at the PV-PM interface (Zumthor et al., 2016). It may therefore be premature to ascribe the enlarged PV phenotype to a division-related defect exclusively.

3.2 Machinery for unconventional secretion at *G. lamblia*'s host-parasite interface

To date, none of the (very few) known subcellular components participating in non-canonical secretion in mammalian and fungal cells have any *in silico* identifiable homologue in *G. lamblia*, suggesting the evolution of highly diverged lineage-specific mechanism/s in this parasite (Touz and Zamponi, 2017). Considering the strong reduction in organellar and molecular complexity in the evolution of *G. lamblia* (Ankarklev et al., 2010; Faso and Hehl, 2011), one could speculate that *un*conventional secretion during trophozoite proliferation in the small intestine is achieved, at least in part, through co-option of conventional secretion components such as COPI/COPII carriers and Arf GTPases. Upon the induction of cyst formation, these components may be re-routed to the canonical secretory pathway for the deposition of cyst wall material, thus inhibiting non-canonical routes during differentiation. Exhaustive testing of this hypothesis requires the identification and functional characterization of the molecular machinery involved in giardial ENO, ADI, OCT and TEF1α trafficking. Recent reports on the variety of surface-exposed yet leader-less secreted proteins have dramatically expanded our catalogue of potential SS substrates (Ma'ayeh et al., 2017), opening up exciting research directions to unveil core conserved US machinery in *G. lamblia* involved in the modulation of host-parasite interactions.

3.3 Gene ablation strategies for functional characterization in *G. lamblia*

Giardia trophozoites in the G1 phase of the cell cycle are tetraploids cells, with each nucleus containing two genome copies. Hence, functional characterization by ablation of any given gene or protein product requires targeting of four distinct loci. In the absence of haploid gametes and a sexual cycle, gene disruption in *G. lamblia* poses a challenge. Approaches to reduce or even abolish gene expression or mRNA translation based on antisense RNA and morpholinos, respectively, were shown to have limited efficacy (Carpenter and Cande, 2009; Rivero et al., 2010a).

By using a combination of sequential recombination and Cre/loxP-mediated antibiotic resistance gene excision (Wampfler et al., 2014), the first *G. lamblia* knock-out line was produced, carrying four non-functional *cwp1* loci (Ebneter et al., 2016). A less time-consuming procedure for gene disruption in *G. lamblia*, based on the *Streptococcus pyogenes* class II CRISPR-Cas9 system, was recently developed and tested. Despite correct nuclear targeting of the Cas9 endonuclease concomitant with *in vivo* sgRNA expression, target gene expression could be significantly decreased but not abolished (Lin et al., 2019). A variant of this system based on a catalytically-inactive Cas9 as a transcription repressor to displace RNA polymerase II complexes yielded similar results (McInally et al., 2019). These data suggest that current CRISPR-Cas9 set-ups are not yet sufficient to obtain complete gene ablation in *G. lamblia*. Further efforts are therefore necessary to harness the full power of the CRISPR-Cas9 tool to perform genomic manipulations in this parasite.

Acknowledgements

T.A. Williams at Bristol University (United Kingdom) and R. Hirt at Newcastle University (United Kingdom) are gratefully acknowledged for help in constructing the *Excavata* dynamin phylogenetic tree.

References

Abodeely, M., DuBois, K.N., Hehl, A., Stefanic, S., Sajid, M., DeSouza, W., Attias, M., Engel, J.C., Hsieh, I., Fetter, R.D., McKerrow, J.H., 2009. A contiguous compartment functions as endoplasmic reticulum and endosome/lysosome in *Giardia lamblia*. Eukaryot. Cell 8 (11), 1665–1676.

Abrahamsen, M.S., Templeton, T.J., Enomoto, S., Abrahante, J.E., Zhu, G., Lancto, C.A., Deng, M., Liu, C., Widmer, G., Tzipori, S., Buck, G.A., Xu, P., Bankier, A.T., Dear, P.H., Konfortov, B.A., Spriggs, H.F., Iyer, L., Anantharaman, V., Aravind, L., Kapur, V., 2004. Complete genome sequence of the apicomplexan, *Cryptosporidium parvum*. Science 304 (5669), 441–445.

Adam, R.D., 2001. Biology of *Giardia lamblia*. Clin. Microbiol. Rev. 14 (3), 447–475.

Adam, R.D., Nigam, A., Seshadri, V., Martens, C.A., Farneth, G.A., Morrison, H.G., Nash, T.E., Porcella, S.F., Patel, R., 2010. The *Giardia lamblia* vsp gene repertoire: characteristics, genomic organization, and evolution. BMC Genomics 11, 424.

Ankarklev, J., Jerlstrom-Hultqvist, J., Ringqvist, E., Troell, K., Svard, S.G., 2010. Behind the smile: cell biology and disease mechanisms of Giardia species. Nat. Rev. Microbiol. 8 (6), 413–422.

Banik, S., Renner Viveros, P., Seeber, F., Klotz, C., Ignatius, R., Aebischer, T., 2013. Giardia duodenalis arginine deiminase modulates the phenotype and cytokine secretion of human dendritic cells by depletion of arginine and formation of ammonia. Infect. Immun. 81 (7), 2309–2317.

Barash, N.R., Nosala, C., Pham, J.K., McInally, S.G., Gourguechon, S., McCarthy-Sinclair, B., Dawson, S.C., 2017. Giardia colonizes and encysts in high-density foci in the murine small intestine. mSphere 2 (3). https://doi.org/10.1128/mSphere.00343-16.

Bingham, A.K., Jarroll Jr., E.L., Meyer, E.A., Radulescu, S., 1979. Giardia sp.: physical factors of excystation in vitro, and excystation vs eosin exclusion as determinants of viability. Exp. Parasitol. 47 (2), 284–291.

Boothroyd, J.C., 1985. Antigenic variation in African trypanosomes. Annu. Rev. Microbiol. 39, 475–502.

Bowers, W.E., 1998. Christian de Duve and the discovery of lysosomes and peroxisomes. Trends Cell Biol. 8 (8), 330–333.

Boxma, B., de Graaf, R.M., van der Staay, G.W., van Alen, T.A., Ricard, G., Gabaldon, T., van Hoek, A.H., Moon-van der Staay, S.Y., Koopman, W.J., van Hellemond, J.J., Tielens, A.G., Friedrich, T., Veenhuis, M., Huynen, M.A., Hackstein, J.H., 2005. An anaerobic mitochondrion that produces hydrogen. Nature 434 (7029), 74–79.

Cabrera-Licona, A., Solano-Gonzalez, E., Fonseca-Linan, R., Bazan-Tejeda, M.L., Raul, A.-G., Bermudez-Cruz, R.M., Ortega-Pierres, G., 2017. Expression and secretion of the Giardia duodenalis variant surface protein 9B10A by transfected trophozoites causes damage to epithelial cell monolayers mediated by protease activity. Exp. Parasitol. 179, 49–64.

Carpenter, M.L., Cande, W.Z., 2009. Using morpholinos for gene knockdown in Giardia intestinalis. Eukaryot. Cell 8 (6), 916–919.

Cavalier-Smith, T., 1987. Eukaryotes with no mitochondria. Nature 326 (6111), 332–333.

Dagley, M.J., Dolezal, P., Likic, V.A., Smid, O., Purcell, A.W., Buchanan, S.K., Tachezy, J., Lithgow, T., 2009. The protein import channel in the outer mitosomal membrane of Giardia intestinalis. Mol. Biol. Evol. 26 (9), 1941–1947.

Dellibovi-Ragheb, T.A., Gisselberg, J.E., Prigge, S.T., 2013. Parasites FeS up: iron-sulfur cluster biogenesis in eukaryotic pathogens. PLoS Pathog. 9 (4), e1003227.

Dolezal, P., Smid, O., Rada, P., Zubacova, Z., Bursac, D., Sutak, R., Nebesarova, J., Lithgow, T., Tachezy, J., 2005. Giardia mitosomes and trichomonad hydrogenosomes share a common mode of protein targeting. Proc. Natl. Acad. Sci. U. S. A. 102 (31), 10924–10929.

Dubourg, A., Xia, D., Winpenny, J.P., Al Naimi, S., Bouzid, M., Sexton, D.W., Wastling, J.M., Hunter, P.R., Tyler, K.M., 2018. Giardia secretome highlights secreted tenascins as a key component of pathogenesis. GigaScience 7 (3), 1–13.

Ebneter, J.A., Heusser, S.D., Schraner, E.M., Hehl, A.B., Faso, C., 2016. Cyst-Wall-Protein-1 is fundamental for Golgi-like organelle neogenesis and cyst-wall biosynthesis in *Giardia lamblia*. Nat. Commun. 7, 13859.

Eckmann, L., Laurent, F., Langford, T.D., Hetsko, M.L., Smith, J.R., Kagnoff, M.F., Gillin, F.D., 2000. Nitric oxide production by human intestinal epithelial cells and competition for arginine as potential determinants of host defense against the lumen-dwelling pathogen *Giardia lamblia*. J. Immunol. 164 (3), 1478–1487.

Elias, E.V., Quiroga, R., Gottig, N., Nakanishi, H., Nash, T.E., Neiman, A., Lujan, H.D., 2008. Characterization of SNAREs determines the absence of a typical Golgi apparatus in the ancient eukaryote *Giardia lamblia*. J. Biol. Chem. 283 (51), 35996–36010.

Emelyanov, V.V., Goldberg, A.V., 2010. Fermentation enzymes of Giardia intestinalis, pyruvate:ferredoxin oxidoreductase and hydrogenase, do not localize to its mitosomes. Microbiology 157 (Pt. 6), 1602–1611.

Evans-Osses, I., Mojoli, A., Monguio-Tortajada, M., Marcilla, A., Aran, V., Amorim, M., Inal, J., Borras, F.E., Ramirez, M.I., 2017. Microvesicles released from Giardia intestinalis disturb host-pathogen response in vitro. Eur. J. Cell Biol. 96 (2), 131–142.

Faso, C., Hehl, A.B., 2011. Membrane trafficking and organelle biogenesis in *Giardia lamblia*: use it or lose it. Int. J. Parasitol. 41 (5), 471–480.

Faso, C., Konrad, C., Schraner, E.M., Hehl, A.B., 2013a. Export of cyst wall material and Golgi organelle neogenesis in *Giardia lamblia* depend on endoplasmic reticulum exit sites. Cell Microbiol. 15 (4), 537–553. https://doi.org/10.1111/cmi.12054. Epub 2012 Dec 2.

Faso, C., Bischof, S., Hehl, A.B., 2013b. The proteome landscape of *Giardia lamblia* encystation. PLoS One 8 (12), e83207.

Feely, D.E., Dyer, J.K., 1987. Localization of acid phosphatase activity in *Giardia lamblia* and Giardia muris trophozoites. J. Protozool. 34 (1), 80–83.

Feliziani, C., Zamponi, N., Gottig, N., Ropolo, A.S., Lanfredi-Rangel, A., Touz, M.C., 2015. The giardial ENTH protein participates in lysosomal protein trafficking and endocytosis. Biochim. Biophys. Acta 1853 (3), 646–659.

Friedman, J.R., Lackner, L.L., West, M., DiBenedetto, J.R., Nunnari, J., Voeltz, G.K., 2011. ER tubules mark sites of mitochondrial division. Science 334 (6054), 358–362.

Furness, B.W., Beach, M.J., Roberts, J.M., 2000. Giardiasis surveillance—United States, 1992–1997. MMWR CDC Surveill. Summ. 49 (7), 1–13.

Gaechter, V., Schraner, E., Wild, P., Hehl, A.B., 2008. The single dynamin family protein in the primitive protozoan *Giardia lamblia* is essential for stage conversion and endocytic transport. Traffic 9 (1), 57–71.

Goldberg, A.V., Molik, S., Tsaousis, A.D., Neumann, K., Kuhnke, G., Delbac, F., Vivares, C.P., Hirt, R.P., Lill, R., Embley, T.M., 2008. Localization and functionality of microsporidian iron-sulphur cluster assembly proteins. Nature 452 (7187), 624–628.

Gottstein, B., Nash, T.E., 1991. Antigenic variation in *Giardia lamblia*: infection of congenitally athymic nude and scid mice. Parasite Immunol. 13 (6), 649–659.

Hehl, A.B., Regos, A., Schraner, E., Schneider, A., 2007. Bax function in the absence of mitochondria in the primitive protozoan *Giardia lamblia*. PLoS One 2 (5), e488.

Hjort, K., Goldberg, A.V., Tsaousis, A.D., Hirt, R.P., Embley, T.M., 2010. Diversity and reductive evolution of mitochondria among microbial eukaryotes. Philos. Trans. R. Soc. Lond. Ser. B Biol. Sci. 365 (1541), 713–727.

Jana, A., Sinha, A., Sarkar, S., 2017. Phosphoinositide binding profiles of the PX domains of *Giardia lamblia*. Parasitol. Int. 66 (5), 606–614.

Jedelsky, P.L., Dolezal, P., Rada, P., Pyrih, J., Smid, O., Hrdy, I., Sedinova, M., Marcincikova, M., Voleman, L., Perry, A.J., Beltran, N.C., Lithgow, T., Tachezy, J., 2011. The minimal proteome in the reduced mitochondrion of the parasitic protist Giardia intestinalis. PLoS One 6 (2), e17285.

Jerlstrom-Hultqvist, J., Einarsson, E., Xu, F., Hjort, K., Ek, B., Steinhauf, D., Hultenby, K., Bergquist, J., Andersson, J.O., Svard, S.G., 2013. Hydrogenosomes in the diplomonad *Spironucleus salmonicida.* Nat. Commun. 4, 2493.

Kochar, N., Chandewal, A., Bakal, R., Kochar, P., 2011. Nitric oxide and the gastrointestinal tract. Int. J. Pharmacol. 7, 10.

Kolios, G., Valatas, V., Ward, S.G., 2004. Nitric oxide in inflammatory bowel disease: a universal messenger in an unsolved puzzle. Immunology 113 (4), 427–437.

Konrad, C., Spycher, C., Hehl, A.B., 2010. Selective condensation drives partitioning and sequential secretion of cyst wall proteins in differentiating *Giardia lamblia.* PLoS Pathog. 6 (4), e1000835.

Kubes, P., 2000. Inducible nitric oxide synthase: a little bit of good in all of us. Gut 47 (1), 6–9.

Li, W., Saraiya, A.A., Wang, C.C., 2012. The profile of snoRNA-derived microRNAs that regulate expression of variant surface proteins in *Giardia lamblia.* Cell. Microbiol. 14 (9), 1455–1473.

Li, W., Saraiya, A.A., Wang, C.C., 2013. Experimental verification of the identity of variant-specific surface proteins in *Giardia lamblia* trophozoites. MBio 4 (3), e00321-00313.

Lill, R., 2009. Function and biogenesis of iron-sulphur proteins. Nature 460 (7257), 831–838.

Lill, R., Kispal, G., 2000. Maturation of cellular Fe-S proteins: an essential function of mitochondria. Trends Biochem. Sci. 25 (8), 352–356.

Lin, Z.Q., Gan, S.W., Tung, S.Y., Ho, C.C., Su, L.H., Sun, C.H., 2019. Development of CRISPR/Cas9-mediated gene disruption systems in *Giardia lamblia.* PLoS One 14 (3), e0213594.

Lloyd, D., Ralphs, J.R., Harris, J.C., 2002. Giardia intestinalis, a eukaryote without hydrogenosomes, produces hydrogen. Microbiology 148 (Pt. 3), 727–733.

Ma'ayeh, S.Y., Liu, J., Peirasmaki, D., Hornaeus, K., Bergstrom Lind, S., Grabherr, M., Bergquist, J., Svard, S.G., 2017. Characterization of the Giardia intestinalis secretome during interaction with human intestinal epithelial cells: the impact on host cells. PLoS Negl. Trop. Dis. 11 (12), e0006120.

Mantel, P.Y., Hoang, A.N., Goldowitz, I., Potashnikova, D., Hamza, B., Vorobjev, I., Ghiran, I., Toner, M., Irimia, D., Ivanov, A.R., Barteneva, N., Marti, M., 2013. Malaria-infected erythrocyte-derived microvesicles mediate cellular communication within the parasite population and with the host immune system. Cell Host Microbe 13 (5), 521–534.

Marti, M., Li, Y., Kohler, P., Hehl, A.B., 2002. Conformationally correct expression of membrane-anchored *Toxoplasma gondii* SAG1 in the primitive protozoan Giardia duodenalis. Infect. Immun. 70 (2), 1014–1016.

Marti, M., Regos, A., Li, Y., Schraner, E.M., Wild, P., Muller, N., Knopf, L.G., Hehl, A.B., 2003a. An ancestral secretory apparatus in the protozoan parasite Giardia intestinalis. J. Biol. Chem. 278 (27), 24837–24848.

Marti, M., Li, Y., Schraner, E.M., Wild, P., Kohler, P., Hehl, A.B., 2003b. The secretory apparatus of an ancient eukaryote: protein sorting to separate export pathways occurs before formation of transient Golgi-like compartments. Mol. Biol. Cell 14 (4), 1433–1447.

Martin, W., 2005. The missing link between hydrogenosomes and mitochondria. Trends Microbiol. 13 (10), 457–459.

Martincova, E., Voleman, L., Pyrih, J., Zarsky, V., Vondrackova, P., Kolisko, M., Tachezy, J., Dolezal, P., 2015. Probing the biology of Giardia intestinalis mitosomes using in vivo enzymatic tagging. Mol. Cell. Biol. 35 (16), 2864–2874.

McInally, S.G., Hagen, K.D., Nosala, C., Williams, J., Nguyen, K., Booker, J., Jones, K., Dawson, S.C., 2019. Robust and stable transcriptional repression in Giardia using CRISPRi. Mol. Biol. Cell 30 (1), 119–130.

Millet, C.O., Williams, C.F., Hayes, A.J., Hann, A.C., Cable, J., Lloyd, D., 2013. Mitochondria-derived organelles in the diplomonad fish parasite *Spironucleus vortens*. Exp. Parasitol. 135 (2), 262–273.

Morf, L., Spycher, C., Rehrauer, H., Fournier, C.A., Morrison, H.G., Hehl, A.B., 2010. The transcriptional response to encystation stimuli in *Giardia lamblia* is restricted to a small set of genes. Eukaryot. Cell 9 (10), 1566–1576.

Morrison, H.G., McArthur, A.G., Gillin, F.D., Aley, S.B., Adam, R.D., Olsen, G.J., Best, A.A., Cande, W.Z., Chen, F., Cipriano, M.J., Davids, B.J., Dawson, S.C., Elmendorf, H.G., Hehl, A.B., Holder, M.E., Huse, S.M., Kim, U.U., Lasek-Nesselquist, E., Manning, G., Nigam, A., Nixon, J.E., Palm, D., Passamaneck, N.E., Prabhu, A., Reich, C.I., Reiner, D.S., Samuelson, J., Svard, S.G., Sogin, M.L., 2007. Genomic minimalism in the early diverging intestinal parasite *Giardia lamblia*. Science 317 (5846), 1921–1926.

Muller, M., 1993. The hydrogenosome. J. Gen. Microbiol. 139 (12), 2879–2889.

Müller, M., 2003. Energy metabolism. Part 1: anaerobic protozoa. In: Marr, J.J., Nilsen, T.W., Komuniecki, R.W. (Eds.), Molecular Medical Parasitology. Academic Press, London, UK, pp. 125–139.

Muller, N., Gottstein, B., 1998. Antigenic variation and the murine immune response to *Giardia lamblia*. Int. J. Parasitol. 28 (12), 1829–1839.

Muller, M., Mentel, M., van Hellemond, J.J., Henze, K., Woehle, C., Gould, S.B., Yu, R.Y., van der Giezen, M., Tielens, A.G., Martin, W.F., 2012. Biochemistry and evolution of anaerobic energy metabolism in eukaryotes. Microbiol. Mol. Biol. Rev. 76 (2), 444–495.

Nash, T.E., 1997. Antigenic variation in *Giardia lamblia* and the host's immune response. Philos. Trans. R. Soc. Lond. Ser. B Biol. Sci. 352 (1359), 1369–1375.

Nash, T.E., Banks, S.M., Alling, D.W., Merritt Jr., J.W., Conrad, J.T., 1990. Frequency of variant antigens in *Giardia lamblia*. Exp. Parasitol. 71 (4), 415–421.

Nyathi, Y., Wilkinson, B.M., Pool, M.R., 2013. Co-translational targeting and translocation of proteins to the endoplasmic reticulum. Biochimica et Biophysica Acta 1833, 2392–2402.

Pfanner, N., Craig, E.A., Honlinger, A., 1997. Mitochondrial preprotein translocase. Annu. Rev. Cell Dev. Biol. 13, 25–51.

Prucca, C.G., Slavin, I., Quiroga, R., Elias, E.V., Rivero, F.D., Saura, A., Carranza, P.G., Lujan, H.D., 2008. Antigenic variation in *Giardia lamblia* is regulated by RNA interference. Nature 456 (7223), 750–754.

Prucca, C.G., Rivero, F.D., Lujan, H.D., 2011. Regulation of antigenic variation in *Giardia lamblia*. Annu. Rev. Microbiol. 65, 611–630.

Pusnik, M., Mani, J., Schmidt, O., Niemann, M., Oeljeklaus, S., Schnarwiler, F., Warscheid, B., Lithgow, T., Meisinger, C., Schneider, A., 2012. An essential novel component of the noncanonical mitochondrial outer membrane protein import system of trypanosomatids. Mol. Biol. Cell 23 (17), 3420–3428.

Pyrihova, E., Motyckova, A., Voleman, L., Wandyszewska, N., Fiser, R., Seydlova, G., Roger, A., Kolisko, M., Dolezal, P., 2018. A single Tim translocase in the mitosomes of Giardia intestinalis illustrates convergence of protein import machines in anaerobic eukaryotes. Genome Biol. Evol. 10 (10), 2813–2822.

Regoes, A., Zourmpanou, D., Leon-Avila, G., van der Giezen, M., Tovar, J., Hehl, A.B., 2005. Protein import, replication, and inheritance of a vestigial mitochondrion. J. Biol. Chem. 280 (34), 30557–30563.

Ringqvist, E., Palm, J.E., Skarin, H., Hehl, A.B., Weiland, M., Davids, B.J., Reiner, D.S., Griffiths, W.J., Eckmann, L., Gillin, F.D., Svard, S.G., 2008. Release of metabolic enzymes by Giardia in response to interaction with intestinal epithelial cells. Mol. Biochem. Parasitol. 159 (2), 85–91.

Rivero, M.R., Kulakova, L., Touz, M.C., 2010a. Long double-stranded RNA produces specific gene downregulation in *Giardia lamblia*. J. Parasitol. 96 (4), 815–819.

Rivero, M.R., Vranych, C.V., Bisbal, M., Maletto, B.A., Ropolo, A.S., Touz, M.C., 2010b. Adaptor protein 2 regulates receptor-mediated endocytosis and cyst formation in *Giardia lamblia*. Biochem. J. 428 (1), 33–45.

Rivero, F.D., Saura, A., Prucca, C.G., Carranza, P.G., Torri, A., Lujan, H.D., 2010c. Disruption of antigenic variation is crucial for effective parasite vaccine. Nat. Med. 16 (5), 551–557.

Rivero, M.R., Miras, S.L., Feliziani, C., Zamponi, N., Quiroga, R., Hayes, S.F., Ropolo, A.S., Touz, M.C., 2012. Vacuolar protein sorting receptor in *Giardia lamblia*. PLoS One 7 (8), e43712.

Rivero, M.R., Jausoro, I., Bisbal, M., Feliziani, C., Lanfredi-Rangel, A., Touz, M.C., 2013. Receptor-mediated endocytosis and trafficking between endosomal-lysosomal vacuoles in *Giardia lamblia*. Parasitol. Res. 112 (4), 1813–1818.

Rout, S., Zumthor, J.P., Schraner, E.M., Faso, C., Hehl, A.B., 2016. An interactome-centered protein discovery approach reveals novel components involved in mitosome function and homeostasis in *Giardia lamblia*. PLoS Pathog. 12 (12), e1006036.

Samuelson, J., Robbins, P., 2011. A simple fibril and lectin model for cyst walls of Entamoeba and perhaps Giardia. Trends Parasitol. 27 (1), 17–22.

Serradell, M.C., Saura, A., Rupil, L.L., Gargantini, P.R., Faya, M.I., Furlan, P.J., Lujan, H.D., 2016. Vaccination of domestic animals with a novel oral vaccine prevents Giardia infections, alleviates signs of giardiasis and reduces transmission to humans. NPJ Vaccines 1, 16018.

Shiflett, A.M., Johnson, P.J., 2010. Mitochondrion-related organelles in eukaryotic protists. Annu. Rev. Microbiol. 64, 409–429.

Simon, M.C., Schmidt, H.J., 2007. Antigenic variation in ciliates: antigen structure, function, expression. J. Eukaryot. Microbiol. 54 (1), 1–7.

Skarin, H., Ringqvist, E., Hellman, U., Svard, S.G., 2011. Elongation factor 1-alpha is released into the culture medium during growth of Giardia intestinalis trophozoites. Exp. Parasitol. 127 (4), 804–810.

Sonda, S., Morf, L., Bottova, I., Baetschmann, H., Rehrauer, H., Caflisch, A., Hakimi, M.A., Hehl, A.B., 2010. Epigenetic mechanisms regulate stage differentiation in the minimized protozoan *Giardia lamblia*. Mol. Microbiol. 76 (1), 48–67.

Stadelmann, B., Merino, M.C., Persson, L., Svard, S.G., 2012. Arginine consumption by the intestinal parasite Giardia intestinalis reduces proliferation of intestinal epithelial cells. PLoS One 7 (9), e45325.

Stefanic, S., Morf, L., Kulangara, C., Regos, A., Sonda, S., Schraner, E., Spycher, C., Wild, P., Hehl, A.B., 2009. Neogenesis and maturation of transient Golgi-like cisternae in a simple eukaryote. J. Cell Sci. 122 (Pt. 16), 2846–2856.

Touz, M.C., Zamponi, N., 2017. Sorting without a Golgi complex. Traffic 18 (10), 637–645.

Touz, M.C., Kulakova, L., Nash, T.E., 2004. Adaptor protein complex 1 mediates the transport of lysosomal proteins from a Golgi-like organelle to peripheral vacuoles in the primitive eukaryote *Giardia lamblia*. Mol. Biol. Cell 15 (7), 3053–3060.

Touz, M.C., Ropolo, A.S., Rivero, M.R., Vranych, C.V., Conrad, J.T., Svard, S.G., Nash, T.E., 2008. Arginine deiminase has multiple regulatory roles in the biology of *Giardia lamblia*. J. Cell Sci. 121 (Pt. 17), 2930–2938.

Touz, M.C., Feliziani, C., Ropolo, A.S., 2018. Membrane-associated proteins in *Giardia lamblia*. Genes (Basel) 9 (8), 404.

Tovar, J., Fischer, A., Clark, C.G., 1999. The mitosome, a novel organelle related to mitochondria in the amitochondrial parasite *Entamoeba histolytica*. Mol. Microbiol. 32 (5), 1013–1021.

Tovar, J., Leon-Avila, G., Sanchez, L.B., Sutak, R., Tachezy, J., van der Giezen, M., Hernandez, M., Muller, M., Lucocq, J.M., 2003. Mitochondrial remnant organelles of Giardia function in iron-sulphur protein maturation. Nature 426 (6963), 172–176.

Twu, O., de Miguel, N., Lustig, G., Stevens, G.C., Vashisht, A.A., Wohlschlegel, J.A., Johnson, P.J., 2013. *Trichomonas vaginalis* exosomes deliver cargo to host cells and mediate hostratioparasite interactions. PLoS Pathog. 9 (7), e1003482.

Voleman, L., Najdrova, V., Astvaldsson, A., Tumova, P., Einarsson, E., Svindrych, Z., Hagen, G.M., Tachezy, J., Svard, S.G., Dolezal, P., 2017. Giardia intestinalis mitosomes undergo synchronized fission but not fusion and are constitutively associated with the endoplasmic reticulum. BMC Biol. 15 (1), 27.

Wampfler, P.B., Faso, C., Hehl, A.B., 2014. The Cre/loxP system in *Giardia lamblia*: genetic manipulations in a binucleate tetraploid protozoan. Int. J. Parasitol. 44 (8), 497–506.

WHO, (Ed.), 2013. World Health Statistics 2013. WHO Press, World Health Organization, Geneva, Switzerland. p.78.

Wink, D.A., Kasprzak, K.S., Maragos, C.M., Elespuru, R.K., Misra, M., Dunams, T.M., Cebula, T.A., Koch, W.H., Andrews, A.W., Allen, J.S., et al., 1991. DNA deaminating ability and genotoxicity of nitric oxide and its progenitors. Science 254 (5034), 1001–1003.

Zamponi, N., Zamponi, E., Mayol, G.F., Lanfredi-Rangel, A., Svard, S.G., Touz, M.C., 2017. Endoplasmic reticulum is the sorting core facility in the Golgi-lacking protozoan *Giardia lamblia*. Traffic 18 (9), 604–621.

Zumthor, J.P., Cernikova, L., Rout, S., Kaech, A., Faso, C., Hehl, A.B., 2016. Static clathrin assemblies at the peripheral vacuole-plasma membrane interface of the parasitic protozoan *Giardia lamblia*. PLoS Pathog. 12 (7), e1005756.

CHAPTER FOUR

Giardia duodenalis: Role of secreted molecules as virulent factors in the cytotoxic effect on epithelial cells

M. Guadalupe Ortega-Pierres*, Raúl Argüello-García
Departamento de Genética y Biología Molecular, Centro de Investigación y de Estudios Avanzados del Instituto Politécnico Nacional, Ciudad de Mexico City, Mexico
*Corresponding author: e-mail address: gortega@cinvestav.mx

Contents

Abstract

During the course of giardiasis in humans and experimental models, *G. duodenalis* trophozoites express and secrete several proteins (ESPs) affecting structural, cellular and soluble components of the host intestinal milieu. These include the toxin-like molecules CRP136 and ESP58 that induce intestinal hyper-peristalsis. After the completion of the *Giardia* genome database and using up-to date transcriptomic and proteomic approaches, secreted 'virulence factors' have also been identified and experimentally characterized. This repertoire includes arginine deiminase (ADI) that competes for arginine, an important energy source for trophozoites, some high-cysteine membrane proteins (HCMPs) and VSP88, a versatile variant surface protein (VSP) that functions as an extracellular protease. Another giardial protein, enolase, moonlights as a metabolic enzyme that interacts with the fibrinolytic system and damages host epithelial cells. Other putative *Giardia* virulence factors are cysteine proteases that degrade multiple

Advances in Parasitology, Volume 106
ISSN 0065-308X
https://doi.org/10.1016/bs.apar.2019.07.003

host components including mucin, villin, tight junction proteins, immunoglobulins, defensins and cytokines. One of these proteases, named giardipain-1, decreases trans-epithelial electrical resistance and induces apoptosis in epithelial cells. A putative role for tenascins, present in the *Giardia*'s secretome, is interfering with the host epidermal growth factor. Based on the roles that these molecules play, drugs may be designed to interfere with their functions. This review presents a comprehensive description of secreted *Giardia* virulence factors. It further describes their cytotoxic mechanisms and roles in the pathophysiology of giardiasis, and then assesses their potential as targets for drug development.

1. Introduction

Giardia duodenalis (syn. *Giardia lamblia, Giardia intestinalis*) is an intestinal protozoan parasite of the order diplomonadida that constitutes a species complex of eight different phylogenetic groups or assemblages characterized by different host specificities (Thompson and Monis, 2012). This parasite causes giardiasis in humans, livestock and wild species, and is considered a leading cause of waterborne diarrheal disease and post-infection, extra-intestinal pathologies. Human giardiasis, with an estimated rate of 280 million cases per year (Thompson and Monis, 2004), is included in the World Health Organization's (WHO) Neglected Disease Initiative (Savioli et al., 2006) and *Giardia* spp. is listed as category B pathogen with potential use in bioterrorism (http://www.bt.cdc.gov/agent/agentlist-category.asp).

During its life cycle, *Giardia* alternates between the active, pathogenic swimming trophozoite and the inactive, resistant cyst. *Giardia* excystation happens after passage through the host's stomach. This gives rise to trophozoites that colonize the duodenum and upper jejunum, then replicate and attach to the intestinal epithelium using their adhesive disc and begin to feed on luminal nutrients. Many of the dividing trophozoites are carried towards the colon, and encyst along the way in response to bile salts and other stimuli. Cysts can appear in the faeces from 3 days to 3 weeks after infection, depending on the host species (Spickler, 2012).

Infections are commonly acquired from parasite cysts in contaminated drinking water, or directly via the faecal-oral route. Although the highest prevalence of *Giardia* infections has been reported in countries with the poorest sanitation, giardiasis is well documented in other countries as well (Cotton et al., 2011; Thompson and Monis, 2004).

A noticeable feature of giardiasis is the spectrum of clinical symptoms in individuals with acute or chronic infections. These include diarrhoea, nausea, weight loss, bloating and abdominal pain. Multiple factors account for the disease variability, including the state of the host immune system, host age and nutritional status, parasite genotype, infectious dose, and the presence of co-infecting pathogens (Buret, 2007; Cotton et al., 2011; Panaro et al., 2007; Troeger et al., 2007).

The pathophysiological consequences of *Giardia* infection are multifactorial, and involve both host and parasite factors, as well as immunological and non-immunological mucosal processes. *G. duodenalis* causes severe malnutrition and diarrhoea from malabsorption. In some cases, especially in young children and in those in developing countries, impaired gain weight and an ultimate *failure to thrive* also occurs (Bartelt and Sartor, 2015). The molecular mechanisms involved in the onset of giardiasis and diarrhoea have not yet been fully described but are typically accompanied by host malabsorption, maldigestion of nutrients, diffuse shortening of brush border microvilli, electrolyte imbalance and increased intestinal peristalsis (Ankarklev et al., 2010; Cotton et al., 2011). Long-term, giardiasis has been related to extra-intestinal consequences including arthritis, skin allergies, myopathy, and diminished cognitive function (Cotton et al., 2011; Thompson and Monis, 2004). In fact, recent evidence has determined that acute *G. duodenalis* infection may also lead to chronic, functional, gastrointestinal disorders including post-infection, irritable bowel syndrome (Halliez and Buret, 2013). *Giardia duodenalis* has also been implicated in the disruption of the host intestinal microbiota during acute infections and as an outcome of chronic symptoms (Amat et al., 2017).

Although giardiasis is usually a self-limiting disease, treatment of confirmed cases is necessary to cure symptoms, shorten the duration of acute infection, reduce the risk of post-infection complications and prevent prolonged excretion of infectious cysts. Currently, no prophylaxis is available for giardiasis, but several drugs are approved for its treatment including 5-nitroimidazoles, benzimidazole derivatives, quinacrine, furazolidone, nitazoxanide and paromomycin (Lalle, 2010). Metronidazole or tinidazole are most often used in humans, but other drugs like furazolidone or paromomycin are also recommended (Spickler, 2012).

2. Transcriptome and secretome changes associated with *G. duodenalis* trophozoites cultured with epithelial cells

To unravel *Giardia* pathogenesis at the molecular level, it is important to examine changes in both the transcriptome and the secretome in *Giardia* trophozoites upon interaction with epithelial cells or their products, since this contact induces trophozoites to secrete virulence factors.

Several studies have analysed the interplay between the host and the parasite (Emery et al., 2016; Ferella et al., 2014; Ma'ayeh and Brook-Carter, 2012; Ringqvist et al., 2008, 2011) while others have examined constitutively produced compounds that are secreted by healthy, growing *Giardia* trophozoites and explored their roles in the host-pathogen interaction (Dubourg et al., 2018) using in vitro models and epithelial cell lines such as Caco-2 cells. During the interaction of *Giardia* trophozoites with Caco-2 epithelial cells, parasites release several metabolic enzymes like arginine deiminase (ADI), enolase (ENO) and ornithine carbamoyl transferase (OCT) (Ringqvist et al., 2008).

One study using subtractive hybridization with IEC-6 cells examined interactions with four isolates of *Giardia duodenalis* (WB, P-1, NF and GS/M) (Ma'ayeh and Brook-Carter, 2012). The study reported that >40 genes were differentially expressed in each of the four *Giardia* isolates. Most of the up-regulated genes were common to the four isolates except for those encoding proteins most likely involved in immune evasion such as VSPs, high-cysteine membrane proteins (HCMp), hypothetical proteins, and oxygen defence proteins (e.g. thioredoxin, peroxiredoxin). These data suggest that while different *Giardia* isolates use the same genetic machinery to infect cells and cause disease, different HCMp and VSPs are expressed in the process conferring antigenic variation that may be responsible for the wide array of symptoms found in giardiasis.

Numerous other techniques have been employed to evaluate changes in gene expression. In one such study, microarrays were used to detect changes in gene expression in *Giardia* trophozoites during interaction with the intestinal colonic cell line Caco-2 (Ringqvist et al., 2011). This study demonstrated that the most highly up-regulated genes encode oxygen defence proteins and several members of the high cysteine membrane protein (HCMp) and Gly-rich repeat (GRREAT) families. In addition, 5S rRNA was slightly down-regulated and small RNAs were up-regulated as were ADI, ENO and cysteine proteinases, previously suggested as important for host-parasite interactions. However, the regulation of these genes was biphasic where transcription increased early during the interaction but was later down-regulated. Cell division and attachment genes were down-regulated at later time-points of interaction.

Serial Analysis of Gene Expression (SAGE) was used to quantify transcriptional changes in *Giardia intestinalis* upon interaction with HT-29 intestinal cells in M199 serum-free medium (Ferella et al., 2014). A total of 90 genes were differentially expressed, many involved in redox homeostasis, metabolism and small molecule transport. Also included were Q3 cysteine proteases and structural proteins of the giardin family.

Tandem mass tag labelling was used to examine trophozoite products secreted early after in vitro exposure to HT-29 cells (Emery et al., 2016). Upon incubating *Giardia* trophozoites with intestinal epithelial cells (IECs) or with host soluble factors (HSF), 45 and 38 differentially expressed proteins were identified, respectively. These included tenascins, cystatin, cathepsin B precursor, uridine phosphorylase 1 (UPL-1), thioredoxin, a HCMP, as well as oxidoreductases, proteins of the ubiquitination pathway, a 14-3-3 protein homologue, a tetratricopeptide (TPR) containing protein and seven hypothetical proteins. These results showed that trophozoites respond to secreted soluble host signals, even before to host intestinal epithelium attachment.

A more recent study on epithelial cells analysed 15 proteins secreted by healthy, growing *Giardia* trophozoites from two human-infective assemblages (Dubourg et al., 2018). Eleven of these proteins had an N-terminal signal sequence, two were of unknown function, five were tenascins, three cathepsin B cysteine proteases and another one was an extracellular nuclease. The most abundant protein was pyridoxamine 5′-phosphate oxidase (PNPO), a flavin mononucleotide-dependent enzyme that fixes molecular oxygen. A complementary electrophysiological analysis in Caco-2 epithelial cells co-cultured with *Giardia* trophozoites or with diluted *Giardia* supernatants, demonstrated that the parasite secretes proteins that adversely affect the homeostasis of enteric epithelia. Thus, *Giardia* trophozoites may counteract host defences by up-regulating antioxidant responses, and damaging the layers of microvilli causing horseshoe-like foci (Emery et al., 2016; Ortega-Pierres et al., 2011).

In summary, the interaction of *Giardia* trophozoites with host products or epithelial cells induces the expression of parasite genes and proteins whose presence is limited or absent in axenic cultures. Among these proteins are virulence factors capable of damaging epithelial cells.

3. Mechanism by which secreted molecules damage epithelial cells

The release of soluble factors by lumen-resident trophozoites causes damage to epithelial cells through the loss of barrier function and induces apoptosis that severely affects intestinal homeostasis. Molecules of *G. duodenalis* excretory/secretory products (ESP)/secretome that trigger cytotoxic and/or cytopathic effects on target cells include catalytic proteins, metabolic enzymes, surface molecules and soluble mediators that bind to host cell receptors and extracellular matrix components. These components are classified into five main groups: toxin-like molecules, energy metabolism enzymes, cysteine-rich surface proteins, cysteine proteases and tenascins (Table 1).

3.1 Toxin-like molecules

In the last two centuries, toxins with deleterious effects on human and vertebrate intestinal tissue have been detected in plant, bacterial and fungal pathogens. Initial attempts to associate giardiasis with the parasite's toxin production and its ability to alter immune responses were done with culture supernatants of isolates obtained from four patients, including one with chronic giardiasis that was cured with quinacrine/metronidazole treatment and from whom the reference strain WB was obtained. However, no evidence of toxin-like factors was obtained from assays done in rabbit ileal-loops, in tests that measure capillary and permeability in the skin, or toxicity to infant mice (Smith et al., 1982). The search for giardial enterotoxins was prompted by in vitro studies in which trophozoite surface antigens were radiolabelled with ^{125}I and labelled proteins were detected by autoradiography in culture supernatants. Further, antibody-based analyses showed inter-strain variability in the ESP repertoire. These studies allowed the classification of isolates into three groups with respect to their high, partial or absent antigenic cross-reactivity (Nash and Keister, 1985; Nash et al., 1983). Ex vivo studies performed in murine brush border membrane vesicles showed that glucose and phenylalanine uptake were impaired along with a Na^+, Cl^- and 3-*O*-methyl-D-glucose leakage in ESP-treated intestinal tissues (Samra et al., 1988).

The first toxin-like molecule derived from *G. duodenalis* trophozoites was identified by genetic analyses of trophozoites from the WB1B strain, assemblage A, exposed first to UV radiation and then to increasing sub-lethal concentrations of metronidazole. The highly expressed mRNA encoded a 136 kDa protein named CRP136 that contained 23.5 copies of a central repeat of 40 amino acids with 57% homology with a sarafotoxin precursor. The latter is strong vasoconstrictor isopeptide toxin present in the venom of burrowing adder *Atractaspis engaddensis* (Chen et al., 1995). CRP136 belongs to the VSP family based on its conserved C-terminal region that contains a membrane-spanning domain, and its characteristic CRGKA cytoplasmic tail which is excised upon release to the extracellular milieu (Papanastasiou et al., 1996).

Table 1 Major virulence factors released by *G. duodenalis* trophozoites upon interaction with intestinal cell monolayers detected by proteomics approaches in secretomes.

Secreted factor	Protein name	Protein ID	Proposed target(s)	Likely pathogenic role	References
Toxin-like	CRP136/VSP188	GL50803_137613	Endothelin receptor A	↑Peristalsis	Chen et al. (1995) and Shant et al. (2002, 2004)
	ESP58	Unknown	Ganglioside M1 receptor	Efflux of water and electrolites	
Energy metabolism enzymes	Enolase	GL50803_11118	Host plasminogen	✓ Epithelial cell damage	Eckmann et al. (2000), Ringqvist et al. (2008), Stadelmann et al. (2012, 2013), Banik et al. (2013), Ma'ayeh et al. (2017), Munoz-Cruz et al. (2018), Barroeta-Echegaray et al. (submitted for publication)
	FBPA	GL50803_11043	Unknown	✓ Modulation of immune system	
	PGM	GL50803_8822	Unknown		
	OCT	GL50803_10311	Arginine?	✓ Recognition and attachment	
	ADI	GL50803_112103	Arginine		
			T-lymphocytes	✓ Competition for arginine?	
			Dendritic cells	✓ ↓Enterocyte proliferation	
			Mast cells	✓ ↓Proliferation	
				✓ ↑TNF-α; ↓IL-10, IL12p40, CD83 and CD86; ↓mTOR S6K	
				✓ IL-6 and TNF-α release	

Continued

Table 1 Major virulence factors released by *G. duodenalis* trophozoites upon interaction with intestinal cell monolayers detected by proteomics approaches in secretomes.—cont'd

Secreted factor	Protein name	Protein ID	Proposed target(s)	Likely pathogenic role	References
Cysteine-rich surface proteins	HCMP TMK-like	GL50803_113319	Extracellular kinase?	Altered cell signaling?	Emery et al. (2014), Ma'ayeh et al. (2017), Dubourg et al. (2018), Cabrera-Licona et al. (2017)
	HCMP Group 2	GL50803_9620	EGF receptor?	Immune evasion	
	HCMP EGF-like	GL50803_113531	Unknown	↓Enterocyte proliferation?	
	HCMP	GL50803_12063	Unknown	Immune evasion	
	HCMP Group 1	GL50803_7715	Unknown	Immune evasion	
	VSP	GL50581_3195	Unknown	Immune evasion	
	VSP9B10A/VSP88	GL50803_101074	Same as cysteine proteases?	Same as cysteine proteases?	
Cysteine proteases	Giardipain-1	GL50803_14019	MUC2, Villin, Claudin-1 and -4, Occludin, ZO-1, E-Cadherin, β-Catenin, Immunoglobulins (IgG, IgAl and -2), Defensins (αDf1, βDf5 and αDf6), Chemokines (CXCL-3, CXCL8, CCL2 and CCL20), Intestinal microbiota biofilms	✓ Epithelial cell damage	Chua et al. (2014), Beatty et al. (2017), Cotton et al. (2014), Gerbaba et al. (2015), Keselman et al. (2016), Amat et al. (2017), Beatty et al. (2017), Ma'ayeh et al. (2017), DuBourg et al. (2018), Ortega-Pierres et al. (2018), Liu et al. (2018, 2019a)
	CP16160	GL50803_16160		✓ Mucus disruption	
	CP16779	GL50803_16779		✓ Microvillus atrophy	
				✓ Breakdown of cell junctions. Impairment of innate and adaptive immune responses	
				✓ Microbiome dysbiosis	
				✓ Apoptosis of enterocytes	
				✓ Relase of pro-inflammatory cytokines	

Tenascins	Tenascin C-like	GL50803_8687	Epidermal growth factor receptor?	✓	Enterocyte separation leading to bacterial translocation and inflammatory responses?	Emery et al. (2016) and Dubourg et al. (2018)
	Tenascin X-like	GL50803_14573				
	Tenascin	GL50803_10330				
	Tenascin	GL50581_4057				
	Tenascin	GL50803_95162				
	Tenascin	GL50803_16468				
	Tenascin-37	GL50803_16477				
	tenascin	GL50803_113038				

Abbreviations are included in the text. Only the most abundant proteins reported are listed and identified on the basis of aminoacid sequences of the clone WBA6 (GL50581) or otherwise isolate GS (GL50581). Hypothetical targets and the mechanisms that are not experimentally defined are indicated with question marks (?). The sign "✓" indicates general pathogenic roles proposed for the identified proteins.

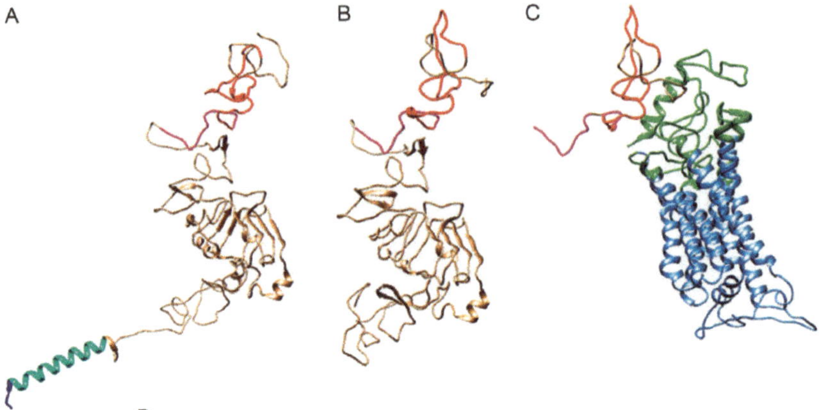

D

```
GdVSP188          TDTKQCTKDPEAPCNVEGCETCVEGNAQQCK-TCRPGYTIN
AeSarafotoxin     -DTKQAARDPSPQRNVEPLCSCKDMSDKECLNFCHQDVIWR
                   ****.::**..  ***    :* : . ::*    *: .   .
```

Fig. 1 (A) Predicted protein structure of VSP188 with the complete sarafotoxin-like repeat in red and the incomplete repeat in magenta; membrane-spanning region is displayed in cyan and the cytoplasmic CRGKA tail is shown in dark blue. (B) Secreted VSP188 form. (C) Protein docking of secreted VSP188 with human endothelin receptor type A (blue) with its extracellular domains (green) interacting with the sarafotoxin-like repeat; the C-terminal region of VSP188 was omitted for clarity. (D) Sequence alignment of giardial repeat and that of *A. engaddensis* sarafotoxin; (*) denotes identity and (.) or (:) indicate semi-conservative or conservative substitutions, respectively.

In The Giardia Genome Project based on the WBA6 clone an open reading frame (GL50803_137613) encodes a 40.5 kDa-sized protein named VSP188 with the highest identity to CRP136 (100% at the 29 amino acid N-terminus and 84.5% identity at the 310 amino acid C-terminus that contains only 1.4 copies of the same sarafotoxin-like repeat) (Fig. 1).

Thus, CRP136 might be an aberrant version of the VSP188 derived from the mutagenic effects of UV rays combined with the genotoxicity of metronidazole that collectively caused errors in DNA replication, e.g., slipped-strand mispairing, and therefore the multiplication of the central 40 amino acid repeat in the metronidazole-resistant line.

Due to its high structural and functional similarity to endothelins expressed in enteric neurons in mammals, sarafotoxins act by binding endothelin receptors A or B ($ET_{A/B}$) which are G protein-coupled receptors. Upon their activation, they could trigger or adversely regulate elevations of intracellular free Ca^{2+} and thereby promote or inhibit intestinal muscle activity (peristalsis) (Luscher and Barton, 2000; Shahbazian and Holzer, 2000). Interestingly, in clinical trials the oral administration of sarafotoxins provokes gastrointestinal disorders such as vomiting and watery, non-bloody diarrhoea in a manner similar to patients diagnosed with acute giardiasis (Solarczyk and Majewska, 2015). Based on these observations, it is hypothesized that giardial sarafotoxin-like CRP136 and VSP188 stimulates intestinal peristalsis through ET_A receptor activation (Fig. 1); however, these observations require further experimental work.

In a series of studies aimed to detect and characterize toxigenic material in ESP from cultures of the Portland-1 strain (assemblage A), a 58 kDa surface glycoprotein (gESP58) was isolated by ammonium sulphate precipitation, affinity chromatography and gel filtration. The purified protein produced: (1) positive skin permeability reaction, (2) severe fluid accumulation in ileal loops of rabbits (a transitory fluid accumulation in sealed gut of mice) and (3) cytopathic effects, from elongated morphology to lysis, when incubated with HEp-2 monolayers. Moreover, it showed hemagglutinating activity and was immunogenic since it was recognized by sera from patients with giardiasis. Further, anti-gESP58 IgGs cross-reacted with cholera and snake (water moccasin and king cobra) toxins (Kaur et al., 2001; Shant et al., 2002) and Western blot analyses using native gESP58 and anti-gESP58 IgGs in the presence of membranes of mouse enterocytes identified a 41 kDa protein as the putative receptor for this enterotoxin. Remarkably, this ligand-receptor interaction was blocked by pre-incubating gESP58 with ganglioside M1 (GM1) in a manner similar to using membranes from duodenum, jejunum or ileum of mice (Shant et al., 2004). GM1 is a sialic acid-ceramide glycolipid that in intestinal cells, is the receptor of the *Vibrio cholerae* toxin B subunits which upon endocytosis allows the release of the enzymatic A subunit. This in turn locks the heterotrimeric protein $G_{S\alpha}$ in an active ADP-ribosylated status inside enterocytes that continuously activates adenylate cyclase and leads to a sustained increase in cAMP. This over activates protein kinase A (PKA) which phosphorylates chloride channels as CFTRs; hence, Cl^- efflux occurs with collateral secretion of water and electrolytes (Na^+, K^+, HCO_3^-) that combine to diminished activity of H_2O/Na^+ cotransporters and ultimately lead to dehydration and diarrhoea (Sanchez and Holmgren, 2011). Nevertheless, recent reports pinpoint that cholera toxin is still able to induce diarrhoea in *gm1*-knocked mice suggesting a role for other host glycoproteins in cholera toxification (Cervin et al., 2018). In the case of mouse enterocytes exposed to gESP58, similar alterations in signal transduction occur within minutes and include decreased GTPase activity, rise of cAMP levels, upregulation of PKA, increased intracellular Ca^{2+} and decreased cytosolic Cl^- concentrations (Shant et al., 2004).

These observations suggest that gESP58 fulfils the mechanistic features of a *bona-fide* enterotoxin. However, its identity has not been unravelled because the small fragment sequenced in these studies (DFVPQVST) has only partial identities in multiple protein sequences in the completed genomes of WB, GS and P15 isolates. Also, the identification of the putative 41 kDa receptor has not yet been addressed.

In this context, advances in the search for giardial enterotoxins and their receptors on the surface of intestinal cells have not been compelling until now because: (a) these have been based on methodologies designed to detect or capture single molecules, (b) the toxin-like molecules identified so far have been derived from cultures modified from or possibly not isogenic to a reference strain with a sequenced genome (e.g. WB) and (c) the presence of Vsp188 or gESP58 in the *Giardia* secretome has not been reported yet. However, the evidence mentioned herein point to the toxigenic potential of the repertoire of molecules secreted by *G. duodenalis* trophozoites.

The development of high throughput sequencing techniques at nucleic acid and protein levels over the last three decades holds an enormous potential in the screening and identification of individual biomolecules from complex biological samples. These 'omics' strategies (i.e. genomics, transcriptomics and proteomics) have been used successfully to characterize proteins secreted by *G. duodenalis* trophozoites in the presence of model epithelial cell monolayers, intestinal explants and intestinal contents of infected animals or patients. As consequence, the former 'forward' protein-based techniques used to isolate toxin-like molecules in trophozoite's ESP have been superseded by 'reverse' proteomics methodologies that focus on functionality (for review see Palcy and Chevet, 2006); hence multiple molecules have been identified and functionally characterized in giardial ESP, now known as the secretome. In the following sections, other examples of *Giardia* molecules that have an effect on epithelial cells are described.

3.2 Energy metabolism enzymes

In recent years, the importance of secreted parasite enzymes, mostly glycolytic, in the host-parasite interface is increasingly recognized. These moonlighting proteins are secreted by pathogens to promote processes such as attachment, invasion, nutrient acquisition, angiogenesis, immuno-modulation and haemostasis. Thus, these can be classified as virulence markers (Gomez-Arreaza et al., 2014; Henderson and Martin, 2011). In these organisms, it has been hypothesized that several factors contribute to the multiple extracellular actions common to glycolytic enzymes including adaptive post-translational modifications. The localization and relative abundance of these glycolytic enzymes in the cytosol and/or organelles facilitates recruitment into secretory vesicles (exosomes) or shedding vesicles and have therefore evolved with interacting targets in the host (Gomez-Arreaza et al., 2014).

The glycolysis/gluconeogenesis pathway, or the prototype Embden-Meyerhof-Parnas route, comprises 10 enzymatic steps that transform glucose into pyruvate. In bacteria it has been shown that virtually all these enzymes have at least one moonlighting function (Henderson and Martin, 2011), while in parasitic protozoa and helminthes six of these enzymes have been shown to have unique extracellular functions which include: hexokinase in nutrient acquisition; glucose-6-phosphate isomerase (G6PI) in angiogenesis; triosephosphate isomerase (TPI) in immune evasion; fructose-bisphosphate aldolase (FBPA), glyceraldehyde-3-phosphate dehydrogenase (G3PDH) and enolase (ENO) in modulation of the immune and hemostatic systems and the two latter together with a phosphoglycerate mutase (PGM) participate in recognition and attachment (Collingridge et al., 2010; Gomez-Arreaza et al., 2014; Guillou et al., 2007; Hewitson et al., 2014).

Transcriptomic studies of *G. duodenalis* trophozoites (strain WB, clone 6, assemblage A) interacting with model human colorectal cell line Caco-2 showed that *eno* and phosphoglycerate kinase (*pgk*) were among the most up-regulated transcripts over short interaction times (1.5 h) but were then down-regulated at 6 and 18 h (Ringqvist et al., 2011). By using representational difference analysis and subtractive hybridizations to identify differentially-expressed mRNAs, *eno, g3pdh* and *fbpa* along with other genes of glycolysis were up-regulated in three assemblage A strains (WB, P-1 and NF) and one assemblage B strain (GS) upon interactions between trophozoites and the murine intestinal cell line IEC-6 (Ma'ayeh and Brook-Carter, 2012). Using 2D-electrophoresis and mass spectrometry (MS) assays to analyse interactions between WB and GS-H7 supernatants of interactions (assemblage B) trophozoite cultures and Caco-2 cells or mouse intestinal loops (Ringqvist et al., 2008) identified *Giardia* ENO (gENO) as the predominant glycolytic enzyme present in the secretome.

Secretome data obtained by analysis of major proteins in interaction supernatants using WB and GS-H7 (assemblage B) trophozoite cultures interacting with Caco-2 cells and in mice intestinal loops by 2D-electrophoresis and mass spectrometry (MS) assays showed that gENO was the predominant glycolytic enzyme identified (Ringqvist et al., 2008). The use of high-throughput

LC/MS to analyse supernatants of WB and GS strains interacting with Caco-2 cell monolayers showed that gENO, gFBPA and gPGM were among the 10 major ESP secreted by trophozoites of both strains; these same proteins were also detected in ESP during axenic culture (Ma'ayeh and Brook-Carter, 2012). Of the three glycolytic enzymes detected so far in the *Giardia* secretome, the crystal structure of gFBPA has been solved (PDB ID: 3GAK) and has been studied at the structural level for inhibitor design and evaluation (see Section 4). The functions of gENO have also been studied in more detail; however, gPGM has not been fully characterized to date.

Several studies have proposed that gENO is a moonlighting enzyme present in the cytosol, flagella and trophozoite membrane and cyst wall. At the intracellular level, studies of some deletions or mutations in the wild type sequence lead to inefficient excystation (Castillo-Romero et al., 2012). At the extracellular level, bioinformatics studies have suggested that dimeric gENO interacts with human plasminogen (HsPLG), a circulating component of the fibrinolytic system which upon activation promotes extracellular matrix degradation. In this process the three lysines of gENO (Lys66 in the open conformation; Lys186 and Lys188 in the closed conformation) could be attracted by Kringle domains K5 and K4 of HsPLG (Aguayo-Ortiz et al., 2017). However, recent experimental studies in our group have shown that endogenous gENO is present as dimer only within the cell and is secreted as a monomer. Further, it can activate HsPLG and thereby generate plasmin activity (i.e. serine protease) by a known binding mechanism involving domains K1 and K4 of HsPLG.

A recombinant form of gENO induced damage in IEC-6 monolayers characterized by increased separation between cells, profuse cell vacuolization and a cell death mechanism distinct from classical apoptosis where the induction of apoptosis inducing factor 1 and expression of tumoural necrosis factor α (TNFα) were observed in the absence of caspase 3 activation (Barroeta-Echegaray et al., submitted for publication). Since TNFα is related to signal transduction pathways leading to programmed necrosis (necroptosis), it is possible that gENO is linked to initial stages of chronic pathologies via the induction of inflammatory bowel disease which is characterized by epithelial *loss of barrier* function and microbiota dysbiosis typically associated with post-giardiasis complications (Allain et al., 2017; Halliez and Buret, 2013).

In addition to glycolysis, *Giardia* uses a prokaryotic-like arginine dihydrolase pathway (ADHP) to generate ATP by substrate level phosphorylation under anaerobic conditions. Another arginine-consuming enzyme is arginase, the fifth enzyme in the urea cycle that converts L-arginine into

L-ornithine and urea. There exist two isoforms (ARG1 and ARG2) which are down-regulated in Caco-2 cells upon interaction with *Giardia* (Stadelmann et al., 2013). Assemblage B of *G. duodenalis* does possesses one sequence annotated as arginase (GSB_152580) and another arginase-like sequence (GSB_155544) but it is unknown if the key function is intra or extracellular. Based on the lack of other enzymes of the urea cycle in *Giardia*, it is likely that the annotated arginase is of mitochondrial origin (type II) (Di Costanzo et al., 2007). It is intriguing why assemblages A and E do not have these sequences but demonstrate a more advantageous use of arginine as an ATP source. In trophozoite cytosol, ADHP carries out the conversions arginine → citrulline → ornithine + carbamoyl phosphate → carbon dioxide + ammonia through the activity of three enzymes: arginine deiminase (gADI), ornithine carbamoyl transferase (gOCT) and carbamate kinase (gCK) (Schofield et al., 1990).

During interactions of trophozoites with Caco-2 monolayers the expression of *ck* gene is always down-regulated while *adi* mRNA exhibits an expression profile similar to *eno* and *pgk*, i.e., up-regulated at 1.5 h post infection then down-regulated by 6 and 18 h (Ringqvist et al., 2011). As noted, gADI and gOCT are major components secreted during interaction of the WB and GS strains of *G. duodenalis* trophozoites with HT-29 and Caco-2 human epithelial cell lines (Ma'ayeh et al., 2017; Ringqvist et al., 2008). These latter observations provide a basis for the 'moonlighting' functions of gADI and gOCT and suggest specific roles for arginine, citrulline and ornithine in the mechanisms promoting damage to epithelial cells.

The depletion of arginine in the gut's extracellular milieu promotes survival of *Giardia* trophozoites by preventing the activity of nitric oxide synthase (NOS) thus it converts arginine into citrulline and NO in intestinal cells decreasing enterocyte proliferation (Banik et al., 2013; Eckmann et al., 2000; Stadelmann et al., 2012, 2013). Arginine depletion within the host cell is supported by estimations of the activity of gADI that suggest at least 20 U of this enzyme (equivalent to >28 mmol of arginine turned over) are produced by trophozoites each day of infection (Stadelmann et al., 2013). As *Giardia* requires arginine for optimal growth and viability, arginine uptake and metabolism by enterocytes provides these cells with a twofold mechanism against trophozoite establishment in the gut. In this '*warginine*', trophozoites have two intervening molecules, namely, a cell surface-located arginine transporter and the secreted gADI. The transporter is an arginine/ornithine antiport (Knodler et al., 1995) that amidst a low intracellular pool of free arginine and provides an extracellular supply to maintain the activity of the ADHP.

Transporter activity might be stimulated by the fast consumption rate of arginine within the trophozoites (97% in 30 s) (Knodler et al., 1995) which implicates an active role in arginine capture for the parasite. In GiardiaDB there is an ABC-type transporter sequence (GL50803_92223) that has seven predicted transmembrane domains and the ability to bind arginine. Moreover, its mRNA levels are increased at 1.5, 6 (peak) and 18 h after initiation of WB-Caco-2 interactions (Ringqvist et al., 2011). Thus, further characterization of this transporter is warranted.

The gADI protein has been related to other non-arginolytic intracellular functions since this enzyme generates citrulline not only from free arginine but also from protein-bound arginine and from arginine located in the cytoplasmic tail (C**R**GKA) of VSPs. Indeed, this enzyme regulates surface protein switching and in encystation gADI, is attached at Lys101 to a Small-Ubiquitin Like Modifier (SUMOylation). Once attached, it is translocated to nucleus where it induces citrullination and down-regulates expression of cyst wall proteins, particularly CWP1 and CWP2 (Touz et al., 2008; Vranych et al., 2014). Outside trophozoites, the secreted gADI could lead to arginine depletion by consumption or capture, i.e., by catalytic conversion of arginine into citrulline or simply by enzyme-substrate binding without catalysis, respectively. In fact, the secretion of a catalytically competent enzyme may occur when cells of the immune system are exposed to purified gADI. In the case of peripheral blood T-lymphocytes from human donors, the proliferative response measured by ^{3}H-thymidine uptake is effectively diminished at 5 μg gADI/mL, a concentration that is physiologically achievable. This effect is completely reversed by the addition of arginine and partially by citrulline (Stadelmann et al., 2013).

In other studies, monocyte-derived human dendritic cells (DCs) stimulated with bacterial LPS in the presence of recombinant, catalytically active gADI showed increased levels of TNFα but decreased levels of IL-10, IL12p40 and surface markers CD83 and CD86 concomitant with inhibition of S6-kinase phosphorylation by mammalian target of rapamycin (mTOR). Therefore, the altered cytokine, mTOR in conjunction with costimulatory surface protein expression in DCs, that in infection are recruited to intestinal epithelium by CCL20 released by enterocytes (Roxstrom-Lindquist et al., 2005), could promote pathogenesis. This is reinforced by the observation that gADI but not gENO is capable of stimulating rat mast cells (HRMC line) in an IgE-independent fashion to release pro-inflammatory cytokines IL-6 and TNFα, an effect more pronounced in the presence of arginine or citrulline but still present under arginine depletion (Munoz-Cruz et al., 2018).

Although TNFα may contribute to trophozoite elimination, the uncontrolled production of this cytokine by DC and mast cells is potentially harmful to epithelial barrier function (Roxstrom-Lindquist et al., 2005; Troeger et al., 2007). These studies highlight the relevance of extracellular gADI as an arginine depleting factor and as a multiple inducer of TNFα production.

When localized, catabolic activities of gOCT in giardial ADHP are a source of L-ornithine that allows trophozoites to import arginine from the extracellular milieu through the aforementioned surface antiport. In this way, the trophozoites compete for free arginine. Although this is one of the predominant enzymes secreted during the interaction of zoonotic assemblages A and B with epithelial cell monolayers (Ma'ayeh et al., 2017; Ringqvist et al., 2008), there is no specific information about its function once secreted. In bacterial infections, for instance, OCT is secreted by *Mycobacterium tuberculosis* and is preferentially recognized by IgG which appears in the urine from patients with active pulmonary tuberculosis. This suggests that MtOCT is a good candidate for developing diagnostic reagents (Napolitano et al., 2008). In support of this, gOCT along with gADI, gENO and gFBPA are recognized by antibodies in human serum and in milk/saliva from giardiasic patients sampled in non-endemic and endemic areas, respectively (Palm et al., 2003; Tellez et al., 2005). It is possible that both glycolytic and arginolytic enzymes secreted by *G. duodenalis* trophozoites while in the presence of intestinal epithelial cells could be processed by antigen sampling, presentation by DC and induction of cytokine secretion by mast cells and T lymphocytes. This, in turn, would induce proliferation of antigen-specific B cells and lead to adaptive antibody production at both local (gut) and systemic levels.

3.3 Cysteine-rich surface proteins

Giardia trophozoites release a variety of surface-exposed proteins, particularly those rich in cysteine, upon interaction with model epithelial intestinal cells. These belong to two main families; the so-called HCMPs and the VSPs. The former constitutes a group of at least 61 proteins about a dozen of which are also secreted during trophozoite-epithelial cell interactions. The VSPs, in contrast, comprise a family of ≈270–303 members of which only one is predominantly expressed and secreted by a given parasite culture or population (Prucca and Lujan, 2009).

The HCMPs contain ≥20 CxxC/CxC motifs and are classified into nine groups based on shared internal motifs (groups 1–6, VSP-like, TMK-like and EGF-like) (Davids et al., 2006). In contrast, VSP sequences which possess 10–12% cysteine, numerous CxxC motifs, one or more conserved GGCY motifs, Zinc finger motif, and hydrophobic and palmitoylated C-termini, are phylogenetically divided into three clades (Adam et al., 2010; Nash, 2002). Among these, a total of 17 mRNAs of distinct HCMPs (groups 1 and 5, VSP-like and EGF-like) were up-regulated in four *Giardia* strains when in the presence of rat IEC-6 cells, whereas VSP123 (WB), VSP8 (P-1), Vsp160 (NF) and GL50581_3335 (GS/M) transcripts exhibited strain-specific up-regulation (Ma'ayeh and Brook-Carter, 2012). However, the repertoire of cysteine-rich surface proteins detected in the secretome is much more restricted: only three HCMPs in the WB strain (one TMK-like, one EGF-like and one of group 2) and one VSP in the GS strain (GL_50581_3195) were up-regulated upon interaction with Caco-2 cells (Ma'ayeh et al., 2017). In other studies, using the same strains and epithelial cell lines, two HCMPs (one of group 1, one of undefined type) that are distinct from the ones mentioned above were found among the 15 more abundant proteins secreted by both WB and GS strains (Dubourg et al., 2018). It is interesting to note that in the latter two studies, multiple HCMPs and one VSP were expressed and surface-exposed by trophozoites though the secretion of different repertoires of surface proteins agrees with the observed 'plasticity' in the biological responses of a given *Giardia* population to stimuli or stress, e.g., susceptibility to anti-giardial drugs (Arguello-Garcia et al., 2004, 2009), and with intrinsic differences in the cellular HCMP and VSP proteomes of isolates belonging to the same assemblage (Emery et al., 2014). Indeed, the versatile dynamics of the trophozoite cell surface that includes antigenic switching by VSPs and the release of several HCMPs, strongly suggest that these components play an important role in evasion of host's immune response and therefore the variable outcomes of human infections by *Giardia*. Nonetheless functional analyses of individual surface molecules are needed to gain insights into their mechanistic contributions to the parasite-host interface.

Because of its reactivity with the Mab 9B10, a particular protein group, VSP9B10, has received special attention and has been analysed using multiple approaches (Nash et al., 2001). The 63 kDa, VSP9B10A-like protein is believed to participate in parasite adhesion given that anti-VSP9B10A antibodies inhibit by 25% the attachment of WB strain trophozoites to MDCK cell monolayers (Bermudez-Cruz et al., 2004). In other studies, Carranza et al. (2002) found that VSP9B10B, a 68 kDa-sized protein, was located at the surface of encysting cells. In more recent studies involving trophozoite-IEC-6 interactions, the 76 kDa protein VSP9B10A (GL_50803_

101074, annotated in GiardiaDB as VSP88) which contains 739 amino acids was identified in the proteolytic secretome of the WB strain. This protease activity was narrowed down to the central region of the protein that spans positions 326–684 and displays similarities in structural folding to typical cathepsin B proteases; the protein also possesses a catalytic triad encompassing Cys30-His80-Asn201. Interestingly, structural alignment of the homology zone of VSP88 with the mature form of giardipain-1 (GL50803_14019) (Ortega-Pierres et al., 2018), the most expressed cysteine protease in *G. duodenalis* trophozoites (DuBois et al., 2006), also displays a similar orientation of catalytic cysteine and histidine residues (Fig. 3A). One might expect distinct substrate affinities/dockings between VSP88 and giardipain-1 because of the larger size of the N-terminal domain (325 amino acids) of the VSP88 and the accessibility of the giardipain-1 to a given protein substrate located in intraepithelial compartments.

In a study aimed to bypass the RNAi silencing mechanism of *all-but-one* VSP expression, VSP9B10A was constitutively expressed by trophozoites transfected with plasmids carrying the entire *vsp9b10a* sequence. When these parasites were co-cultured with IEC-6 monolayers, cytopathic damage consisting in cell-cell and cell-substrate detachments was observed (Cabrera-Licona et al., 2017). These observations indicate the direct effect of VSP88 on the integrity of intercellular molecules at tight and adherens junctions in a manner similar to that observed with cysteine proteases in the trophozoite secretome (see Section 3.4). In fact, five out of the six closest relatives of VSP88 (VSPs 77, 92, 160, 162.1 and 169) exhibit a semiconservative change in the catalytic triad (Asp80 instead His80) and only VSP8, the last of the six closest relatives to VSP88, retains His80. This suggests that VSP8 could function in a manner similar to VSP88 if expressed and secreted. Some of these surface proteins, namely, VSP8 and VSP160, were transcriptionally up-regulated in the P-1 and NF strains, respectively, upon interaction with IEC-6 monolayers (Ma'ayeh and Brook-Carter, 2012).

Based on the studies reported so far, continuing the functional characterization of VSPs will further elucidate the role of a given VSP secreted by a parasite culture or population (strain, isolate or clone) in the cytotoxic effects on epithelial cells and whether this occurs by a VSP-specific mechanism or by biological activities that are redundant or concurrent with other virulence factors secreted by trophozoites. As example, the presence of VSP188 as a sarafotoxin-like molecule in conjunction withVSP8 and VSP88 as cysteine protease-like molecules may provide a promising landscape in the discovery of other non-immunological functions carried out by secreted giardial VSPs and that may be related to clinical spectrum, zoonotic transmission and host specificity. This also applies for HCMPs due to the existence of multiple common and genotype-specific members of this surface protein family in assemblages (A, B and E) and even sub-assemblages of known genomic background (Ankarklev et al., 2015; Jerlstrom-Hultqvist et al., 2010).

3.4 Cysteine proteases

The presence of extracellular proteases is well documented in parasitic infections as these molecules participate in parasite invasion, migration, nutrient digestion and immunomodulation. Among these proteases, cysteine proteases are closely related to cytotoxic and cytopathic damage caused by anaerobic protozoa such as *Trichomonas*, *Entamoeba* and *Giardia* that are endowed with a sulphur-containing amino acid metabolism (Ali and Nozaki, 2007). The genome of *G. duodenalis* (reference clone WBA6) contains up to 25 cysteine protease genes, of which 21 are cathepsin type: 8 cathepsin-L, 9 cathepsin-B with endopeptidase activity, 3 cathepsin-B with endopeptidase and dipeptidyl peptidase activity (associated to the presence of an 'occluding loop') and 1 cathepsin-C-like (the encystation-specific cysteine protease, ESCP) (Touz et al., 2002). The cathepsin-like gene repertoire varies between strains and assemblages. Thus, in assemblage B the strain GS has 17 homologue while strain GS-B has 23 homologues, and in assemblage E the strain P15 contains 23 homologues. These proteases are predominantly synthesized as inactive precursors that following proteolytic removal of the N-terminal pro-domain become activated. These molecules have a catalytic site containing the typical Cys-His-Asn triad and a S2-binding pocket. In addition, they display a catalytic mechanism involving nucleophilic attack on substrate's carbonyl carbon group by deprotonated Cys with the formation of an intermediate thioester that is further hydrolysed to generate a carboxylic acid moiety in the remaining portion of the substrate. This mechanism, common to cysteine-type proteases, engenders cumulative and coordinated effects on target (host) proteins when the enzymes are expressed or secreted by the trophozoites. However, differential expression of these proteases occurs during trophozoite growth and encystation, where the cathepsins-B-like proteases formerly named as CP2, CP4 and CP5, and the cathepsin-L-like protease CP17 (Ward et al., 1997), are the most abundantly expressed (DuBois et al., 2006). These observations indicate that this family of enzymes has both individual and overlapping roles in the function of the biological processes and cellular compartment in which they are involved.

In this context, during trophozoite-epithelial cell interactions, a restricted repertoire of cysteine-type proteases, with gelatinolytic as well as collagenolytic activities, is expressed and released by parasites as shown in zymography analyses of ESP (Jimenez et al., 2000; Rodriguez-Fuentes et al., 2006). At the mRNA level, cathepsin-L-like proteins GL50803_137680 or GL_50803_3099 were found to be up-regulated in trophozoites of WB strain (Ringqvist et al., 2011) and in trophozoites of four strains (WB, P-1, GS/M and NF) (Ma'ayeh and Brook-Carter, 2012) when interacting with IEC-6 monolayers. In proteomic analyses of secretomes from trophozoite culture or in trophozoite-Caco-2 interactions, a set of three cathepsin B-like proteases from the WB strain (GL50803_16160, _16468 and _16779) and their identical homologue (e-value = 0.0) in the GS strain (GL50581_2946, _438 and _78, respectively) were detected along with a different cathepsin B (GL50803_14019 and GL50581_2036) (Ma'ayeh et al., 2017). In the other proteomic study on secretomes using the same strains and cell line, a different repertoire of three cathepsin B-like proteases was identified for the WB strain (GL50803_15564, _16468 and _17516) along with their closest homologue in the GS strain (GL50581_2036, _438 and _2318) (Dubourg et al., 2018). These data suggest that trophozoites of zoonotic assemblages A and B release a restricted but very similar pattern of cysteine proteases into culture medium and when in the company of viable epithelial cells; however, greater amounts or proteases are released when epithelial cells are present (Rodriguez-Fuentes et al., 2006).

All these proteases may become catalytically competent outside trophozoites by the absence of an occluding loop and the intracellular excision of pro-domains. The latter is best exemplified in giardipain-1 (GL50803_14019, formerly named as CP2) where its precursor (33 kDa) is 8 kDa larger and 76 amino acids longer than the mature protein (25 kDa) which possess gelatinolytic activity and exhibits pro-apoptotic effects on IEC-6 and MDCK epithelial monolayers (Ortega-Pierres et al., 2018). The exposure of IEC-6 epithelial cell monolayers to the purified, mature and secreted form of giardipain-1 displayed membrane blebbing which is coincident with apoptosis (Fig. 2).

The harm induced by secreted giardial proteases on epithelial cell indicates that these proteases target several important host proteins and that the process is not monophasic but involves a multifactorial and stepwise mechanism that disrupts intestinal homeostasis and damages the host intestine.

To accomplish this, the secreted cathepsins must initially interact with physiological barriers such as the mucus layer present on the brush border of intestinal epithelium which is among the first barriers encountered by

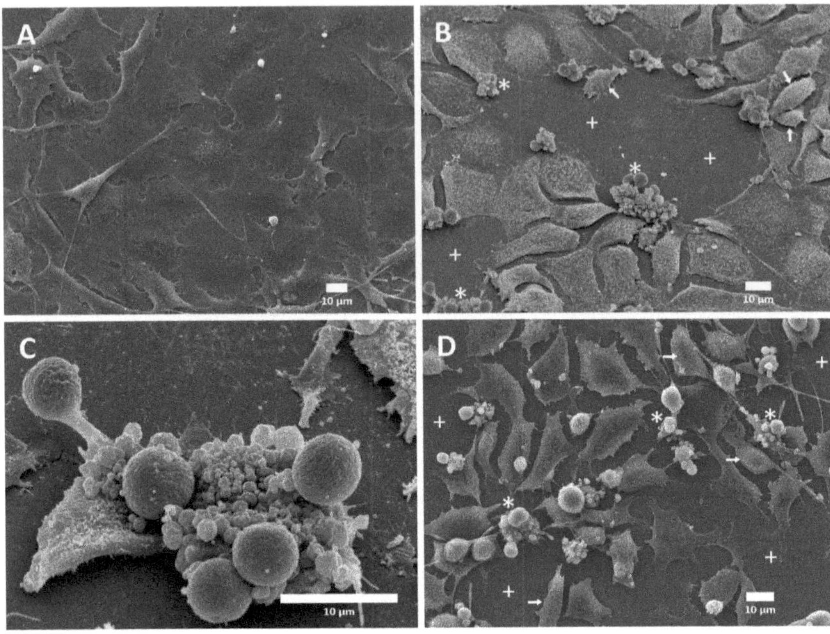

Fig. 2 Effect of purified giardipain-1 in IEC-6 epithelial monolayer integrity. (A) Confluent control monolayer. (B) By 60 min exposure to 8 μg/mL giardipain-1, there are zones with cells displaying shrinking (arrows) or multiple membrane blebbing processes (asterisks) and zones without attached cells (crosses). (C) Magnified view of a shrinked epithelial cell with multiple blebbing. (D) By 120 min of exposure to giardipain-1, multiple foci of apoptotic cells appear in monolayers. Scale bars are as indicated.

infecting trophozoites. This layer is mainly composed by membrane-bound mucins such as MUC4 and MUC16, and gel-forming mucins as MUC2 which is the predominant isoform in the gastrointestinal tract (Johansson and Hansson, 2016). Given that giardiasis patients exhibit a thinner mucus layer that covers the colon, experiments that exposed the mucin from a human mucus-producing colonic cell line (LS174T) to ESPs from strains NF (assemblage A) and GS/M (Assemblage B) revealed a concentration-dependent degradation of MUC2 that was abrogated by pretreatment with the cysteine protease inhibitor E64. This finding was further supported in experiments on transgenic Muc2 −/− mice where an increase in trophozoite numbers and weight loss in infected mice were observed, in addition to enlarged goblet cells and bacterial translocation in the jejunum and colon relative to uninfected controls (Amat et al., 2017). These results provided direct evidence that secreted cysteine proteases have mucolytic activity in the host.

The next barrier for the parasite to cross is the brush border at the apical surface of enterocytes. In acute giardiasis, trophozoites adhere to the microvilli lining of the enterocytes, induce structural alterations, and decrease the net absorptive area of the intestinal epithelial (Troeger et al., 2007). Villin, an actin-binding protein expressed in the gut and renal epithelia of mammals, regulates microfilament assembly/disassembly by means of its six gelsolin-like domains. Data showed that villin was degraded and redistributed by the action of surface-exposed giardial cysteine proteases. This was inferred from the conservation of villin structure in Caco-2 monolayers when in the presence of trophozoites that had been pre-incubated with E64 or ML-9, a known inhibitor of myosin light chain phosphorylation (i.e. MLCK) (Bhargava et al., 2015). This was an indirect study and the direct effect of giardial ESPs on villin integrity was not assessed. Thus, the use of purified cysteine protease(s) will shed light in this point by circumventing the villin remodelling activity in vivo carried out by T-lymphocyte CD4+/CD8+-mediated immune responses (Solaymani-Mohammadi and Singer, 2013).

The next step in the pathophysiology of giardiasis occurs when secretory proteases of *G. duodenalis* trophozoites disturb the organization of the intercellular epithelial barrier. This involves transmembrane, plaque and filamentous proteins intervening in apical junctional complexes (AJCs) known as tight junctions (claudins, occludins, zonula occludens or ZO proteins), and adherens junctions (E-cadherin, β-catenin). Under experimental conditions, giardial ESPs alter the distribution of AJC components such as claudin-1, occludin, ZO-1 and even intracellular F-actin in Caco-2 cells (Liu et al., 2018). The mature form of the cysteine protease giardipain-1 (so named by its 'papain-like' structural, functional and E64-inhibition features) was shown to be secreted by trophozoites and deposited on the epithelial cell surface. When added to IEC-6 monolayers, giardipain-1 co-localized with claudin-1, occludin and E-cadherin at cell junctions as early as 5 min following treatment and long before the IEC-6 monolayer was damaged (≈120 min). The interaction of giardipain-1 with occludins, which affects claudin distribution in the IEC-6 monolayers and diminishes these proteins in epithelial monolayers, was further demonstrated by immunoprecipitation and Western blots, respectively (Ortega-Pierres et al., 2018).

In a recent study, three major secreted cysteine proteases, namely, GL50803_14019 (giardipain-1), GL50803_16160 and GL50803_16779 (formerly CP3) (Ma'ayeh et al., 2017) were generated in recombinant form. When added separately to Caco-2 monolayers in their auto-activated mature states, a redistribution of AJC proteins was observed (Liu et al., 2018). Degradation of E-cadherin and occludin also occurred in the presence of these recombinant proteins and, as was previously demonstrated, E64 reduced these effects (Liu et al., 2018). Additionally, the three proteases degraded claudin-1 and -4 and β-catenin in situ. These data collectively indicate that the limited set of cysteine proteases released by trophozoites have redundant activities on target JAC proteins presumably to insure a thorough degradation of substrates responsible for barrier function of the epithelial cell layer. Redundancy among disparate proteases may also allow the secreted proteins to target a broader range of epithelial cell sources and expand the range of host infectivity.

Recently, the use of recombinant proteins and bioinformatics have advanced a better understanding of the proteolytic mechanisms displayed by cysteine proteases secreted by *G. duodenalis* trophozoites, and further expanded the repertoire of in vivo target proteins beyond those located at mucus, microvilli and cell junction barriers. To characterize the substrate specificity of the major secreted cysteine proteases, recombinant proteins identified via a phage display library screened with GL50803_16160 were expressed in a two-thioredoxin system and exposed to recombinant giardipain-1, GL50803_16160 and GL50803_16779. Similar substrate selectivities were observed for giardipain-1 and GL50803_16160; however, these differed from GL50803_16779 (Liu et al., 2019a,b). This discrepancy may have foundations in the cysteine-histidine catalytic mechanism described above and in the results of comparative protein modelling that predict the C26 and H170 residues in giardipain-1 and in GL50803_16160 have orientations similar to one another but remarkably different from the corresponding residues in GL50803_16779. This may translate not only to different docking positions with a same substrate but also to distinct substrate affinities (Fig. 3A).

In predictive bioinformatics analyses, the screening of a human small intestinal proteome with the cleavage consensus sequence of GL50803_16779 identified immunoglobulins (Ig), defensins (Df) and chemokines (Ck) as targets among the many cell junction proteins, mucins and novel potential substrates. First, recombinant IgG, IgA1 and IgA2 (heavy and light chains) were similarly cleaved by the three cysteine proteases except for the IgG light chain which was cleaved only by GL50803_16779. These data suggest that trophozoite secreted molecules are capable of interfering with and avoiding adaptive immune responses. Second, these three proteases exhibited distinct abilities to degrade recombinant human defensins αDf1, βDf5 and αDf6 where the activity of giardipain-1was noticeably higher than the other

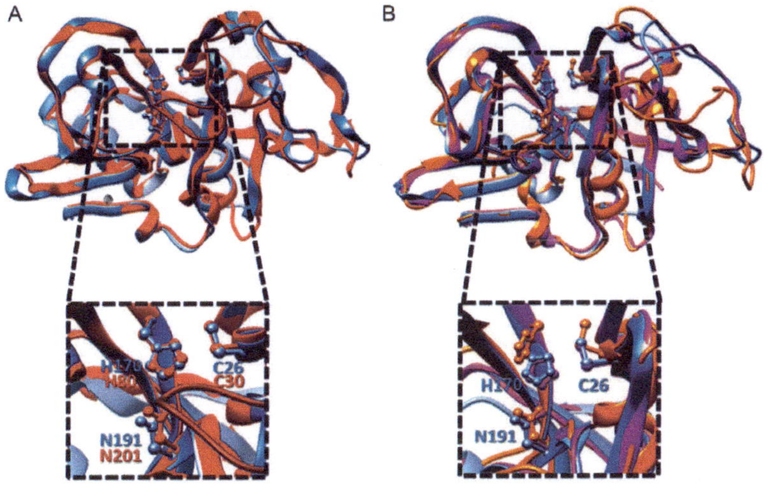

Fig. 3 (A) Protein structure alignment of the cysteine protease-homology zone (amino acids 326–684) of VSP88 (red) with mature giardipain-1 (blue). The catalytic triad C26-H170-N191 (giardipain-1) and C30-H80-N201 (VSP88) are displayed in *ball-and-stick* conformation. In these, all catalytic residues have a similar orientation. (B) Structure alignment of three major, mature cysteine proteases secreted by *G. duodenalis* trophozoites: giardipain-1 (blue), GL50803_16160 (purple) and GL50803_16779 (orange). The catalytic triad C26-H170-N191 of giardipain-1 is taken as reference and displayed in *ball-and-stick* conformation. In GL50803_16779 catalytic cysteine and adjacent histidine display a strikingly different orientation.

proteases (Liu et al., 2019a,b). This activity could be responsible for the cytotoxicity of some Df against trophozoites (Aley et al., 1994). As example, these proteases help neutralize the innate response engendered by Paneth cell-derived Dfs. Third, epithelial cells produce soluble immune mediators known as chemokines/cytokines including CXCL1–3 that are up-regulated upon exposure to trophozoites (Roxstrom-Lindquist et al., 2005). In the case of interleukin-8 (CXCL8), the gene is up-regulated by 1.5 h after infection but declines significantly by 4.5 h after infection (Ma'ayeh et al., 2018) where eventually giardial cysteine proteases post-transcriptionally degrade CXCL8 and decrease neutrophil recruitment and inflammatory responses (Cotton et al., 2014). Interestingly, recombinant (and up-regulated) CXCL1–3, CXCL8, CCL2 and CCL20 were cleaved by either ESPs or recombinant GL-50803_16160 albeit CXCL3 was the only chemokine not degraded by giardipain-1 and GL50803_16779 (Liu et al., 2018). Taken together, these potential in vivo targets of *Giardia* cysteine proteases underlying not only the impact of ESP on controlling host immune responses, but also favour the onset and establishment of infection.

Assays performed with laboratory device-isolated biofilms and microbiota-free mice showed that giardial secreted cysteine proteases are also involved in the interplay of *Giardia* with the commensal microbiota communities residing in the gut as biofilm-forming planktonic bacteria. Using *Caenorhabditis elegans* to model *Giardia*-microbiota interactions, it was shown that commensal human microbiota experimentally-exposed to *Giardia* induced lethal paralysis in this nematode (Gerbaba et al., 2017). Further studies on human colonic biofilms from healthy donors that were exposed to *Giardia* trophozoites (strain NF) or spent medium (i.e. ESP), exhibited biofilm disruption, decrease in thickness and an altered bacterial composition (dysbiosis) with an over-representation of *Clostridiales*. The transfer of these microbiota biofilms to germ-free mice also led to an increase in *Clostridiales* and other unclassified Firmicutes, and to a decrease in *Phascolarctobacterium*. Remarkably, biofilm-released bacteria provoked the disruption of the cell junction protein ZO-1, apoptosis and the expression of pro-inflammatory molecules TLR4 and CXCL8 in epithelial cells (Caco-2). In addition, upregulation was observed among mucosal pro-inflammatory cytokines (IL-6, IL-1β, IL-17, TNFα and IFNγ) and bacterial translocation in mice. Collectively, these data suggest that the planktonic bacteria became pathobionts as observed in other pathogen-microbiota interactions (Beatty et al., 2017; Chua et al., 2014). These effects were decreased by the addition of E-64, which implicates cysteine proteases in this dysbiotic process via a mechanism that involves proteolytic action on components of the biofilm's extracellular matrix such as biofilm-associated protein (bap), pili or fimbriae.

Based on these studies, the sustained pro-inflammatory response at the gut mucosa, even in the absence of *Giardia*, provides an in-force hypothesis on an association between cysteine proteases in giardial ESP and intestinal diseases such as post-infection, irritable bowel syndrome (PI-IBS) (Beatty et al., 2017; Keselman et al., 2016). Further studies on species-specific inhibition of giardial cysteine proteases, the effects of isolated proteases (e.g. giardipain-1, GL50803_16160 and GL50803_16779) on microbiota communities, parasite-derived perturbation to intestinal bacterial communities, and elucidation of changes to intestinal homeostasis in infection and post-infection models, are warranted.

3.5 Tenascins

The wide range of molecules secreted by *Giardia* trophozoites in the presence or the absence of epithelial cells, leads to in vivo damage of intestinal mucosa at the structural and molecular levels. A recent hypothesis has emerged that relates the pathogenesis of giardiasis to components of the giardial secretome that affect intestinal tissue repair; in particular, tenascins (Dubourg et al., 2018). In vertebrates, tenascins are trimeric or hexameric proteins of the extracellular matrix (ECM) present in developing tissues such as embryonic, healing and tumourigenic tissues and are classified into four paralogue groups: C (founder group), R, X and W. Their primary structures contain an N-terminal heptad repeat, approximately 14 epidermal growth factor (EGF)-like repeats, 8 or more fibronectin III-like repeats and a C-terminal fibrinogen-like globular domain (Hsia and Schwarzbauer, 2005). In GiardiaDB there are approximately 20 different tenascin-encoding genes encoded in strains WB (10), GS (9) and P15 (11). Among these, some are annotated as tenascin-X (4 in WB and P15, 3 in GS) or tenascin-37 (1 per clone/assemblage). In proteomic studies on the secretome of trophozoites from an Australian isolate (BRIS/95/HEPU/2041) exposed to soluble factors collected from HT-29 cells, two tenascins (GL50803_8687, [C-like] and GL50803_14573, [X-like]) were detected (Emery et al., 2016). Similarly, one tenascin was reported in each of the WB (GL50803_10330) and GS (Gl50581_4057) trophozoites when in the presence of Caco-2 cells (Ma'ayeh et al., 2017). In another study, a 2-mass spectrometry method to examine the secretomes of WB and GS trophozoites interacting with Caco-2 cells identified seven distinct tenascins secreted by the WB strain, four of which were found in the GS strain (Dubourg et al., 2018).

To date, the role of giardial tenascins in pathogenic damage to intestinal tissues has not been elucidated. However, from evolutionarily, these molecules could have evolved from HCMPs and/or VSPs and molecular mimicry with vertebrate EGF receptor. In the process, giardial tenascins apparently would have lost or failed to acquire fibronectin III domains and retained only some EGF-like domains (e.g. 3–4 in the tenascins C- and X-like secreted by WB strain) (Dubourg et al., 2018; Emery et al., 2016). These domains (30–40 amino acids in length) usually contain cysteine residues that form disulphide bridges within a two stranded β-sheet followed by a loop towards a short, C-terminal, two-stranded sheet. In this way, once secreted tenascins could ligate EGF receptors exposed at the surface of intestinal cells through its EGF-like domains thus competing with endogenous EGF (Theocharis et al., 2016); however, EGF receptor exposure must be facilitated by an earlier action of cathepsins B and an extracellular nuclease secreted by trophozoites that degrade the mucus layer that covers epithelial cells (Dubourg et al., 2018). This mechanism is thought to induce separation between the enterocytes and exacerbate intestinal damage together with bacterial translocation and pro-inflammatory responses. Despite tenascins being present in

Giardia secretomes and being linked to epithelial cell damage, there remains a need for in vivo and in vitro experimental studies using purified native and recombinant tenascins in model systems to further elucidate the mechanisms of action. This will help to unravel the specific role of these molecules in pathogenesis, disease onset and post-infection complications caused by *Giardia*.

4. Secreted virulence factors: Potential therapeutic agents?

Control of *G. duodenalis* relies on the use of six classes of pharmacological agents that have a primary and direct action on parasite molecules such as DNA (e.g. quinacrine), rRNA and ribosomes (e.g. paromomycin) and β-tubulin (e.g. albendazole), or that are activated within trophozoites to form adducts with nucleic acids and/or proteins (e.g. 5-nitroheterocyclic drugs including metronidazole, furazolidone and nitazoxanide) (Gardner and Hill, 2001; Lalle and Hanevik, 2018).

Proposals for alternative therapies include phytochemicals, probiotics (e.g. *Lactobacillus*) and nanotechnology (Vivancos et al., 2018). One promising approach for treating giardiasis is to evaluate and further characterize previously identified agents that target virulence factors. Targeting virulent factors have specific advantages. First, toxin-like components of pathogens are often species-specific molecules that are intracellularly synthesized, and then transported and exposed to the trophozoite's surface which makes them available for binding exogenous drugs. Second, most virulence factors evolved to preserve parasite viability (e.g. cysteine proteases and 'moonlighting' enzymes). This strategy has been used in the search for compounds that target secreted bacterial toxins or enzymes such as phosphatases and secreted fungal aspartic proteases (Gauwerky et al., 2009; Ivarsson et al., 2012). Indeed, the design of drugs that can neutralize, inhibit or degrade virulence factors intra- or extracellularly would not only compromise trophozoites´ proliferation, but would also neutralize their pathogenic potential and in so doing, ameliorate some post-giardiasis complications as PI-IBS.

Rational drug design has become an approachable way to find new drug candidates that will interact with virulence factors of *Giardia*. Structure-based drug design (SBDD) (Merz et al., 2010) is based on using computational analyses of molecules denoted as protein ligands that are conformationally and electrostatically complementary to a given target biomolecule. The availability of target crystal structures from known databases (e.g. Protein Data Bank, PDB) can be a significant help in such an endeavour. To date, the crystal structures of only two possible *Giardia* virulent factors of the ADHP (gOCT and gCK) and one glycolytic enzyme (gFBPA) have been solved and most of these have been evaluated by SBDD strategies.

The recombinant form of gFBPA, the fourth enzyme in catabolic glycolysis, has been generated and the structure of its predominant dimeric conformation (with one or two Zn^{2+} atoms) has been experimentally determined by X-ray diffraction of orthorhombic and hexagonal crystals in complex with the transition state (enediolate) analog phosphoglycolohydroxamate (PGH). This protein is a possible target for SBDD because: (a) gene silencing by antisense RNA (RNAi) techniques is lethal for trophozoites, and (b) significant differences exist among the human and *Giardia* FBPAs to diminish the potential for overlapping activities. While human FBPAs are type I aldolases, which have a Lysine in the active site that promotes cleavage of the C (3)–C (4) bond in the substrate, gFBPA is a type II aldolase. Type II aldolases possess a C-terminal catalytic site where a Zn^{2+} cofactor coordinates the imidazole rings of His110, His226 and His264 residues with the C (2)-carbonyl and C (3)-hydroxyl oxygen atoms of the substrate. Also, the Asp83 has an essential role in catalysis as determined by site-directed mutagenesis (Galkin et al., 2007). The inhibitor for PGH may inhibit type II FBPAs as well, since these enzymes do not have significant amino acid sequence homology with type I aldolases; however, this inhibitor is active against the TPI glycolytic enzyme precluding its use in humans. The C (4) epimer of FBP, tagatose-1,6-bisphosphate (TBP), is a selective inhibitor of gFBPA (Galkin et al., 2007).

In other work, the crystal structure of gFBPA was used as a template for in silico (SBDD) design and synthesis of nine dihydroxypyridinones (DHP1 to DHP9). These are first-generation inhibitors that interact with phosphate binding residues on putative substrates and function as hydrogen bond donors to Asn83 and Zn^{2+}-binding groups (Li et al., 2011). Among this group of potential inhibitors, DHP8 displayed higher affinity for gFBPA; however, the interactions determined by synchrotron radiation in gFBPA-DHP8 crystals showed a rather weak coordination of the inhibitor with Zn^{2+} which is otherwise strong with the enediolate intermediate (Li et al., 2011). Another SBDD strategy used chemical synthesis and in vitro screening to examine the anti-giardial activity of four 5-nitrothiazole (nitazoxanide) analogs and four 6-benzonitrothiazole acetamides. Results demonstrated giardicidal efficacy which was more pronounced on the recombinant gFBPA. Two 5-nitrothiazole acetamide compounds, 5NTA-1 and 5NTA-4, displayed high cytotoxicity against *G. duodenalis* trophozoites when compared to VERO cells, and a greater inhibitory effect on gFBPA activity than nitazoxanide. This was explained by a closer interaction of the nitrogen in the thiazole moiety of these compounds with the Zn^{2+} cofactor, and by the catalytic activity of Asn253 as assessed by docking studies (Navarrete-Vazquez et al., 2015).

A recent study examined the anti-giardial efficacy of tiliroside, a flavonoid isolated from the aerial parts of the flowering plant *Sphaeralcea angustifolia*. Docking analyses suggest that tiliroside could interact with an allosteric moiety of gFBPA. This differentiates it from metronidazole activity which is predicted to interact with gFBPA at its active site (Calzada et al., 2017). In light of these studies with synthetic and natural compounds targeting gFBPA, current bioinformatics as well as experimental evidence indicate that DHP8, 5NTA-1 and 5NTA-4 could be leading candidates for preclinical evaluation.

As noted above, the crystal structure of two enzymes of the ADHP have been the focus of drug screening studies. Similar to the urotelic human OCT, the gOCT exists as a trimer and possesses similar activity; however, its low sequence identity with the human homologue (30%) and the differences at several key positions in the so-called disordered loops 1 and 2 suggest that selective inhibitors can be designed (Galkin et al., 2009). In contrast, gCK is also an essential enzyme for trophozoite survival that is absent in the human host. Three crystal structures of gCK have been determined: (a) in complex with the non-hydrolysable ATP analog, AMP-PNP; (b) in complex with citric acid, a carbamate phosphate analog; and (c) in the unbound state (Galkin et al., 2010; Lim et al., 2013). Functional screening of two drug libraries using both bioluminescent detection of ATP production by trophozoites and gCK activity, it was determined that disulfiram (tetraethylthiuram, Antabuse™) is a highly effective compound against gCK activity ($IC_{50} = 0.58\,\mu M$) and is high in giardicidal activity ($IC_{50} = 0.90\,\mu M$). This compound is an FDA-approved drug commonly used for long term treatment of chronic alcoholism; however, in *Giardia*, it acts by a semi-allosteric mechanism where the Cys242 located at the edge of active site is thiocarbamoylated. This prevents the conformational transition of the loop adjacent to ADP/ATP binding site that is needed for catalysis as assessed by the gCK-disulfiram crystallography. This effect is shared by simpler analogs such as thiuram disulphide (Thiram), Interestingly, these compounds have cytotoxic activity against metronidazole-resistant *Giardia* (Galkin et al., 2014).

The other ADHP enzyme, a multifunctional dimeric gADI, has been experimentally analysed in mechanistic studies as a possible drug target using

Cys-modifying substrate analogs. In one approach, based on the crystal structures of bacterial ADIs from *Pseudomonas aeruginosa* and *Bacillus cereus*, the catalytic mechanism involving the participation of Cys400 was analysed in detail. The Cys400 together with L-arginine formed an initial Cys-thiolate which, upon elimination of ammonia, gave rise to a Cys-alkyl-thiouronium ion intermediate, which was hydrolysed to form L-citrulline. This study was advanced because L-canavanine, a non-proteinogenic amino acid that differs from L-arginine by the substitution of a methylene bridge by an oxa group, irreversibly inhibits recombinant BcADI but reversibly inhibits recombinant PaADI and gADI. It was proposed that the reversible inhibition results from the formation of a less electrophilic Cys-alkyl-thiourea adduct which reacts more slowly with water than does the Cys-alkyl-thiouronium intermediate which forms O-ureido-L-homoserine in the active enzyme. In contrast, the covalent modification of BcADI by L-canavanine involves the formation of a thiocarbamate adduct that permanently renders the enzyme inactive (Li et al., 2008). Even though gADI is a proven target for L-canavanine, and L-canavanine occurs naturally in alfalfa and in the seeds of leguminous plants as a biological defence against herbivores, toxicological studies have revealed that its consumption may cause lupus-like reactions in mice and humans (Akaogi et al., 2006; Montanaro and Bardana, 1991). Consequently, these findings have hampered clinical evaluation of the natural product.

Other mechanistic studies have been performed on several L-arginine derivatives that were shown to be substrates of gADI. N^{ω}-cyano L-arginine is an irreversible BcADI inhibitor but it had no effect on gADI. On the other hand, S-nitroso-L-homocysteine, an endogenous carrier of NO, irreversibly inhibited gADI by a mechanism apparently involving S-nitroso and N-thiosulphoximide adducts at catalytic and allosteric cysteines (Li et al., 2009). A recent bioinformatics study was based on homology modelling of gADI followed by docking and molecular dynamics simulations using two sets of benzimidazole derivatives BZDs: 3196 from the commercial ZINC database and 19 synthesized *in house*. Once screened, three synthetic derivatives, BZD1, BZD10 and BZD19, that harbour a 1-methyl group and ethoxy or ester moieties resulted in theoretically viable interactions with the active site of gADI (Trejo-Soto et al., 2016). Collectively, these studies provide insights into mechanistic and drug design strategies for gADI; however, better experimental studies are required to define candidates for evaluation in giardiasis.

Based on the importance of secreted cysteine proteases in giardial pathogenicity, the screening of compounds capable of interacting with and modifying their catalytic or allosteric cysteines is a promising approach to drug design. This strategy is different from the mechanism displayed by the endogenous protease inhibitor cystatin, which was recently identified in *Giardia* (GL50803_27918). Cystatin binds papain-like cysteine proteases likely by its QxVxG motif, and belongs to the type 1 cystatins (stefins) (Liu et al., 2019b). Even though the crystal structures of the major giardial secreted cysteine proteases, i.e., giardipain-1, GL50803_CP16160 and GL50803_16779, have not yet been solved, homology modelling using the human cathepsin B precursor (PDB ID: 1GMY) has provided reliable information for docking studies. These data explain not only the interactions between cathepsin B and its inhibitors such as CA-074 or E64 (Ortega-Pierres et al., 2018), but also predict inhibition by natural compounds such as diallyl thiosulphinate, commonly known as allicin (Arguello-Garcia et al., 2018). This compound is a thioallyl derivative enzymatically formed when garlic bulbs or cloves are macerated or crushed in water. Alternatively, allicin can be generated in the lab by chemical oxidation of diallyl disulphide. Synthetic allicin was found to have giardicidal activity in vitro mediated by cysteine thioallylation. When administered intragastrically, it eliminated trophozoites from the intestines of experimentally infected Mongolian gerbils. Allicin also inhibited some cysteine protease activities including giardipain-1 when used in zymography assays and abolished the cytopathic and pro-apoptotic effects of giardipain-1 on epithelial cell monolayers when preincubated with the purified protease (Arguello-Garcia et al., 2018). These data strongly support testing allicin in clinical trials to treat giardiasis and to advance its natural benefits to human health.

5. Conclusions

Studies on the interplay of epithelial cells with *G. duodenalis* have provided useful information regarding the roles that parasite molecules play in giardial pathogenesis. Identification and characterization of these molecules have been fine-tuned using techniques such as microarrays, representational difference analysis, SAGE, tandem mass tag labelling, Q-Exactive and Orbitrap MS, and next-generation sequencing. In some cases, these molecules have been further evaluated for their abilities to directly or indirectly interact with structural and molecular targets in host cells including mucus, microbiota biofilms, microvilli, cell surface sensors (endothelin receptor, arginine transporter, EGF receptor), cell junctions, the fibrinolytic system (plasminogen, fibrinogen) and soluble immune mediators (Ig, Df, Ck). These data present an important platform upon which to advance studies that better define the roles of these molecules during trophozoite infection of the intestine. Although old challenges remain, new challenges are looming such as identifying strain or assemblage 'specific' molecules, better characterizing the intestinal immune responses that are activated during infection, clarifying the relationship between giardiasis and dysbiosis, and elucidating the long lasting inflammatory responses that cause post-infection disorders such as irritable bowel disease. In spite of its genetic minimalism, *Giardia* provides holistically a wonderful model system to advance discovery and control in the fight against inflammatory bowel diseases as well as in the knowledge of host-microbiota changes during and after parasitic diseases.

Acknowledgements

The authors wish to express special thanks to Lorenza González Mariscal for her valuable comments and suggestions on the manuscript. We are immensely grateful to Dante Zarlenga for his comments, technical and language editing of the manuscript. We thank Silvia Espinosa-Matías and Bibiana Chávez Munguía for their skillful assistance in obtaining scanning electron microscopy micrographs and Arturo Pérez-Taylor for the art work. We would like to acknowledge support from Miguel Alemán Foundation and Cinvestav.

References

Adam, R.D., Nigam, A., Seshadri, V., Martens, C.A., Farneth, G.A., Morrison, H.G., Nash, T.E., Porcella, S.F., Patel, R., 2010. The Giardia lamblia vsp gene repertoire: characteristics, genomic organization, and evolution. BMC Genomics 11, 424. https://doi.org/10.1186/1471-2164-11-424.

Aguayo-Ortiz, R., Meza-Cervantez, P., Castillo, R., Hernandez-Campos, A., Dominguez, L., Yepez-Mulia, L., 2017. Insights into the Giardia intestinalis enolase and human plasminogen interaction. Mol. BioSyst. 13 (10), 2015–2023. https://doi.org/10.1039/c7mb00252a.

Akaogi, J., Barker, T., Kuroda, Y., Nacionales, D.C., Yamasaki, Y., Stevens, B.R., Reeves, W.H., Satoh, M., 2006. Role of non-protein amino acid L-canavanine in autoimmunity. Autoimmun. Rev. 5 (6), 429–435. https://doi.org/10.1016/j.autrev.2005.12.004.

Aley, S.B., Zimmerman, M., Hetsko, M., Selsted, M.E., Gillin, F.D., 1994. Killing of Giardia lamblia by cryptdins and cationic neutrophil peptides. Infect. Immun. 62 (12), 5397–5403.

Ali, V., Nozaki, T., 2007. Current therapeutics, their problems, and sulfur-containing-amino-acid metabolism as a novel target against infections by "amitochondriate" protozoan parasites. Clin. Microbiol. Rev. 20 (1), 164–187. https://doi.org/10.1128/cmr.00019-06.

Allain, T., Amat, C.B., Motta, J.P., Manko, A., Buret, A.G., 2017. Interactions of Giardia sp. with the intestinal barrier: epithelium, mucus, and microbiota. Tissue Barriers 5 (1), e1274354. https://doi.org/10.1080/21688370.2016.1274354.

Amat, C.B., Motta, J.-P., Fekete, E., Moreau, F., Chadee, K., Buret, A.G., 2017. Cysteine protease-dependent mucous disruptions and differential mucin gene expression in giardia duodenalis infection. Am. J. Pathol. 187 (11), 2486–2498. https://doi.org/10.1016/j.ajpath.2017.07.009.

Ankarklev, J., Jerlstrom-Hultqvist, J., Ringqvist, E., Troell, K., Svard, S.G., 2010. Behind the smile: cell biology and disease mechanisms of Giardia species. Nat. Rev. Microbiol. 8 (6), 413–422. https://doi.org/10.1038/nrmicro2317.

Ankarklev, J., Franzen, O., Peirasmaki, D., Jerlstrom-Hultqvist, J., Lebbad, M., Andersson, J., Andersson, B., Svard, S.G., 2015. Comparative genomic analyses of freshly isolated Giardia intestinalis assemblage A isolates. BMC Genomics 16, 697. https://doi.org/10.1186/s12864-015-1893-6.

Arguello-Garcia, R., Cruz-Soto, M., Romero-Montoya, L., Ortega-Pierres, G., 2004. Variability and variation in drug susceptibility among Giardia duodenalis isolates and clones exposed to 5-nitroimidazoles and benzimidazoles in vitro. J. Antimicrob. Chemother. 54 (4), 711–721. https://doi.org/10.1093/jac/dkh388.

Arguello-Garcia, R., Cruz-Soto, M., Romero-Montoya, L., Ortega-Pierres, G., 2009. In vitro resistance to 5-nitroimidazoles and benzimidazoles in Giardia duodenalis: variability and variation in gene expression. Infect. Genet. Evol. 9 (6), 1057–1064. https://doi.org/10.1016/j.meegid.2009.05.015.

Arguello-Garcia, R., de la Vega-Arnaud, M., Loredo-Rodriguez, I.J., Mejia-Corona, A.M., Melgarejo-Trejo, E., Espinoza-Contreras, E.A., Fonseca-Linan, R., Gonzalez-Robles, A., Perez-Hernandez, N., Ortega-Pierres, M.G., 2018. Activity of thioallyl compounds from garlic against Giardia duodenalis trophozoites and in experimental Giardiasis. Front. Cell. Infect. Microbiol. 8, 353. https://doi.org/10.3389/fcimb.2018.00353.

Banik, S., Renner Viveros, P., Seeber, F., Klotz, C., Ignatius, R., Aebischer, T., 2013. Giardia duodenalis arginine deiminase modulates the phenotype and cytokine secretion of human dendritic cells by depletion of arginine and formation of ammonia. Infect. Immun. 81 (7), 2309–2317. https://doi.org/10.1128/iai.00004-13.

Bartelt, L.A., Sartor, R.B., 2015. Advances in understanding Giardia: determinants and mechanisms of chronic sequelae. F1000Prime Rep. 7, 62. https://doi.org/10.12703/p7-62.

Beatty, J.K., Akierman, S.V., Motta, J.P., Muise, S., Workentine, M.L., Harrison, J.J., Bhargava, A., Beck, P.L., Rioux, K.P., McKnight, G.W., Wallace, J.L., Buret, A.G., 2017. Giardia duodenalis induces pathogenic dysbiosis of human intestinal microbiota biofilms. Int. J. Parasitol. 47 (6), 311–326. https://doi.org/10.1016/j.ijpara.2016.11.010.

Bermudez-Cruz, R.M., Ortega-Pierres, G., Ceja, V., Coral-Vazquez, R., Fonseca, R., Cervantes, L., Sanchez, A., Depardon, F., Newport, G., Montanez, C., 2004. A 63 kDa VSP9B10A-like protein expressed in a C-8 Giardia duodenalis Mexican clone. Arch. Med. Res. 35 (3), 199–208. https://doi.org/10.1016/j.arcmed.2003.12.005.

Bhargava, A., Cotton, J.A., Dixon, B.R., Gedamu, L., Yates, R.M., Buret, A.G., 2015. Giardia duodenalis surface cysteine proteases induce cleavage of the intestinal epithelial cytoskeletal protein villin via myosin light chain kinase. PLoS One 10 (9), e0136102. https://doi.org/10.1371/journal.pone.0136102.

Buret, A.G., 2007. Mechanisms of epithelial dysfunction in giardiasis. Gut 56 (3), 316–317. https://doi.org/10.1136/gut.2006.107771.

Cabrera-Licona, A., Solano-Gonzalez, E., Fonseca-Linan, R., Bazan-Tejeda, M.L., Arguello-Garcia, R., Bermudez-Cruz, R.M., Ortega-Pierres, G., 2017. Expression and secretion of the Giardia duodenalis variant surface protein 9B10A by transfected trophozoites causes damage to epithelial cell monolayers mediated by protease activity. Exp. Parasitol. 179, 49–64. https://doi.org/10.1016/j.exppara.2017.06.006.

Calzada, F., Basurto, J.C., Barbosa, E., Velazquez, C., Hernandez, N.G., Ordonez Razo, R.M., Luna, D.M., Mulia, L.Y., 2017. Antiprotozoal activities of tiliroside and other compounds from sphaeralcea angustifolia (Cav.) G. Don. Pharm. Res. 9 (2), 133–137. https://doi.org/10.4103/0974-8490.204644.

Carranza, P.G., Feltes, G., Ropolo, A., Quintana, S.M., Touz, M.C., Lujan, H.D., 2002. Simultaneous expression of different variant-specific surface proteins in single Giardia lamblia trophozoites during encystation. Infect. Immun. 70 (9), 5265–5268. https://doi.org/10.1128/iai.70.9.5265-5268.2002.

Castillo-Romero, A., Davids, B.J., Lauwaet, T., Gillin, F.D., 2012. Importance of enolase in Giardia lamblia differentiation. Mol. Biochem. Parasitol. 184 (2), 122–125. https://doi.org/10.1016/j.molbiopara.2012.04.011.

Cervin, J., Wands, A.M., Casselbrant, A., Wu, H., Krishnamurthy, S., Cvjetkovic, A., Estelius, J., Dedic, B., Sethi, A., Wallom, K.L., Riise, R., Backstrom, M., Wallenius, V., Platt, F.M., Lebens, M., Teneberg, S., Fandriks, L., Kohler, J.J., Yrlid, U., 2018. GM1 ganglioside-independent intoxication by Cholera toxin. PLoS Pathog. 14 (2), e1006862. https://doi.org/10.1371/journal.ppat.1006862.

Chen, N., Upcroft, J.A., Upcroft, P., 1995. A Giardia duodenalis gene encoding a protein with multiple repeats of a toxin homologue. Parasitology 111 (Pt 4), 423–431.

Chua, S.L., Liu, Y., Yam, J.K., Chen, Y., Vejborg, R.M., Tan, B.G., Kjelleberg, S., Tolker-Nielsen, T., Givskov, M., Yang, L., 2014. Dispersed cells represent a distinct stage in the transition from bacterial biofilm to planktonic lifestyles. Nat. Commun. 5, 4462. https://doi.org/10.1038/ncomms5462.

Collingridge, P.W., Brown, R.W., Ginger, M.L., 2010. Moonlighting enzymes in parasitic protozoa. Parasitology 137 (9), 1467–1475. https://doi.org/10.1017/s0031182010000259.

Cotton, J.A., Beatty, J.K., Buret, A.G., 2011. Host parasite interactions and pathophysiology in Giardia infections. Int. J. Parasitol. 41 (9), 925–933. https://doi.org/10.1016/j.ijpara.2011.05.002.

Cotton, J.A., Bhargava, A., Ferraz, J.G., Yates, R.M., Beck, P.L., Buret, A.G., 2014. Giardia duodenalis cathepsin B proteases degrade intestinal epithelial interleukin-8 and attenuate interleukin-8-induced neutrophil chemotaxis. Infect. Immun. 82 (7), 2772–2787. https://doi.org/10.1128/iai.01771-14.

Davids, B.J., Reiner, D.S., Birkeland, S.R., Preheim, S.P., Cipriano, M.J., McArthur, A.G., Gillin, F.D., 2006. A new family of giardial cysteine-rich non-VSP protein genes and a novel cyst protein. PLoS One 1, e44. https://doi.org/10.1371/journal.pone.0000044.

Di Costanzo, L., Moulin, M., Haertlein, M., Meilleur, F., Christianson, D.W., 2007. Expression, purification, assay, and crystal structure of perdeuterated human arginase I. Arch. Biochem. Biophys. 465 (1), 82–89. https://doi.org/10.1016/j.abb.2007.04.036.

DuBois, K.N., Abodeely, M., Sajid, M., Engel, J.C., McKerrow, J.H., 2006. Giardia lambia cysteine proteases. Parasitol. Res. 99 (4), 313–316. https://doi.org/10.1007/s00436-006-0149-4.

Dubourg, A., Xia, D., Winpenny, J.P., Al Naimi, S., Bouzid, M., Sexton, D.W., Wastling, J.M., Hunter, P.R., Tyler, K.M., 2018. Giardia secretome highlights secreted tenascins as a key component of pathogenesis. Gigascience 7 (3), 1–13. https://doi.org/10.1093/gigascience/giy003.

Eckmann, L., Laurent, F., Langford, T.D., Hetsko, M.L., Smith, J.R., Kagnoff, M.F., Gillin, F.D., 2000. Nitric oxide production by human intestinal epithelial cells and competition for arginine as potential determinants of host defense against the lumen-dwelling pathogen Giardia lamblia. J. Immunol. 164 (3), 1478–1487. https://doi.org/10.4049/jimmunol.164.3.1478.

Emery, S.J., van Sluyter, S., Haynes, P.A., 2014. Proteomic analysis in Giardia duodenalis yields insights into strain virulence and antigenic variation. Proteomics 14 (21-22), 2523–2534. https://doi.org/10.1002/pmic.201400144.

Emery, S.J., Mirzaei, M., Vuong, D., Pascovici, D., Chick, J.M., Lacey, E., Haynes, P.A., 2016. Induction of virulence factors in Giardia duodenalis independent of host attachment. Sci. Rep, 6. https://doi.org/10.1038/srep20765.

Ferella, M., Davids, B.J., Cipriano, M.J., Birkeland, S.R., Palm, D., Gillin, F.D., McArthur, A.G., Svard, S., 2014. Gene expression changes during Giardia-host cell interactions in serum-free medium. Mol. Biochem. Parasitol. 197 (1-2), 21–23. https://doi.org/10.1016/j.molbiopara.2014.09.007.

Galkin, A., Kulakova, L., Melamud, E., Li, L., Wu, C., Mariano, P., Dunaway-Mariano, D., Nash, T.E., Herzberg, O., 2007. Characterization, kinetics, and crystal structures of fructose-1,6-bisphosphate aldolase from the human parasite, Giardia lamblia. J. Biol. Chem. 282 (7), 4859–4867. https://doi.org/10.1074/jbc.M609534200.

Galkin, A., Kulakova, L., Wu, R., Gong, M., Dunaway-Mariano, D., Herzberg, O., 2009. X-ray structure and kinetic properties of ornithine transcarbamoylase from the human parasite Giardia lamblia. Proteins 76 (4), 1049–1053. https://doi.org/10.1002/prot.22469.

Galkin, A., Kulakova, L., Wu, R., Nash, T.E., Dunaway-Mariano, D., Herzberg, O., 2010. X-ray structure and characterization of carbamate kinase from the human parasite Giardia lamblia. Acta Crystallogr. Sect. F. Struct. Biol. Cryst. Commun. 66 (Pt 4), 386–390. https://doi.org/10.1107/s1744309110004665.

Galkin, A., Kulakova, L., Lim, K., Chen, C.Z., Zheng, W., Turko, I.V., Herzberg, O., 2014. Structural basis for inactivation of Giardia lamblia carbamate kinase by disulfiram. J. Biol. Chem. 289 (15), 10502–10509. https://doi.org/10.1074/jbc.M114.553123.

Gardner, T.B., Hill, D.R., 2001. Treatment of giardiasis. Clin. Microbiol. Rev. 14 (1), 114–128. https://doi.org/10.1128/cmr.14.1.114-128.2001.

Gauwerky, K., Borelli, C., Korting, H.C., 2009. Targeting virulence: a new paradigm for antifungals. Drug Discov. Today 14 (3-4), 214–222. https://doi.org/10.1016/j.drudis.2008.11.013.

Gerbaba, T.K., Gupta, P., Rioux, K., Hansen, D., Buret, A.G., 2015. Giardia duodenalis-induced alterations of commensal bacteria kill Caenorhabditis elegans: a new model to study microbial-microbial interactions in the gut. Am. J. Physiol. Gastrointest. Liver Physiol. 308 (6), G550–G5561. https://doi.org/10.1152/ajpgi.00335.201.

Gerbaba, T.K., Green-Harrison, L., Buret, A.G., 2017. Modeling host-microbiome interactions in caenorhabditis elegans. J. Nematol. 49 (4), 348–356.

Gomez-Arreaza, A., Acosta, H., Quinones, W., Concepcion, J.L., Michels, P.A., Avilan, L., 2014. Extracellular functions of glycolytic enzymes of parasites: unpredicted use of ancient proteins. Mol. Biochem. Parasitol. 193 (2), 75–81. https://doi.org/10.1016/j.molbiopara.2014.02.005.

Guillou, F., Roger, E., Mone, Y., Rognon, A., Grunau, C., Theron, A., Mitta, G., Coustau, C., Gourbal, B.E., 2007. Excretory-secretory proteome of larval Schistosoma mansoni and Echinostoma caproni, two parasites of Biomphalaria glabrata. Mol. Biochem. Parasitol. 155 (1), 45–56. https://doi.org/10.1016/j.molbiopara.2007.05.009.

Halliez, M.C., Buret, A.G., 2013. Extra-intestinal and long term consequences of Giardia duodenalis infections. World J. Gastroenterol. 19 (47), 8974–8985. https://doi.org/10.3748/wjg.v19.i47.8974.

Henderson, B., Martin, A., 2011. Bacterial virulence in the moonlight: multitasking bacterial moonlighting proteins are virulence determinants in infectious disease. Infect. Immun. 79 (9), 3476–3491. https://doi.org/10.1128/iai.00179-11.

Hewitson, J.P., Ruckerl, D., Harcus, Y., Murray, J., Webb, L.M., Babayan, S.A., Allen, J.E., Kurniawan, A., Maizels, R.M., 2014. The secreted triose phosphate isomerase of Brugia malayi is required to sustain microfilaria production in vivo. PLoS Pathog. 10 (2), e1003930. https://doi.org/10.1371/journal.ppat.1003930.

Hsia, H.C., Schwarzbauer, J.E., 2005. Meet the tenascins: multifunctional and mysterious. J. Biol. Chem. 280 (29), 26641–26644. https://doi.org/10.1074/jbc.R500005200.
Ivarsson, M.E., Leroux, J.C., Castagner, B., 2012. Targeting bacterial toxins. Angew. Chem. Int. Ed. Eng. 51 (17), 4024–4045. https://doi.org/10.1002/anie.201104384.
Jerlstrom-Hultqvist, J., Franzen, O., Ankarklev, J., Xu, F., Nohynkova, E., Andersson, J.O., Svard, S.G., Andersson, B., 2010. Genome analysis and comparative genomics of a Giardia intestinalis assemblage E isolate. BMC Genomics 11, 543. https://doi.org/10.1186/1471-2164-11-543.
Jimenez, J.C., Uzcanga, G., Zambrano, A., Di Prisco, M.C., Lynch, N.R., 2000. Identification and partial characterization of excretory/secretory products with proteolytic activity in Giardia intestinalis. J. Parasitol. 86 (4), 859–862. https://doi.org/10.1645/0022-3395(2000)086[0859:iapcoe]2.0.co;2.
Johansson, M.E., Hansson, G.C., 2016. Immunological aspects of intestinal mucus and mucins. Nat. Rev. Immunol. 16 (10), 639–649. https://doi.org/10.1038/nri.2016.88.
Kaur, H., Ghosh, S., Samra, H., Vinayak, V.K., Ganguly, N.K., 2001. Identification and characterization of an excretory-secretory product from Giardia lamblia. Parasitology 123 (Pt 4), 347–356.
Keselman, A., Li, E., Maloney, J., Singer, S.M., 2016. The microbiota contributes to CD8+ T cell activation and nutrient malabsorption following intestinal infection with Giardia duodenalis. Infect. Immun. 84 (10), 2853–2860. https://doi.org/10.1128/iai.00348-16.
Knodler, L.A., Schofield, P.J., Edwards, M.R., 1995. L-arginine transport and metabolism in Giardia intestinalis support its position as a transition between the prokaryotic and eukaryotic kingdoms. Microbiology 141 (Pt 9), 2063–2070. https://doi.org/10.1099/13500872-141-9-2063.
Lalle, M., 2010. Giardiasis in the post genomic era: treatment, drug resistance and novel therapeutic perspectives. Infect. Disord. Drug Targets 10 (4), 283–294.
Lalle, M., Hanevik, K., 2018. Treatment-refractory giardiasis: challenges and solutions. Infect. Drug Resist. 11, 1921–1933. https://doi.org/10.2147/idr.s141468.
Li, L., Li, Z., Chen, D., Lu, X., Feng, X., Wright, E.C., Solberg, N.O., Dunaway-Mariano, D., Mariano, P.S., Galkin, A., Kulakova, L., Herzberg, O., Green-Church, K.B., Zhang, L., 2008. Inactivation of microbial arginine deiminases by L-canavanine. J. Am. Chem. Soc. 130 (6), 1918–1931. https://doi.org/10.1021/ja0760877.
Li, Z., Kulakova, L., Li, L., Galkin, A., Zhao, Z., Nash, T.E., Mariano, P.S., Herzberg, O., Dunaway-Mariano, D., 2009. Mechanisms of catalysis and inhibition operative in the arginine deiminase from the human pathogen Giardia lamblia. Bioorg. Chem. 37 (5), 149–161. https://doi.org/10.1016/j.bioorg.2009.06.001.
Li, Z., Liu, Z., Cho, D.W., Zou, J., Gong, M., Breece, R.M., Galkin, A., Li, L., Zhao, H., Maestas, G.D., Tierney, D.L., Herzberg, O., Dunaway-Mariano, D., Mariano, P.S., 2011. Rational design, synthesis and evaluation of first generation inhibitors of the Giardia lamblia fructose-1,6-biphosphate aldolase. J. Inorg. Biochem. 105 (4), 509–517. https://doi.org/10.1016/j.jinorgbio.2010.12.012.
Lim, K., Kulakova, L., Galkin, A., Herzberg, O., 2013. Crystal structures of carbamate kinase from Giardia lamblia bound with citric acid and AMP-PNP. PLoS One 8 (5), e64004. https://doi.org/10.1371/journal.pone.0064004.
Liu, J., Ma'ayeh, S., Peirasmaki, D., Lundstrom-Stadelmann, B., Hellman, L., Svard, S.G., 2018. Secreted Giardia intestinalis cysteine proteases disrupt intestinal epithelial cell junctional complexes and degrade chemokines. Virulence 9 (1), 879–894. https://doi.org/10.1080/21505594.2018.1451284.
Liu, J., Fu, Z., Hellman, L., Svard, S.G., 2019a. Cleavage specificity of recombinant Giardia intestinalis cysteine proteases: degradation of immunoglobulins and defensins. Mol. Biochem. Parasitol. 227, 29–38. https://doi.org/10.1016/j.molbiopara.2018.10.004.

Liu, J., Svard, S.G., Klotz, C., 2019b. Giardia intestinalis cystatin is a potent inhibitor of papain, parasite cysteine proteases and, to a lesser extent, human cathepsin B. FEBS Lett. 593 (12), 1313–1325. https://doi.org/10.1002/1873-3468.13433.

Luscher, T.F., Barton, M., 2000. Endothelins and endothelin receptor antagonists: therapeutic considerations for a novel class of cardiovascular drugs. Circulation 102 (19), 2434–2440.

Ma'ayeh, S.Y., Brook-Carter, P.T., 2012. Representational difference analysis identifies specific genes in the interaction of Giardia duodenalis with the murine intestinal epithelial cell line, IEC-6. Int. J. Parasitol. 42 (5), 501–509. https://doi.org/10.1016/j.ijpara.2012.04.004.

Ma'ayeh, S.Y., Liu, J., Peirasmaki, D., Hornaeus, K., Bergstrom Lind, S., Grabherr, M., Bergquist, J., Svard, S.G., 2017. Characterization of the Giardia intestinalis secretome during interaction with human intestinal epithelial cells: the impact on host cells. PLoS Negl. Trop. Dis. 11 (12), e0006120. https://doi.org/10.1371/journal.pntd.0006120.

Ma'ayeh, S.Y., Knorr, L., Skold, K., Garnham, A., Ansell, B.R.E., Jex, A.R., Svard, S.G., 2018. Responses of the differentiated intestinal epithelial cell line caco-2 to infection with the giardia intestinalis GS isolate. Front. Cell. Infect. Microbiol. 8, 244. https://doi.org/10.3389/fcimb.2018.00244.

Merz, K.M., Ringe, D., Reynolds, C.H., 2010. Drug Design: Structure- and Ligand-Based Approaches. Cambridge University Press, Cambridge.

Montanaro, A., Bardana Jr., E.J., 1991. Dietary amino acid-induced systemic lupus erythematosus. Rheum. Dis. Clin. N. Am. 17 (2), 323–332.

Munoz-Cruz, S., Gomez-Garcia, A., Matadamas-Martinez, F., Alvarado-Torres, J.A., Meza-Cervantez, P., Arriaga-Pizano, L., Yepez-Mulia, L., 2018. Giardia lamblia: identification of molecules that contribute to direct mast cell activation. Parasitol. Res. 117 (8), 2555–2567. https://doi.org/10.1007/s00436-018-5944-1.

Napolitano, D.R., Pollock, N., Kashino, S.S., Rodrigues Jr., V., Campos-Neto, A., 2008. Identification of mycobacterium tuberculosis ornithine carboamyltransferase in urine as a possible molecular marker of active pulmonary tuberculosis. Clin. Vaccine Immunol. 15 (4), 638–643. https://doi.org/10.1128/cvi.00010-08.

Nash, T.E., 2002. Surface antigenic variation in Giardia lamblia. Mol. Microbiol. 45 (3), 585–590.

Nash, T.E., Keister, D.B., 1985. Differences in excretory-secretory products and surface antigens among 19 isolates of Giardia. J. Infect. Dis. 152 (6), 1166–1171. https://doi.org/10.1093/infdis/152.6.1166.

Nash, T.E., Gillin, F.D., Smith, P.D., 1983. Excretory-secretory products of Giardia lamblia. J. Immunol. 131 (4), 2004–2010.

Nash, T.E., Lujan, H.T., Mowatt, M.R., Conrad, J.T., 2001. Variant-specific surface protein switching in Giardia lamblia. Infect. Immun. 69 (3), 1922–1923. https://doi.org/10.1128/iai.69.3.1922-1923.2001.

Navarrete-Vazquez, G., Chavez-Silva, F., Colin-Lozano, B., Estrada-Soto, S., Hidalgo-Figueroa, S., Guerrero-Alvarez, J., Mendez, S.T., Reyes-Vivas, H., Oria-Hernandez, J., Canul-Canche, J., Ortiz-Andrade, R., Moo-Puc, R., 2015. Synthesis of nitro (benzo)thiazole acetamides and in vitro antiprotozoal effect against amitochondriate parasites Giardia intestinalis and Trichomonas vaginalis. Bioorg. Med. Chem. 23 (9), 2204–2210. https://doi.org/10.1016/j.bmc.2015.02.059.

Ortega-Pierres, G., Bazan-Tejeda, M.L., Fonseca-Linan, R., Bermudez-Cruz, R.M., Arguello-Garcia, R., 2011. Interaction of Giardia with host cells. In: Lujan, H.D., Svard, S. (Eds.), Giardia: A Model Organism. Springer-Verlag Wien, Vienna, pp. 261–274.

Ortega-Pierres, G., Arguello-Garcia, R., Laredo-Cisneros, M.S., Fonseca-Linan, R., Gomez-Mondragon, M., Inzunza-Arroyo, R., Flores-Benitez, D., Raya-Sandino, A.,

Chavez-Munguia, B., Ventura-Gallegos, J.L., Zentella-Dehesa, A., Bermudez-Cruz, R.M., Gonzalez-Mariscal, L., 2018. Giardipain-1, a protease secreted by Giardia duodenalis trophozoites, causes junctional, barrier and apoptotic damage in epithelial cell monolayers. Int. J. Parasitol. 48 (8), 621–639. https://doi.org/10.1016/j.ijpara.2018.01.006.

Palcy, S., Chevet, E., 2006. Integrating forward and reverse proteomics to unravel protein function. Proteomics 6 (20), 5467–5480. https://doi.org/10.1002/pmic.200600211.

Palm, J.E., Weiland, M.E., Griffiths, W.J., Ljungstrom, I., Svard, S.G., 2003. Identification of immunoreactive proteins during acute human giardiasis. J. Infect. Dis. 187 (12), 1849–1859. https://doi.org/10.1086/375356.

Panaro, M.A., Cianciulli, A., Mitolo, V., Mitolo, C.I., Acquafredda, A., Brandonisio, O., Cavallo, P., 2007. Caspase-dependent apoptosis of the HCT-8 epithelial cell line induced by the parasite Giardia intestinalis. FEMS Immunol. Med. Microbiol. 51 (2), 302–309. https://doi.org/10.1111/j.1574-695X.2007.00304.x.

Papanastasiou, P., Hiltpold, A., Bommeli, C., Kohler, P., 1996. The release of the variant surface protein of Giardia to its soluble isoform is mediated by the selective cleavage of the conserved carboxy-terminal domain. Biochemistry 35 (31), 10143–10148. https://doi.org/10.1021/bi960473b.

Prucca, C.G., Lujan, H.D., 2009. Antigenic variation in Giardia lamblia. Cell. Microbiol. 11 (12), 1706–1715. https://doi.org/10.1111/j.1462-5822.2009.01367.x.

Ringqvist, E., Palm, J.E.D., Skarin, H., Hehl, A.B., Weiland, M., Davids, B.J., Reiner, D.S., Griffiths, W.J., Eckmann, L., Gillin, F.D., Svard, S.G., 2008. Release of metabolic enzymes by Giardia in response to interaction with intestinal epithelial cells. Mol. Biochem. Parasitol. 159 (2), 85–91. https://doi.org/10.1016/j.molbiopara.2008.02.005.

Ringqvist, E., Avesson, L., Soderbom, F., Svard, S.G., 2011. Transcriptional changes in Giardia during host-parasite interactions. Int. J. Parasitol. 41 (3-4), 277–285. https://doi.org/10.1016/j.ijpara.2010.09.011.

Rodriguez-Fuentes, G.B., Cedillo-Rivera, R., Fonseca-Linan, R., Arguello-Garcia, R., Munoz, O., Ortega-Pierres, G., Yepez-Mulia, L., 2006. Giardia duodenalis: analysis of secreted proteases upon trophozoite-epithelial cell interaction in vitro. Mem. Inst. Oswaldo Cruz 101 (6), 693–696. https://doi.org/10.1590/s0074-02762006000600020.

Roxstrom-Lindquist, K., Ringqvist, E., Daniel, P., Svard, S., 2005. Giardia lamblia-induced changes in gene expression in differentiated Caco-2 human intestinal epithelial cells. Infect. Immun. 73 (12), 8204–8208. https://doi.org/10.1128/iai.73.12.8204-8208.2005.

Samra, H.K., Ganguly, N.K., Garg, U.C., Goyal, J., Mahajan, R.C., 1988. Effect of excretory-secretory products of Giardia lamblia on glucose and phenylalanine transport in the small intestine of Swiss albino mice. Biochem. Int. 17 (5), 801–812.

Sanchez, J., Holmgren, J., 2011. Cholera toxin—a foe & a friend. Indian J. Med. Res. 133, 153–163.

Savioli, L., Smith, H., Thompson, A., 2006. Giardia and cryptosporidium join the 'neglected diseases initiative'. Trends Parasitol. 22 (5), 203–208. https://doi.org/10.1016/j.pt.2006.02.015.

Schofield, P.J., Costello, M., Edwards, M.R., O'Sullivan, W.J., 1990. The arginine dihydrolase pathway is present in Giardia intestinalis. Int. J. Parasitol. 20 (5), 697–699.

Shahbazian, A., Holzer, P., 2000. Regulation of guinea pig intestinal peristalsis by endogenous endothelin acting at ET(B) receptors. Gastroenterology 119 (1), 80–88.

Shant, J., Bhattacharyya, S., Ghosh, S., Ganguly, N.K., Majumdar, S., 2002. A potentially important excretory-secretory product of Giardia lamblia. Exp. Parasitol. 102 (3-4), 178–186.

Shant, J., Ghosh, S., Bhattacharyya, S., Ganguly, N.K., Majumdar, S., 2004. The alteration in signal transduction parameters induced by the excretory-secretory product from Giardia lamblia. Parasitology 129 (Pt 4), 421–430.

Smith, P.D., Gillin, F.D., Spira, W.M., Nash, T.E., 1982. Chronic giardiasis: studies on drug sensitivity, toxin production, and host immune response. Gastroenterology 83 (4), 797–803.

Solarczyk, P., Majewska, A.C., 2015. Implications of Giardia taxonomic controversies and genetic diversity. Probl. Hig. Epidemiol. 96 (3), 7.

Solaymani-Mohammadi, S., Singer, S.M., 2013. Regulation of intestinal epithelial cell cytoskeletal remodeling by cellular immunity following gut infection. Mucosal Immunol. 6 (2), 369–378. https://doi.org/10.1038/mi.2012.80.

Spickler, A.R., 2012. Giardiasis. Available: The Center for Food Security and Public Health, Iowa State University Digital Repository. http://www.cfsph.iastate.edu/DiseaseInfo/factsheets.php.

Stadelmann, B., Merino, M.C., Persson, L., Svard, S.G., 2012. Arginine consumption by the intestinal parasite Giardia intestinalis reduces proliferation of intestinal epithelial cells. PLoS One 7 (9), e45325. https://doi.org/10.1371/journal.pone.0045325.

Stadelmann, B., Hanevik, K., Andersson, M.K., Bruserud, O., Svard, S.G., 2013. The role of arginine and arginine-metabolizing enzymes during Giardia—host cell interactions in vitro. BMC Microbiol. 13, 256. https://doi.org/10.1186/1471-2180-13-256.

Tellez, A., Palm, D., Weiland, M., Aleman, J., Winiecka-Krusnell, J., Linder, E., Svard, S., 2005. Secretory antibodies against Giardia intestinalis in lactating Nicaraguan women. Parasite Immunol. 27 (5), 163–169. https://doi.org/10.1111/j.1365-3024.2005.00758.x.

Theocharis, A.D., Skandalis, S.S., Gialeli, C., Karamanos, N.K., 2016. Extracellular matrix structure. Adv. Drug Deliv. Rev. 97, 4–27. https://doi.org/10.1016/j.addr.2015.11.001.

Thompson, R.C.A., Monis, P.T., 2004. Variation in Giardia: implications for taxonomy and epidemiology. Adv. Parasitol. 58 (58), 69–137. https://doi.org/10.1016/s0065-308x(04)58002-8.

Thompson, R.C.A., Monis, P., 2012. Giardia-from genome to proteome. In: Rollinson, D., Hay, S.I. (Eds.), Advances in Parasitology. In: vol. 78. Elsevier Academic Press Inc, San Diego, pp. 57–95.

Touz, M.C., Nores, M.J., Slavin, I., Carmona, C., Conrad, J.T., Mowatt, M.R., Nash, T.E., Coronel, C.E., Lujan, H.D., 2002. The activity of a developmentally regulated cysteine proteinase is required for cyst wall formation in the primitive eukaryote Giardia lamblia. J. Biol. Chem. 277 (10), 8474–8481. https://doi.org/10.1074/jbc.M110250200.

Touz, M.C., Ropolo, A.S., Rivero, M.R., Vranych, C.V., Conrad, J.T., Svard, S.G., Nash, T.E., 2008. Arginine deiminase has multiple regulatory roles in the biology of Giardia lamblia. J. Cell Sci. 121 (Pt 17), 2930–2938. https://doi.org/10.1242/jcs.026963.

Trejo-Soto, P.J., Aguayo-Ortiz, R., Yepez-Mulia, L., Hernandez-Campos, A., Medina-Franco, J.L., Castillo, R., 2016. Insights into the structure and inhibition of Giardia intestinalis arginine deiminase: homology modeling, docking, and molecular dynamics studies. J. Biomol. Struct. Dyn. 34 (4), 732–748. https://doi.org/10.1080/07391102.2015.1051115.

Troeger, H., Epple, H.-J., Schneider, T., Wahnschaffe, U., Ullrich, R., Burchard, G.-D., Jelinek, T., Zeitz, M., Fromm, M., Schulzke, J.-D., 2007. Effect of chronic Giardia lamblia infection on epithelial transport and barrier function in human duodenum. Gut 56 (3), 328–335. https://doi.org/10.1136/gut.2006.100198.

Vivancos, V., Gonzalez-Alvarez, I., Bermejo, M., Gonzalez-Alvarez, M., 2018. Giardiasis: characteristics, pathogenesis and new insights about treatment. Curr. Top. Med. Chem. 18 (15), 1287–1303. https://doi.org/10.2174/1568026618666181002095314.

Vranych, C.V., Rivero, M.R., Merino, M.C., Mayol, G.F., Zamponi, N., Maletto, B.A., Pistoresi-Palencia, M.C., Touz, M.C., Ropolo, A.S., 2014. SUMOylation and deimination of proteins: two epigenetic modifications involved in Giardia encystation. Biochim. Biophys. Acta 1843 (9), 1805–1817. https://doi.org/10.1016/j.bbamcr.2014.04.014.

Ward, W., Alvarado, L., Rawlings, N.D., Engel, J.C., Franklin, C., McKerrow, J.H., 1997. A primitive enzyme for a primitive cell: The protease required for excystation of Giardia. Cell 89 (3), 437–444. https://doi.org/10.1016/s0092-8674(00)80224-x.

CHAPTER FIVE

Recent insights into innate and adaptive immune responses to *Giardia*

Steven M. Singer*, Marc Y. Fink, Vanessa V. Angelova
Department of Biology, Georgetown University, Washington, DC, United States
*Corresponding author: e-mail address: steven.singer@georgetown.edu

Contents

Abstract

Infection with *Giardia* produces a wide range of clinical outcomes. Acutely infected patients may have no overt symptoms or suffer from severe cramps, diarrhea, nausea and even urticaria. Recently, post-infectious irritable bowel syndrome and chronic fatigue syndrome have been identified as long-term sequelae of giardiasis. Frequently, recurrent and chronic *Giardia* infection is considered a major contributor to stunting in children from low and middle income countries. Perhaps the most unusual outcome of infection with *Giardia* is the apparent reduced risk of developing moderate-to-severe

Advances in Parasitology, Volume 106
ISSN 0065-308X
https://doi.org/10.1016/bs.apar.2019.07.004

diarrhea due to other enteric infections which has been noted in several recent studies. The goal of understanding immune responses against *Giardia* is therefore to identify protective mechanisms which could become targets for vaccine development, but also to identify mechanisms whereby infections lead to these other diverse outcomes.

Giardia induces a robust adaptive immune response in both humans and animals. It has been known for many years that there is production of large amounts of parasite-specific IgA following infection and that $CD4^+$ T cell responses contribute to this IgA production and control of the infection. In the past decade, there have been advances in our understanding of the non-antibody effector mechanisms used by the host to fight *Giardia* infections, in particular the importance of the cytokine interleukin (IL)-17 in orchestrating these responses. There have also been major advances in understanding how the innate response to *Giardia* infection is initiated and how it contributes to the development of adaptive immunity. Finally, there here have been significant increases in our knowledge of how the resident microbial community influences the immune response and how these responses contribute to the development of some of the symptoms of giardiasis. In this article, we will focus on data generated in the last 10 years and how it has advanced our knowledge about this important parasitic disease.

1. Protective immune responses against *Giardia*

1.1 Interleukin 17

The most notable change in our understanding of the immune response to *Giardia* in the last decade has been the discovery of the role of interleukin 17 (IL-17). IL-17 has been shown to be an important component of mucosal immunity to fungal pathogens such as *Candida albicans* and to promote neutrophil responses and anti-microbial expression by epithelial cells (Li et al., 2018a). IL-17 production was first reported in giardiasis by Solaymani-Mohammadi and Singer in supernatants of *Giardia* extract-stimulated splenocytes obtained from mice seven days following *G. duodenalis* infection (Solaymani-Mohammadi and Singer, 2011). In contrast, a microarray analysis in calves found a down-regulation of IL-17 transcripts in the jejunum three weeks post-infection with *G. duodenalis* (Dreesen et al., 2012). Peroxisome proliferator-activated receptors alpha and gamma (PPAR-α and PPAR-γ) were shown to be increased in this same infection, which the authors hypothesized could lead to downregulation of NF-κB and activator protein 1 (AP1) and thus, a decrease in cytokine production.

In contrast to the calves infected with *G. duodenalis*, IL-17 seems to play an important role in the mouse response to *G. muris* (Dreesen et al., 2012, 2014). Infected mice had significantly increased levels of IL-17 mRNA in the small intestine three weeks post infection (Dreesen et al., 2014). Importantly, mice lacking the IL-17A receptor exhibited increased cyst shedding in feces compared to wild-type mice (Dreesen et al., 2014). Interestingly, PPARα knockout mice did not seem to have significantly altered cyst counts or IL-17 levels, although the data for IL-17 were not shown (Dreesen et al., 2014). This report clearly showed that IL-17A was important for elimination of *G. muris* infections.

In a similar study of mice infected with *G. muris*, mucosal IL-17A transcripts were elevated in the first week of infection, reached a maximum level by week 2, and decreased in week 3 (Dann et al., 2015). Tissue levels of cytokines were also significantly elevated at 2 weeks in this study. IL-17A was also shown to be expressed following *G. duodenalis* infection in wild-type mice, and IL-17A deficient mice had a defect in clearance of *G. duodenalis* as well as *G. muris*. Trophozoite numbers in the small intestine were greater in IL-17A deficient mice than wild-type controls at 2, 3 and 7 weeks post-infection with *G. muris*. Parasite numbers appeared to be decreasing slowly with time, even in the absence of IL-17A, consistent with a multi-factorial control of *Giardia*.

Several immune cell types may be contributing to IL-17 production during a *Giardia* infection. Analysis of infections in bone marrow chimeric mice indicated that hematopoietic cells are the important source of IL-17A in this model (Dann et al., 2015). Flow cytometry demonstrated an upregulation of $CD4^+$ T cells producing IL-17 in the lamina propria of *G. muris* infected mice, which likely represent Th17 cells (Dann et al., 2015). This is consistent with increased detection of the transcription factor RORγt reported by Dreesen et al. (2014). Dann et al. also reported an increase in IL-17 producing intraepithelial lymphocytes in *G. muris* infected mice (Dann et al., 2015). Interestingly, $CD4^{-/-}$ and $Rag2^{-/-}$ mice still exhibited elevated numbers of IL-17 producing cells and IL-17 mRNA within the epithelial layer, indicating that Th17 cells are not the only cells responsible for the production of IL-17, and suggesting an innate lymphocyte population might be involved (Dann et al., 2015). Further work is needed to determine if these are type 3 innate lymphoid cells (ILC3s), γδ17 cells or another cell type. The role of this innate production of IL-17 is also unclear since both $CD4^{-/-}$ and SCID mice exhibit prolonged infections with *Giardia* (Dann et al., 2015; Fink and Singer, 2017; Singer and Nash, 2000b).

The importance of IL-17 in human giardiasis has also been examined. Peripheral blood mononuclear cells (PMBCs) isolated from humans were stimulated with *G. duodenalis* and cytokine expression from

$CD4^+CD197^-CD45RA^-$ cells (markers for effector memory T cells) was analyzed using flow cytometry. These studies revealed an upregulation of IL-17A and a combination of IL-17A and TNF-α in samples from individuals previously exposed to *Giardia* (Saghaug et al., 2016). Interestingly, stratification of patients into those whose infections resolved in fewer than 8 weeks and those who required longer than 8 weeks to eliminate their infections showed that more rapid parasite elimination was associated with a more pronounced IL-17A and TNF-α expression profile (Saghaug et al., 2016). These data are consistent with IL-17 having a protective role in human giardiasis as well as in mouse models.

As might be expected, given the importance of IL-17A, mice lacking the cognate IL-17A receptor (IL-17RA) also exhibited a defect in parasite elimination (Dann et al., 2015). Interestingly, bone marrow chimera studies demonstrated that IL-17RA expression by bone marrow derived cells, but not from epithelial cells or other radiation-resistant cells, was necessary and sufficient for parasite elimination (Dann et al., 2015). IL-17A is known to recruit neutrophils and induce anti-microbial peptide expression in the mucosa (Li et al., 2018a). IL-17A deficient mice were shown to have a near complete absence of fecal IgA, although serum IgA levels were normal in these mice (Dann et al., 2015). These data suggest that transport of IgA is lacking in IL-17A deficient mice, consistent with a role for IL-17 in enhancing expression of the poly-immunoglobulin receptor (polyIgR) on epithelial cells (Cao et al., 2012; Paerewijck et al., 2017). Given the outcome of infections in bone marrow chimeras, however, this regulation may be indirect as IL-17RA on epithelial cells was not needed for parasite control. Other changes seen in IL-17RA deficient mice infected with *G. muris* included reduced expression of genes for numerous anti-microbial peptides and the mannose binding lectin (Dann et al., 2015).

1.2 Immunoglobulin A

Immunoglobulin A (IgA) is the primary antibody in the intestinal mucosa, making it a popular candidate for giardiasis research. Studies focusing on the role of IgA in controlling infection have shown different effects for *G. duodenalis* and *G. muris* infections. Mice deficient in IgA and infected with *G. muris* showed significantly delayed clearance of primary and secondary infections. A similar observation is made for mice lacking pIgR (Davids et al., 2006). In contrast, lack of pIgR had no significant effect on *G. duodenalis* infection. Mice with a deletion in the μ exons of the immunoglobulin heavy chain locus (μMT mice) lack mature B cells. μMT mice primed with *G. duodenalis* and then re-infected showed much lower parasite burdens 5 days post-infection compared to mice which were not primed against the parasite, despite the absence of B cells (Li et al., 2014). These data do not rule out a potential role for antibodies in protection against re-infection with *Giardia,* but they do indicate that antibodies are not essential and that other mechanisms are sufficient for protection in this model.

Several studies in the last decade have further documented that infection with *Giardia* does induce a robust IgA response. IgA levels were found to be increased in the saliva and serum of individuals infected with *Giardia* (El-Gebaly et al., 2012; Zarebavani et al., 2012). Studies have looked at IgA stimulation by excretory/secretory products (ESP) derived from *Giardia* and soluble *Giardia* extract, as well as the response to variant surface specific proteins on the parasite surface (Hjøllo et al., 2018; Jimenez et al., 2014). Mice given weekly oral administration of *Giardia* ESP exhibited increased anti-*Giardia* antibodies in the serum, including IgA (Jimenez et al., 2014). IgA in the feces was also elevated, although not until 100 days from the start of the inoculations. Another target of anti-*Giardia* IgA is the family of variant-specific surface proteins (VSPs) on the surface of trophozoites. VSPs have a variable region, a semi-conserved region, and a region anchoring them to the parasite (Hjøllo et al., 2018). Hjøllo et al. followed IgA levels in patients' sera against two semi-conserved VSP regions (VSP3 and VSP5) prior to treatment and then at 6 weeks, 6 months, and 12 months post-treatment (Hjøllo et al., 2018). They noted that IgA levels were high prior to treatment but fell dramatically by the follow up 6 weeks later (Hjøllo et al., 2018). The rapid fall in IgA levels against conserved portions of the VSP could contribute to the abundance of reinfections seen in individuals residing in endemic areas.

1.3 Mast cells

Mast cells have an important role in controlling infections with both *G. muris* and *G. duodenalis* (Li et al., 2004, 2007). Upon infection, mast cells are recruited to the intestine where they degranulate. In addition to releasing histamines and mouse mast cell protease-1 (MMCP-1), previous work has shown that they may interact with cholecystokinin (CCK), which in turn leads to increased intestinal contractility. Treating tissues with compounds inhibiting mast cell degranulation (ketotifen) or depleting them of granule contents (compound 48/80) removes the effects of CCK (Li et al., 2007).

One potential mechanism of mast cell recruitment is via activation of complement via the lectin pathway. Mannose-binding lectin (MBL) has been shown to bind to *Giardia duodenalis* in vitro (Li et al., 2016). This relationship was disrupted by adding soluble N-acetylglucosamine (GlcNAc), suggesting that MBL binds to GlcNAc on the surface of the parasite (Li et al., 2016). Complement activation is known to contribute to recruitment of immune cells, specifically mast cells, and indeed mast cell recruitment was severely diminished in MBL2 and C3aR knockout mice models (Li et al., 2016). As noted above, increased intestinal expression of MBL2 was shown to depend on IL-17 following *Giardia* infection (Paerewijck et al., 2017). Interestingly, unlike Tako et al. (2013) who identified significant upregulation of mast cell transcripts in the mucosa 10 days following *G. duodenalis* infection, Paerewijck et al. (2017) did not identify any mast cell related transcripts in their transcriptomic analysis of *G. muris* infected mice, 21 days post-infection. This might reflect differences between the parasite species or the different time points analyzed in the two studies.

Mast cells may also contribute to resistance to reinfection with *Giardia*. Mice that were infected with *Giardia*, treated with metronidazole, and then reinfected exhibited a rapid recruitment of mast cells to the mucosa along with greatly reduced parasite loads compared with mice challenged with *Giardia* but not pre-infected (Li et al., 2014). Interestingly, mast cell recruitment and activation were not dependent on IgE as serum levels of the mast cell protease MMCP-1 were similarly elevated in wild-type and μMT mice following infection (Li et al., 2014). Thus, mast cells clearly contribute protection against *Giardia*, but may also be involved in its pathophysiology, especially defects in intestinal motility such as the severe cramps noted in some patients (Solaymani-Mohammadi and Singer, 2010).

1.4 Nitric oxide and anti-microbial peptides

In 2000, Eckman showed that nitric oxide (NO) inhibited replication of *G. duodenalis* and that the parasite production of arginine deiminase (ADI) may reduce the amount of arginine available for intestinal epithelial cells, thus reducing their ability to produce NO (Eckmann et al., 2000). Interestingly, the depletion of arginine may not just block production of NO, but may also have an effect on the proliferation of intestinal epithelial cells (Stadelmann et al., 2012). Growing CaCo2 cells in arginine-free media decreased the number of cells when compared to media supplemented with arginine or with citrulline (Stadelmann et al., 2012). Co-culturing *Giardia* and CaCo2 cells similarly reduced epithelial cell counts, a phenotype which could be partially restored by supplementing with additional arginine (Stadelmann et al., 2012). WB strain *Giardia* overexpressing ADI further decreased cell counts in co-culture experiments (Stadelmann et al., 2012). Host macrophages expressing arginase (Arg1) have recently been shown to accumulate in the lamina propria of mice infected with *G. duodenalis* (Maloney et al., 2015). Thus, at least three enzymes, ADI from the parasite and arginase (Arg1) and inducible nitric oxide synthase (NOS2) from the host, may all compete for available arginine during *in vivo* infections.

During *G. duodenalis* infection in mice, Nitric oxide, produced by NOS2, functions in a redundant pathway alongside α-defensins to help eliminate infections (Tako et al., 2013). Tako and colleagues found elevated mRNA expression for the matrix metalloprotease MMP7 in the mucosa of *Giardia* infected mice. MMP7 is involved in activating α-defensins during their synthesis and release from Paneth cells. Mice lacking MMP7 had slightly increased parasite counts on day 7 and on day 13 compared with wild-type mice (Tako et al., 2013). In contrast, mice with a deletion in the NOS2 gene or wild-type mice treated with *N*-iminoethyl-L-lysine (L-NIL), a NOS2-selective inhibitor, had parasite levels indistinguishable from control mice following infection (Tako et al., 2013). Double deficient, $MMP7^{-/-}$ $NOS2^{-/-}$ mice, however, had significantly higher parasite counts both on day 5 and on day 13 (Tako et al., 2013). Furthermore, $MMP7^{-/-}$ mice treated with L-NIL also had significantly increased parasite counts on 10 days post-infection compared to untreated controls (Tako et al., 2013). Together these data suggest that NO and α-defensins may be functioning in redundant pathways to contribute to *Giardia* control.

The importance of antimicrobial peptides during giardiasis has been the subject of investigation for many years. In 1994, Aley et al. showed that culturing *G. duodenalis* with defensins and other antimicrobial peptides was destructive to cell morphology and decreased the viability of trophozoites (Aley et al., 1994). Human neutrophil peptide (HNP)-1, rabbit neutrophil peptide NP-2, bovine indolicidin, and the murine Paneth cell α-defensins cryptdins 2 and 3 all significantly decreased trophozoite viability *in vitro* (Aley et al., 1994). As alluded to above, cryptdins in mice are synthesized as propeptides that require proteolytic cleavage by MMP-7 in order to mature into active molecules and data from MMP7 deficient mice indicate that cryptdins contribute to parasite control in vivo (Tako et al., 2013). As noted in the discussion of the importance of IL-17, mice lacking IL-17A or its receptor have been shown to express less mRNA for several members of the β-defensin family (Dann et al., 2015). However, direct demonstrations that these peptides can kill *Giardia in vitro* or that they are important *in vivo* is lacking. Recently, lactoferrin and lactoferricin have also been shown to affect parasite growth *in vitro* and promote the encystation to futile cysts (Frontera et al., 2018). The process seems to require the endocytosis of lactoferrin and lactoferricin into the parasite through a *G. duodenalis* low-density lipoprotein receptor (GlLPR) (Frontera et al., 2018). It seems likely that the full range of host effector mechanisms involved in controlling *Giardia* infections has not been identified.

Similar to its ability to inhibit production of NO, *Giardia* appears to protect itself from the actions of antimicrobial peptides. The dose-dependent cleavage of Human β-Defensin 1 (β-HD1) and α-Human Defensin 6 (α-HD6) by *Giardia*-released cysteine proteases has recently been demonstrated *in vitro* (Liu et al., 2019). Specifically, β-HD1 is cleaved by the parasite proteases CP16160, CP14019, and CP16779. α-HD6 is cleaved by CP14019 and CP16779 but not CP16160 (Liu et al., 2019).

Interestingly, antimicrobial peptides might play a part in the protective role of *Giardia* during co-infection with *Citrobacter rodentium* (Manko et al., 2017). *C. rodentium* is a commonly used murine model for enteropathogenic *E. coli* (EPEC), and co-infection with *Giardia* alleviated some of the symptoms seen during *C. rodentium* infection alone, including weight loss and bacterial translocation. Co-infection also resulted in increased expression of murine β-defensin 3 (MBD-3) and Trefoil factor 3 (TFF3) (Manko et al., 2017). A similar result was also observed *in vitro* in CaCo2 cells where co-incubation was associated with an increase in human β-defensin 2 (HBD-2) and TFF3 (Manko et al., 2017). The increased expression of these antimicrobial peptides was blocked using inhibitors of cysteine proteases, suggesting that parasite proteases might be involved in this response (Manko et al., 2017). Given the large numbers of antimicrobial peptides present in the intestinal mucosa, obtaining solid *in vivo* evidence for their role during infections and co-infections will be a significant challenge. However, given reports of reduced severe disease during *Giardia* coinfections with other enteropathogens in humans, further studies exploring how *Giardia* infections interact during co-infections are clearly warranted.

1.5 Mucous

Anti-microbial peptides and IgA are thought to be embedded within the mucous layer which covers the epithelium. Recent work has shown that

Giardia cysteine proteases have effects on host mucins and that mucous helps protect the host during infection (Amat et al., 2017). Incubation of biopsied human colon tissue with *G. duodenalis* resulted in a decrease of the mucous-positive area per crypt as indicated by histology and staining of the mucous (Amat et al., 2017). The thickness of the mucous layer was also decreased during mouse infections with the GS strain of *G. duodenalis* (Amat et al., 2017). Furthermore, incubation of a goblet cell-like cell line (LS174T) with parasites reduced the amount of mucin stored in cells, and inhibition of cysteine protease, protein kinase C and phosphoinositide-3 kinase activities all could block this effect (Amat et al., 2017). At the same time, mRNA for Muc2 was increased in LS174T cells exposed to parasites. Induction of Muc2 and Muc5Ac mRNA levels was observed in the colons of mice infected with GS on day 7, although only Muc5Ac was induced in the small intestine (Amat et al., 2017). The importance of mucous in responding to the infection was seen in Muc2$^{-/-}$ mice. Mice lacking this mucin exhibited weight loss when infected with GS, while wild-type control mice did not. Mice lacking Muc2 also had thinner colonic mucous layers than wild-type mice and also had significantly higher parasite burdens in the small intestine at day 7 following infection (Amat et al., 2017). Whether immune responses such as IL-13 production (see below) contribute to goblet cell production of mucous during infections has not been studied.

2. Activation of the immune response during giardiasis

2.1 The complement system

One fundamental challenge for the field of *Giardia* immunology is identifying the specific initial interactions with innate immune cells and the mechanisms that are used to activate downstream effector cells, such as T cells. Indeed, various reports involving early activation and protective mechanisms have begun to reveal how anti-*Giardia* immunity is initiated. In the past, the role of the complement system has been somewhat overlooked as both an effector mechanism as well as an initiator of immunity. This chemical death squad plays a role in not only microbial killing, but also contains molecules that serve as recruiters of immune cells. A role for the complement system in protective *Giardia* immunity was established by Hill et al., when trophozoite killing was observed following exposure of trophozoites to human sera that had no history of prior *Giardia* infection. Killing was lost when complement components were blocked, suggesting parasite killing was complement-dependent. Furthermore, this killing was dependent on structures found on the parasite's surface, as trophozoites treated with neuraminidase or trypsin did not activate the complement pathway (Hill et al., 1984). At this point in time, the authors credited the activation of complement to the alternative pathway, however the lectin pathway had not been identified and several more recent reports have described a role for this pathway in *Giardia* protection.

The lectin pathway is initiated through the binding of mannose binding lectin (MBL), a C-type lectin, to carbohydrates such as mannose and *N*-acetylglucosamine (GlcNAc), the latter being commonly found on *Giardia* trophozoites (Ratner et al., 2008; Ward et al., 1988). It was shown *in vitro* that MBL is able to bind to trophozoites and cause cell lysis through the complement system (Evans-Osses et al., 2010). Moving forward, the Singer group reported that MBL was expressed in the murine small intestine during *Giardia* infection (Tako et al., 2013) and that MBL-deficient mice exhibited a delay in the clearance of *Giardia* parasites and recruitment of mast cells to the small intestine (Li et al., 2016). This defect in clearance and recruitment was also dependent on C3a signaling via C3a receptor as mice lacking C3aR exhibited the same delayed-clearance phenotype as infected MBL-deficient mice. Moreover, significantly reduced T-cell cytokine responses against parasite antigens following infection were observed in C3aR deficient mice, although IgA levels within the small intestine were unaffected (Li et al., 2016). These results have been generally confirmed using the *G. muris* infection model (Paerewijck et al., 2017) suggesting that this pathway may also be relevant to human giardiasis. Despite the evidence provided, it is still unclear if other canonical cellular recognition strategies leading to the activation of the immune system are in play during *Giardia* infections.

2.2 Toll-like receptors, macrophages, and dendritic cells

The lamina propria of the small intestine is considered one of the largest sites of immune cell localization in the human body; this layer contains not only myeloid cells that are primarily responsible for initiating downstream effector immune mechanisms, but also T cells that mediate protection (Singer and Nash, 2000b) and pathology (Keselman et al., 2016; Scott et al., 2004) during *Giardia* infection. Several mechanisms are known to allow macrophages and dendritic cells (DCs) in the lamina propria to interact with antigens in the intestinal lumen (e.g., M cell transport or dendritic cell "periscopes"). *Giardia* is well-known to induce epithelial barrier breakdown and to promote microbial translocation out of the lumen (Chen et al., 2013;

Scott et al., 2002; Zhou et al., 2007). Thus, macrophages and DCs could act as sentinels during giardiasis and interact with conserved microbial-associated molecular patterns (e.g., lipopolysaccharide [LPS] from gram negative bacteria) as well as with antigens from *Giardia*.

The role of DCs in the immune system is thought mainly to be involved in the activation of the adaptive immune response through presentation of antigen:MHC complexes to T cells, expression of co-stimulatory molecules such as CD80 and CD86, and the provision of cytokines that help direct the differentiation of naïve T cells into mature effector cells. Several studies have reported that the DC cytokine response is able to be modulated through a combined treatment of *Giardia* protein extract and lipopolysaccharide (LPS) which leads to the inhibition of pro-inflammatory cytokine production (Kamda and Singer, 2009; Obendorf et al., 2013; Summan et al., 2018). Murine bone marrow derived DCs (BMDCs) exposed to *Giardia* alone led to poor cytokine induction and only slightly increasing expression of the costimulatory molecules, CD80 and CD86; yet, the combination of Toll-like Receptor (TLR) agonists and parasite extract led to the reduction of IL-6, IL-12, and TNFα while enhancing IL-10 production when compared to LPS controls (Kamda and Singer, 2009). This report further showed that blocking IL-10R and phosphoinositide-3 kinase (PI-3K) restores production of IL-12, which suggests that *Giardia* may activate PI-3K in DCs and that *Giardia* may restrict development of Th1 cells via IL-12 inhibition (Kamda and Singer, 2009). This reduction of pro-inflammatory cytokines was also recapitulated in TLR4-stimulated cell cultures using human monocyte-derived DCs (mo-DCs) and the report also suggested a reduction in IL-12/23p40, IL-12p70, and IL-23 (Obendorf et al., 2013; Summan et al., 2018). However, when these cells were stimulated with parasite antigen plus a TLR2 agonist, PAM3CSK4, an increase in IL-12/23p40 and IL-23 production occurred (Obendorf et al., 2013). Human mo-DC survival was also reduced when exposed to *Giardia* extract or live parasites, and the number of apoptotic DCs increased when compared to controls. Moreover, this effect was *Giardia* specific as mo-DC cultures solely exposed to helminth products did not lead to a reduction in viability, yet co-incubation with both *Giardia* and helminth extract did (Summan et al., 2018).

Members of the TLR family are often the main receptors used for detecting microbial patterns and activating innate immune responses. Currently, only two reports have suggested that TLRs may play a role in the recognition of *Giardia*; the HSP70 immunoglobulin binding protein, BiP, from *Giardia* was found to be a TLR4 agonist using both TLR4 reporter HEK 293 cells and primary cells from TLR4-deficient BALB/c mice (Lee et al., 2014). Immature murine (BMDCs) treated with anti-TLR4 blocking antibody had reduced TNF-α cytokine production in response to recombinant BIP (rBIP) when compared to controls. Furthermore, when TLR4-expressing HEK 293 cells were treated with rBIP, a NF-κB-dependent response was induced, similar to what was seen with for LPS-stimulated controls. Using BMDCs, it was found that rBIP was able to induce greater production of canonical DC maturation and expression of surface molecules, MHCII, CD80, and CD86, to levels that resembled LPS-induced stimulation. The production of cytokines in rBIP-activated BMDCs was also measured using ELISAs; IL-12, TNF-α, IL-6, and IL-4 concentrations were all increased in response to rBIP. However, the production of both IL-6 and IL-4 was decreased at the highest concentration of rBIP. BMDCs cultured from TLR4-deficent mice were unable to reproduce this cytokine response and most cytokines had drastically reduced concentrations when compared to wild-type mice (Lee et al., 2014). Recent work from Serradell et al. (2019) indicates that VSPs may also signal through TLR4.

A role for TLR2 has also recently been described in recognition of *Giardia* and, interestingly, it suggests that TLR2 may have a detrimental role for protective immunity (Li et al., 2017). Using C57BL/6J peritoneal macrophages, quantitative reverse transcription polymerase chain reaction (qRT-PCR) revealed that TLR2 gene expression was greatly increased in these cells in response to *Giardia* WB trophozoites. Immunohistochemical staining of duodenum tissues from mice infected with WB cysts also indicated increased levels of TLR2. The production of IL-6, IL-12p40, and TNF-α in response to live trophozoites was increased in peritoneal macrophages that were treated with TLR2 blocking antibody or if the macrophages were obtained from mice deficient for TLR2 and compared to wild-type controls. Moreover, the concentration of IFN-γ was also reduced in TLR2-deficient cells. Western blot analysis of macrophages exposed to trophozoites revealed the phosphorylation of both p38 and ERK (MAP kinases) along with AKT; phosphorylation of p38, ERK, and AKT as well as the production of cytokines that were reduced in TLR2-deficient macrophages. These data suggest that TLR-2 signaling in response to *Giardia* activates AKT, p38 and ERK and results in enhanced expression of pro-inflammatory cytokines. However, inhibition of AKT via chemical or siRNA methods instead increased the production of IL-6, IL-12p40, and

TNF-α, suggesting that the signaling mechanisms involved are not straightforward. In murine infections using WB cysts, parasite burden and typical *Giardia*-associated pathologies were found to be drastically decreased in both TLR2-knockout and AKT-inhibited mice when compared to wild-type or vehicle-treated controls; however, this infection model relied on the use of antibiotics for stable infection which may play a role in the presentation of pathologies and immune cell response (Keselman et al., 2016). Additionally, it is unclear if littermate control mice were used in the infection model comparisons as different intestinal microbiota may provide protection during *Giardia* infections (Singer and Nash, 2000a). Taken together these data suggest that *Giardia* mediates the reduction of cytokines via TLR2 by activating AKT, p38, and ERK (Li et al., 2017).

Downstream of the TLRs are cytosolic adaptor proteins that enable the transmission of TLR signals that eventually reach the nucleus; MyD88, along with TRIF, are the main link between the TLRs and downstream signaling proteins to initiate an immune response. However, at this point, it is still not fully understood if MyD88 or TRIF truly plays a meaningful biological role in protective *Giardia* immunity. BMDCs derived from MyD88-deficient mice stimulated with rBIP were unable to produce cytokines when compared to wild-type controls, suggesting a role for a TLR-MyD88 interaction leading to cytokine production (Lee et al., 2014). *G. muris* infections in MyD88$^{-/-}$, IL-10$^{-/-}$ double knockout mice cleared parasites equally as well as IL-10$^{-/-}$ controls (and similar to wild-type controls) suggesting the TLR pathway is dispensable for protection (Dann et al., 2018). Lastly, TLRs are not solely found on antigen presenting cells and are also found on intestinal epithelial cells (Abreu, 2010); thus, it is unclear if receptors found on these cells have a role in protection or coordinate any immune responses during infection.

The interaction of DCs with *Giardia* has been mainly studied *in vitro* and only a few reports have analyzed their function during *in vivo* infections. IL-6 deficient mice have a defect in parasite control and DCs have been shown to be a significant source of IL-6 during infection (Bienz et al., 2003; Kamda et al., 2012; Zhou et al., 2003). Interleukin-6 helps to drive the differentiation of IL-17 producing (Th17) T cells *in vitro* (Weaver et al., 2006), and as such, mice that lack IL-6 ought to have reduced IL-17 expression. However, this has not been directly demonstrated during *Giardia* infection.

Studies of macrophage responses during giardiasis are also sparse. The Singer lab recently reported an increase in a population of intestinal macrophages, following infection, that expresses both nitric oxide synthase 2

(NOS2) and arginase 1 (ARG1) (Maloney et al., 2015). During *G. muris* infection in IL-10-deficient mice, an expansion of $CD11b^{+}$, $CD11c^{-}$ macrophages was observed in the colon, yet not in the small intestine. This expansion led to colonic inflammation in IL-10-deficient mice, although no such inflammation was seen in wild-type mice. This suggests a regulatory role for these cells in limiting inflammatory signals (Dann et al., 2018). Peritoneal macrophages also were reported to release extracellular traps in response to *Giardia* trophozoites to ensnare parasites. However these macrophages were collected, and consequently activated, using thioglycollate which ultimately may not describe the true biological macrophage function (Li et al., 2018b).

Overall, it is clear that the cytokine production of DCs and macrophages is able to be directed by *Giardia* towards a less inflammatory state within the gut; yet this shift may require other accessory signals that are commonly found in the lumen of the intestine—highlighting the importance of maintaining the integrity of the intestinal epithelial barrier. While cytokines are able to dictate the differentiation of activated T-cells and other immune responses, it is still unclear *Giardia* infection stimulates the immune system to produce a robust immune response while simultaneously limiting inflammation. Understanding the mechanisms whereby *Giardia* limits inflammation could be valuable for developing therapeutics for chronic intestinal inflammation and for understanding how environmental enteropathy leads to poor vaccine efficacy.

3. *Giardia* and the intestinal microbiome

Since the turn of the millennium, there has been a rapid increase in the number of reports regarding the interactions between the intestinal microbiome and *Giardia* (Fink and Singer, 2017). However, the foundation for these reports was first reported in 1994, when the Nash group identified that Assemblage A strains, such as WB, could not colonize adult mice while Assemblage B strains like GS could (Byrd et al., 1994). Singer and Nash followed up on this observation and next reported that infection outcomes in the adult mouse model of giardiasis were dependent on the vendor source of the animals. Mice purchased from Taconic Farms were resistant to *Giardia* infections while mice of the same immunodeficient strain from Jackson Laboratories were susceptible. Treatment with antibiotics made mice from either vendor susceptible to infection, while cohousing animals made them all resistant, suggesting that the composition of microbes within the gut determined susceptibility to this parasitic infection (Singer and Nash, 2000a). The same year, a group from Brazil reported that duodenal microbes were required to stimulate *Giardia* pathogenicity during infection. Conventional mice, germ-free mice, and germ-free mice reconstituted with microbiota derived from symptomatic giardiasis patients, were all infected with *Giardia* trophozoites. Infected conventional mice showed the greatest signs of intestinal pathology among the three groups, with the reconstituted germ-free mice showing moderate pathology. However, the most intriguing observation from this report was that infected germ-free mice did not develop intestinal pathology as compared to the other groups, suggesting a need for intestinal microbes to stimulate *Giardia*-induced pathology (Torres et al., 2000).

The interactions between intestinal microbiota and *Giardia* are not unexpected, as both reside in the same environmental niche along the lumen of the epithelial barrier during *Giardia* colonization (Adam, 2001). However, it is quite interesting that this parasite is able to affect the composition of the intestinal microbiota and the virulence of other microbes, while also being susceptible to various commensal bacterial secretions.

The Singer and Dawson groups first described the influence of *Giardia* on the architecture and abundance of the intestinal microbiota during *in vivo* murine infections (Barash et al., 2017). Significant shifts in microbial ecology were observed following *G. duodenalis* strain GS infection in mice pre-treated with antibiotics, as well as in non-antibiotic treated infected mice. Decreases in overall microbial diversity and the abundance of the obligate anaerobic Firmicutes occurred, while an increase in the abundance of aerobic taxa such as Rhodocyclaceae, Moraxellaceae, Flavobacteriales, and Comamonadaceae was reported (Barash et al., 2017). These enriched taxa are all considered to be metabolically flexible, and prosper with increased oxygen tension, lipid availability, and competition for arginine.

During the same year, Bartelt et al. (2017) also reported an alteration of the intestinal microbiota in mice fed a protein-deficient diet, prior to and continuously throughout, an infection with commercially obtained *Giardia* H3 cysts (Assemblage B). Quantitative PCR analysis of the 16S rRNA revealed that infected mice had greater duodenal bacterial abundance and an increase in the Firmicutes:Bacteroidetes ratio, with *Giardia* infections leading to increases in the population of Firmicutes while reducing the number of Bacteroidetes. Moreover, stool qPCR also revealed a large increase in the relative abundance of Enterobacteriaceae 14 days post infection, which was considered a better predictor of growth impairment than *Giardia* burden in stool or duodenum. This shift in the duodenal microbial composition of mice fed a protein-deficient diet also coincided with the persistence of the parasite within the gut rather than clearance (Bartelt et al., 2017). Interestingly, antibiotic treatment of mice with ampicillin, vancomycin, and neomycin prevented *Giardia*-induced growth impairment which suggests that *Giardia* interaction with intestinal microbes is a critical factor for the determination of growth outcome. Growth impairment was also exacerbated in mice that were co-infected with a pathogen commonly isolated from malnourished children, enteroaggregative *Escherichia coli* (EAEC) (Bartelt et al., 2017).

In a human study of the intestinal microbiome of children from Medellin, Columbia the diversity and composition of the microbiome was compared between uninfected children and groups infected with either *Cryptosporidium* alone, *Giardia* alone, or co-infected with both helminths and protozoans (Toro-Londono et al., 2019). Using 16S rDNA sequencing, *Giardia*-only infected children (mixed-gender, 5 years or younger) had an enrichment of *Prevotella* along with a drastic reduction in *Bacteroides* when compared to uninfected controls, and this alteration was also seen in children co-infected with both helminths and protozoans. The most abundant groups observed in *Giardia*-only infected children were *Ruminococcus* of the phylum Firmicutes followed by *Prevotella*. The authors suggest that in this case, *Giardia* is able to shift the intestinal microbiome from a *Bacteroides*-dominant composition (type 1 enterotype), which was associated with the uninfected control children group, to a *Prevotella*-dominant composition (type 2 enterotype), which was seen in both *Giardia*-only and co-infected children (Toro-Londono et al., 2019). Although a *Giardia*-mediated shift in the composition of the young human intestinal microbiome is clearly evident, it must be noted that different regions of the world may not express the same type 1 enterotype as seen in uninfected controls, as diet is clearly a significant factor determining the composition of the microbiome. Thus, more human clinical studies examining microbiome composition and changes in giardiasis will be needed in the future to elucidate the role and effect of *Giardia* in mediating shifts of the human intestinal microbiome. Nevertheless, these data suggest that *Giardia* colonization leads to a compositional and metabolic shift among the intestinal microbial community, which could contribute to both microbial-mediated protection and variation seen in the clinical manifestations of giardiasis.

The Buret group has also described several studies that further suggest the ability of *Giardia* infections to induce damage in infected host may result from changes in the resident microbiota. When *Giardia* was exposed to laboratory strains of *Escherichia coli* or human intestinal microbiota each bacterial group were converted to a toxic state that was deadly to *Caenorhabditis elegans* (Gerbaba et al., 2015). Moreover, the Buret lab has also demonstrated that *Giardia* not only induced microbial dysbiosis in human mucosal biofilms, but also increased the virulence of commensal microbes towards human epithelial cells *in vitro*. An increase in the levels of inflammatory markers, TLR4 and CXCL-8, were also reported in germ-free mice that were reconstituted with human microbes that had been exposed to *Giardia* products, yet was not induced during exposure to the living parasite. It was found that *Giardia* cysteine proteases [described in greater detail in the next section] were required for the induction of intestinal permeability that also mediated the disruption of microbial biofilms (Beatty et al., 2017).

While *Giardia* clearly has effects on the commensal microbiota, it is also clear that the microbiota impacts the ability of the parasite to colonize the host. Several microbial probiotic therapies involving various strains of *Lactobacilli* have been examined to shield the host from the detrimental effects mediated by *Giardia* during infection. The proliferative ability of the WB strain (assemblage A) of *Giardia* was inhibited when trophozoites were exposed to supernatants of *Lactobacillus johnsonii* culture medium (Perez et al., 2001), and this effect was confirmed *in vivo* using a gerbil model that evaded WB colonization when treated with *L. johnsonii* (Humen et al., 2005). The cause for this toxicity to *Giardia* trophozoites was attributed to the generation of deconjugated bile salts produced by *L. johnsonii* (Travers et al., 2016). Three Bile-Salt-Hydrolase-like (BSH) genes were recently identified in this probiotic microbe and were cloned into *E. coli* in order to assess the ability to be used as an anti-giardial agent (Allain et al., 2018). Two recombinant BSH proteins, rBSH47 and rBSH56, were purified from transgenic *E. coli* cultures and incubated with *Giardia* WB trophozoites. A dose-dependent inhibition of *Giardia* growth was reported when compared to non-BSH controls with concentrations of 1 μg/mL or greater resulting in 100% parasite killing. Scanning electron microscopy revealed significant structural damage to the parasite surface with several protrusions and perforations seen along the parasite plasma membrane. Using a murine infection model, the protective effects of rBSH47 were tested *in vivo* with *Giardia*-infected OF1 suckling mice. After infection with 1×10^5 trophozoites, groups of mice were administered different (but increasing) dosages of rBSH47 for five consecutive days post-infection. Parasite burden analysis revealed an increase in parasite numbers in PBS-treated controls (1×10^6

parasites/intestine); rBSH47-treated groups contained lesser numbers of parasites with the highest dosage group having the fewest parasites in the intestine (Allain et al., 2018).

In murine models used by the Shukla and Goyal group, *Lactobacillus casei* was able to reduce parasite-mediated mucosal damage and lessen both trophozoite burden and cyst shedding (Shukla et al., 2008). *Giardia*-mediated immunopathologies were also reduced with *Lactobacillus rhamnosus* treatments as infected mice treated with *L. rhamnosus* had increased antioxidants and brush-border disaccharidases levels, while oxidant concentrations were decreased in the small intestine (Goyal et al., 2013). Using BALB/c mice, prior treatment with *L. rhamnosus* led to a significant increase in secretory IgA antibody concentration and in the percentage of $CD4^+$ T cells in the small intestine following *Giardia* infection. Moreover, they also observed a decrease in the percentage of $CD8^+$ T cells (Goyal and Shukla, 2013), which are required to mediate the hallmark pathology seen during infection (Keselman et al., 2016). This effect was recapitulated in C57BL6/J mice where probiotic administration of *Enterococcus faecium* lessened parasite burdens and induced a stronger IgA antibody immune response (Benyacoub et al., 2005). Recently, a reduction in *Giardia*-mediated pathology, decreased duration of parasite burden, and an increase in anti-*Giardia* IgA and nitric oxide were seen in infected mice that were treated with killed probiotics or probiotic proteins (Shukla et al., 2019). Whether manipulation of the microbiome presents a viable strategy for reducing the impact of giardiasis clinically remains to be determined.

4. *Giardia* proteases and host chemokines

The interface between the intestinal lumen and the epithelial barrier is the site of attachment for *Giardia* trophozoites (Adam, 2001); thus, it is a critical area for initiating both parasite colonization and host immunity. At this point, it can be agreed upon that *Giardia* induces a breakage in this barrier which allows luminal contents to exit into the intestinal lamina propria to activate immune cells (Fig. 1), however the actual mechanisms leading to barrier breakdown are still uncertain. Early studies examining the ability of *Giardia* to colonize the intestinal lumen revealed that trophozoites use a variety of excretory-secretory products (ESPs) to aid in the colonization of the intestine (Nash et al., 1983; Nash and Keister, 1985; Samra et al., 1988). The Svärd lab was able to identify the major ESPs from both WB and GS strains of *Giardia* using proteomic methods, and revealed that both

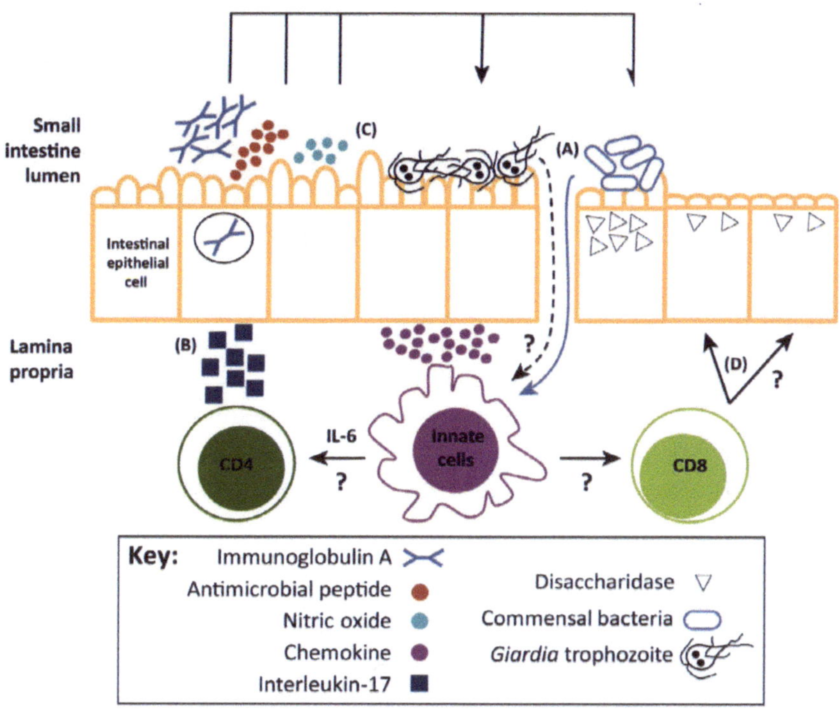

Fig. 1 Model of the interactions among *Giardia*, the microbiota and the host that can result in activation of protective, IL-17 dependent immune responses and also pathogenic $CD8^+$ T cell dependent responses. *Reprinted with permission from Fink, M.Y., Singer, S.M., 2017. The intersection of immune responses, microbiota, and pathogenesis in giardiasis. Trends Parasitol. 33, 901–913.*

serine (alanyl dipeptidyl peptidases) and cysteine (cathepsins B and L) proteases are among the most abundant proteins secreted by either strain of this parasite (Ma'ayeh et al., 2017). Similarly, the Tyler lab reported that tenascins were abundant in the ESP from *Giardia* (Dubourg et al., 2018). *Giardia*-secreted cysteine proteases have been extensively studied throughout the history of *Giardia* research (de Carvalho et al., 2008; Jiménez et al., 2000; Rodriguez-Fuentes et al., 2006), yet most importantly, it seems that this protease class are critical mediators in *Giardia* pathogenicity.

In vitro studies suggest that cysteine proteases mediate the degradation or rearrangement of tight junction proteins such as ZO-1, occludin, and claudin-1 following co-culture with *Giardia* (Bhargava et al., 2015; Chin et al., 2002; Liu et al., 2018; Ma'ayeh et al., 2017; Ortega-Pierres et al., 2018; Scott et al., 2002) and infections in humans have been shown to produce increases in the lactulose:mannitol ratio, a common marker of epithelial permeability and degradation of claudin-1 (Troeger et al., 2007). Furthermore, in animal models, increased rates of microbial translocation and decreased transepithelial electrical resistance have also been observed, which provides further evidence that cysteine proteases induce breakages in the intestinal epithelial barrier (Chen et al., 2013; Ortega-Pierres et al., 2018; Scott et al., 2002; Zhou et al., 2007).

Interestingly, the Ortega-Pierres group has characterized two proteases in cell culture with rat epithelial cell (IEC6) monolayers and Madin-Darby canine kidney (MDCK) cells (Cabrera-Licona et al., 2017; Ortega-Pierres et al., 2018). A variable surface protein, VSP9B10A, was identified during a screen of the WB *Giardia* secretome and bioinformatic analysis identified a cysteine protease-like domain within this VSP. When IEC6 and MDCK cell cultures were exposed to *Giardia* trophozoites that constitutively expressed VSP9B10A, greater disruption of the monolayer and atypical morphology of cells were reported when compared to parasites transfected with empty vector or to non-transfected *Giardia*. Moreover, this effect was lost when polyclonal antibodies specific for VSP9B10A were added to the transfected *Giardia* co-cultures. However, trophozoite supernatants could not mediate this proteolytic effect, suggesting that VSP9B10A is generated during the initial stages of contact with epithelial cells (Cabrera-Licona et al., 2017). More recently, a secreted protease that structurally resembles a papain-like cysteine protease was characterized and named giardipain-1 (Ortega-Pierres et al., 2018). IEC6 and MDCK monolayers were both severely damaged and had altered morphology when exposed to purified giardipain-1 and giardipain-1 expressing trophozoites; these changes were reversed when cell cultures were incubated with trophozoites that expressed antisense RNA complementary to giardipain-1 or in the presence of the protease inhibitor, E-64. Additionally, induction of Caspase-3 mediated apoptosis and degradation of occludin-1 and claudin-1 were reported in IEC6 and MDCK cell cultures, respectively, when exposed to purified giardipain-1. Together, these results describe possible mechanisms for the pathology seen in human biopsies (Troeger et al., 2007) and identify two candidate proteins that should be further studied to prevent *Giardia*-induced intestinal breakdown.

Following disruption of the epithelial barrier, chemokines are released by intestinal epithelial cells to recruit immune cells to the barrier and to initiate protective immune responses. Microarray analysis revealed that exposure of human colon carcinoma, CaCo2 cells, to *Giardia* parasites resulted in increased expression of numerous chemokines, including CXCL1-3,

CCL2, and CCL20 (Ma'ayeh et al., 2018; Roxstrom-Lindquist et al., 2005). However, the immunomodulatory effects of *Giardia* ESPs were seen in the degradation of these chemokine signals as the Buret group reported that cathepsin B protease degrades CXCL8 (IL-8) in both cell culture and *ex vivo* models (Cotton et al., 2014a). Chemotaxis of neutrophils was reduced when supernatants were used from CaCo2 cells incubated with *Giardia*, but this downregulation was alleviated upon addition of a cysteine protease inhibitor (Cotton et al., 2014b). Since IL-8 is a chemoattractant for neutrophils, these data suggest that degradation of chemokines by *Giardia* can limit neutrophil recruitment. Interestingly, the effects of the parasite on IL-8 and neutrophil chemotaxis were often dose- and *Giardia* strain-dependent (Cotton et al., 2014b). Furthermore, the Svärd group also reported that CXCL1-3, CCL2, and CCL20 protein can also be degraded when exposed to *Giardia*-secreted cysteine proteases (Liu et al., 2018; Ma'ayeh et al., 2018). Given the large number of proteases present within the ESP of *Giardia*, additional studies of their roles in modulation of the epithelial barrier and induction of immune responses are definitely required.

5. Vaccines

A major goal of understanding immune responses in *Giardia* is to develop a vaccine. GiardiaVAX is approved for veterinary use, but does not have great efficacy, despite being able to induce good IgA responses against the vaccine. Several *Giardia* antigens have been examined for their potential to establish an immune response, especially as this pertains to developing a vaccine. Potential immunogens include variant-specific surface proteins (VSPs), the immunoglobulin binding protein (BIP), excretory-secretory products (ESPs), the annexin homolog α1-giardin, and cell wall protein 2 (CWP-2) (Feng et al., 2016; Jimenez et al., 2014; Lee et al., 2014; Lopez-Romero et al., 2017; Quintero et al., 2013, 2017; Rivero et al., 2010; Serradell et al., 2016, 2018).

Variant-specific proteins (VSPs) are the dominant protein expressed on the surface of *Giardia* parasites. Normally, each parasite will only express one type of VSP at a time. Trophozoites periodically undergo antigenic variation and express one of the other ~150 VSP genes in the genome to evade immune responses (Prucca et al., 2011). Monoclonal antibodies (mAb) against specific VSPs often exhibit cytotoxicity against parasites expressing that VSP, prompting Rivero et al. to suggest that generating an antibody response against a diverse set of VSPs may allow for protection (Rivero et al., 2010).

The Lujan group developed an siRNA-based approach to generate strain WB trophozoites that simultaneously expressed multiple VSPs (Prucca et al., 2008). They also used a combination of limiting dilution and mAb screening to isolate several trophozoite populations that expressed unique VSP molecules on the trophozoite surface. Gerbils infected with *Giardia* that simultaneously expressed multiple VSPs had fewer excreted cysts upon a secondary infection (Rivero et al., 2010). Gerbils were also resistant to secondary infection when the same single-VSP expressing *Giardia* clone was used in both primary and secondary infections; however resistance was lost when a different single-VSP clone was used for the secondary infection. Taken together, these infection studies suggest that a primary infection with *Giardia* expressing multiple VSPs may be protective against secondary infections with *Giardia* expressing individuals VSPs (Rivero et al., 2010). Furthermore, culturing parasites with serum containing antibodies from gerbils infected with the multi-VSP expressing parasite revealed that the serum antibodies can cause agglutination of a number of different VSP-expressing clones (Rivero et al., 2010). In contrast, gerbils that were initially infected with parasites expressing a single VSP were then only protected against re-infection with parasites expressing the same VSP (Rivero et al., 2010). These data suggest that mounting a response to a collection of VSPs may be protective against future exposure to parasites with diverse VSP profiles (Rivero et al., 2010).

In simulating a potential vaccine, Rivero et al. administered to gerbils VSPs purified from trophozoites simultaneously expressing multiple VSPs and then challenged them with live parasites two months later (Rivero et al., 2010). Animals receiving the immunization had a lower fecal cyst count (Rivero et al., 2010). Later studies indicated that immunization with purified VSPs in gerbils did not induce the same increase in size and number of Peyer's patches as an actual infection did; immunization also maintained the weight of the mesenteric lymph nodes which normally increased by day 4 post-infection before going down (Serradell et al., 2018). Serum IgG and fecal IgA also increased post-immunization and were high in infection with different VSP clones (Serradell et al., 2018).

In addition to gerbils, 6–8 week-old dogs and 5–8 week-old cats were similarly protected from a secondary infection regardless of the specific VSP being expressed if they were initially infected with *Giardia* expressing the full VSP repertoire or received an immunization with VSPs purified from multi-VSP expressing parasites (Serradell et al., 2016). Following this study, cats and dogs from a community in Cordoba, Argentina where cats, dogs, and children are almost universally infected were vaccinated and followed over 2 years (Serradell et al., 2016). *Giardia* was not observed in any vaccinated animals over this time period (Serradell et al., 2016). Together, these data suggest that the VSPs are a promising target for vaccine development in giardiasis.

Quintero et al. characterized a 71 kDa potential immunogen (5G8) which was seen intracellularly and, to a lesser extent, on the cell surface (Quintero et al., 2013). Trophozoites expressing 5G8 were agglutinated after treatment with antibodies for 5G8 (Quintero et al., 2013). Further studies suggested that 5G8 was a member of the VSP family, but not the VSP-H7 nor the immunoglobulin binding protein (BIP) which are both similar in size (Lopez-Romero et al., 2017; Quintero et al., 2017).

The *G. duodenalis* immunoglobulin binding protein (GlBIP) has been shown to have strong immunogenic properties (Lee et al., 2014). As noted earlier, GlBIP activates DCs through TLR4. GlBIP itself is composed of two domains; the Hsp70 domain seems to be the immunoreactive one (Lee et al., 2014). The isolated Hsp70 domain was able to induce production of IL-12 and TNF-α, while the other domain was not successful at doing so (Lee et al., 2014). Similarly, dendritic cells stimulated with the Hsp70 domain were then able to promote IL-2 and IFN-γ production from $CD4^+$ T cells, which was not observed with the other domain (Lee et al., 2014). On the other hand, using C3H/HeN mice, it was reported that rBIP was not a potent stimulator of proliferation in cell culture using the splenocytes of infected mice, yet this variance could be attributed to the differing mouse strains used. However, rBIP did seem to be immunogenic as the serum of C3H/HeN mice, which were re-infected with GS *Giardia* trophozoites 6-week post infection, had greater binding to rBIP protein *in vitro* when compared to non-re-infected samples. Furthermore, when mice were infected and re-infected with a culture of GS trophozoites containing greater numbers of parasites that expressed the immunodominant antigen 5G8 (Quintero et al., 2013), IgG binding to rBIP protein was even greater than infections using standard GS cultures (Lopez-Romero et al., 2017).

The effects of ESP and their proteases were described earlier in this chapter. Jimenez et al. showed that after infection with *G. duodenalis* in mice, serum IgG1, IgG2, IgA, IgE and secretory IgA against ESP and *Giardia* extract were increased, although the increase was only significant for some of the antibodies (Jimenez et al., 2014). Furthermore, restimulation of spleens from infected mice with ESP led to an increase in spleen cell proliferation and an increase in the amount of cytokines produced

(Jimenez et al., 2014). ESP restimulation increased IL-4 responses at day 7 post-infection, while increased IFN-γ was seen 14 days post-infection, increased IL-5 21 days post-infection, and increased IL-10 at 21 and 28 days post-infection. Overall, this research supports the immunogenicity of E/S products (Jimenez et al., 2014).

Finally, α1-giardin and cyst wall proteins (CWPs) have also been examined as potential antigens to generate vaccines (Feng et al., 2016). A bivalent DNA vaccine with both α1-giardin and CWP2 DNA leads to both decreased trophozoite and fecal cyst numbers (79% reduction in trophozoites and 93% reduction in cysts) (Feng et al., 2016). In contrast, univalent α1-giardin vaccines generated a strong trophozoite decrease (74.2%) but a lower cyst output decrease (28%), while a univalent CWP2 vaccine generated decreased cyst output only (89%) (Feng et al., 2016). A combined vaccine allowed for dual targeting of the parasite, both its trophozoite and cyst form (Feng et al., 2016). Additionally, the bivalent vaccine led to an increase of both anti-α1-giardin IgG2 and anti-CWP2 IgG2, as well as an increase in both anti-α1-giardin IgA and anti-CWP2 IgA (Feng et al., 2016).

6. Pathogenic responses

While the perfect immune response would succeed in eliminating infections without producing concomitant damage in the host, it is clear that most actual immune responses produce significant ancillary pathology. Early work from our lab and others showed that intestinal transit rates were accelerated in wild-type mice infected with *Giardia*, but not in SCID mice (Andersen et al., 2006; Li et al., 2006), that smooth muscle hypercontractility was dependent on mast cell function (Li et al., 2004, 2007) and that disaccharidase deficiency involved $CD8^+$ T cells (Keselman et al., 2016; Scott et al., 2004). More recent work has focused on understanding regulation of these immune responses in order to help understand the variability seen in the outcomes of infections in humans.

6.1 IFN-γ

Previous work has indicated that neither Th1 (IFN-γ) nor Th2 (IL-4, IL-5) response is required for control of *Giardia* infections (Singer and Nash, 2000b). IFN-$\gamma^{-/-}$ mice cleared the infection as well as wild-type controls. Recently, Babaei et al. (2016) measured IFN-γ levels in symptomatic and asymptomatic patients infected with *Giardia*, along with uninfected controls (Babaei et al., 2016). IFN-γ levels were increased in the symptomatic patient group compared to the uninfected controls. The difference in IFN-γ levels between symptomatic and asymptomatic patients was not statistically significant, although there was a trend toward more IFN-γ in the symptomatic group. (Babaei et al., 2016). Studies with larger sample sizes should be conducted in order to further test this hypothesis.

Additional information regarding the role of IFN-γ has recently come from a study of children in Ecuador infected with the soil-transmitted helminth, *Ascaris lumbrocoides, G. duodenalis*, or both (Weatherhead et al., 2017). Children who were co-infected with *Ascaris* and *Giardia* had reduced serum levels of IL-2, IL-12, and TNF-α compared to children infected with only *Giardia* (Weatherhead et al., 2017). While each of these, is associate with Th1 responses, the level of IFNγ was not found to be reduced. Interestingly, the IL-10/IFN-γ ratio was higher in children with co-infections compared to children infected with *Giardia* alone (Weatherhead et al., 2017). Levels of the Th2 cytokines IL-4, IL-5 and IL-13 were also not different among groups in this study. Whether children with co-infection exhibited differences in acute symptoms like diarrhea or chronic symptoms including stunting was not investigated. In a different cohort of children in Venezuela, *Giardia* infection in children with a light concurrent *Ascaris* infection (<5000 eggs/g feces) exhibited increased serum IFN-γ levels compared to children with similar *Ascaris*-only infections (Hagel et al., 2011). However, in children where the *Ascaris* infection was more intense, the levels of IFN-γ between *Giardia* co-infected and *Ascaris*-only infected individuals were not significantly different (Hagel et al., 2011). Given that polyparasitism is common in children in low and middle income countries, additional analyses of co-infections are clearly warranted.

6.2 Other cytokines

In addition to IFN-γ and IL-17, other cytokines play important roles during a *Giardia* infection. While IL-17 appears to be the most important cytokine for controlling infections, it was actually among the least abundant cytokines produced when splenocytes or mesenteric lymph node cells from infected mice were stimulated in vitro with parasite extracts (Solaymani-Mohammadi and Singer, 2011). Data suggest that IL-4, IL-5, IL-6, IL-10, IL-13, IL-17, IL-22, IFN-γ and TNF-α are all produced following *Giardia* infections in mice (Bartelt et al., 2017; Dann et al., 2015; Li et al., 2014; Solaymani-Mohammadi and Singer, 2011; Zhou et al., 2003). Recent data from gerbils infected with *G. duodenalis* strain WB1267 also indicated a mixed cytokine response to infection. Messenger RNA for almost all of the cytokines queried were elevated in mesenteric lymph nodes at day 14. IL-5 mRNA was not elevated at day 14, although it was seen at day 28. (Serradell et al., 2018). The changes in cytokines observed over time likely reflect evolution of the immune response as the majority of parasites are eliminated between days 7 and 14 in this model.

The abundant production of IL-13 was reported for spleen cells from mice infected with either GS or WB strain *Giardia* after *in vitro* stimulation with parasite extracts (Solaymani-Mohammadi and Singer, 2011). Bartelt et al., also reported elevated IL-13 mRNA in mice infected with cysts of strain H3 (Bartelt et al., 2017). While the role of this cytokine has not been tested directly, it is intriguing to speculate that it may be involved in the goblet cell responses, including increased expression of Muc2, TFF3 and RELMβ that has been reported (Amat et al., 2017; Paerewijck et al., 2017).

Interleukin-10 (IL-10) is an anti-inflammatory cytokine involved in limiting chronic inflammation to commensal microbial antigens and self-proteins. Mucosal IL-10 mRNA levels were shown to increase between weeks 2–4 post infection in mice infected with *G. muris* (Dann et al., 2018). IL-10 mRNA was also increased in mesenteric lymph nodes of gerbils infected with *G. duodenalis* (Serradell et al., 2018) and spleen cells from mice infected with *G. duodenalis* produced IL-10 after *in vitro* stimulation with parasite extracts (Solaymani-Mohammadi and Singer, 2011). In the *G. muris* model, IL-10 mRNA levels peaked in the mucosa at week 3 corresponding with the major decrease in trophozoites in the small intestine (Dann et al., 2018). However, IL-$10^{-/-}$ mice were not deficient in clearing the parasite, indicating that this cytokine is not required for protective immunity.

Intriguingly, mice lacking IL-10 developed more severe symptoms from the infection including diarrhea and colonic inflammation (Dann et al., 2018). In IL-$10^{-/-}$ mice, the colon which is not the major site for *Giardia* infection showed increased inflammation as early as 1 week post infection, with increasing crypt depth and lamina propria cell accumulation in weeks 4 and 7 post infection (Dann et al., 2018). Neutrophil recruitment was also increased in the IL-$10^{-/-}$ infected mice (Dann et al., 2018). The mRNA levels of the CXCL5 neutrophil chemokine were high on days 5 and 12 post-infection; MPO mRNA levels increased by day 12 (Dann et al., 2018). Dann et al. concluded that these symptoms resemble the colitis IL-$10^{-/-}$ mice develop naturally as they age (Dann et al., 2018). TCR$\alpha^{-/-}$ mice similarly develop colitis-like symptoms as they age; *G. muris* infection in TCRα$^{-/-}$ mice led to similarly high histological scores, increased crypt depth, and lamina propria cell accumulation, although unlike the IL-10 deficient mice, these mice failed to control trophozoite counts (Dann et al., 2018).

T cells seem to play a role in developing post-infectious colitis in IL10$^{-/-}$ mice (Dann et al., 2018). Infected IL10$^{-/-}$Rag2$^{-/-}$ mice had a reduced histological score compared to infected IL10$^{-/-}$ mice, although there was significantly more inflammation than in infected wild-type mice or Rag2$^{-/-}$ mice (Dann et al., 2018). This suggests that both T cells and non-T cells contribute to colitis in this model. Indeed, the authors demonstrated dependence on CD11c^{+} cells (most likely dendritic cells), the intestinal microbiota and the MyD88 adaptor protein. These data are consistent with a model in which *Giardia* infection leads to epithelial barrier defects and microbial translocation that initiates an inflammatory response that is normally controlled by IL-10 dependent homeostatic mechanisms.

T cells are clearly not the only source of cytokines during a *Giardia* (or any) infection. Interleukin-6 was the first cytokine demonstrated to have a significant role in parasite clearance, since IL-6$^{-/-}$ mice take significantly longer to clear the infection compared to wild-type controls (Bienz et al., 2003; Zhou et al., 2003). While many cell types can produce IL-6, bone marrow chimera experiments have demonstrated that IL-6 from bone marrow derived cells is necessary and sufficient for control of *Giardia* (Kamda et al., 2012). Furthermore, transferring spleen T cells from IL-6$^{-/-}$ donors into TCRβ$^{-/-}$ mice allowed these mice to control infections, suggesting that T cell production of IL-6 is not crucial (Kamda et al., 2012). Interestingly, dendritic cells were identified as a potent source of IL-6 (Kamda et al., 2012). Adoptive transfer of IL-6 competent dendritic cells, pulsed with *Giardia* antigens prior to transfer into IL-6$^{-/-}$ mice, reduced parasite counts following infections compared to transfers of just extract or dendritic cells which were not pulsed with antigens (Kamda et al., 2012). Furthermore, since IL-6 in combination with TGF-β is able to drive differentiation of naïve T cells into IL-17 producing cells (Weaver et al., 2006), these data suggest that IL-6 from dendritic cells helps drive development of IL-17 producing CD4^{+} T cells, leading to successful control of infections. Direct demonstration of a role for IL-6 in Th17 development during giardiasis remains to be demonstrated.

Lee et al. looked at cytokine expression from human PBMCs and the monocytic cell line THP-1 stimulated with GS and WB (Lee et al., 2012). PMBCs from naïve donors produced TNF-α, IL-6, IL-8, IL-1β and IFN-γ, with GS stimulation facilitating higher levels of cytokine production than WB (Lee et al., 2012). THP-1 cells were also more responsive to GS, but only secreted TNF- α, IL-1β, IL-8, and IFN-γ in response (Lee et al., 2012). A similar experiment was performed with HT-29 cells which were physically separated from the live *Giardia*, so the effects of excretory/secretory antigens could be assessed (Lee et al., 2012). While stimulation of HT-29 cells with live *G. duodenalis* increased production of TNF-α, IL-6, and IL-1β, IL-8 responses decreased with increasing numbers of *Giardia* trophozoites (Lee et al., 2012). A potential explanation is that IL-8 is cleaved/degraded by cysteine proteases released from the parasite (Liu et al., 2019; Ma'ayeh et al., 2018). Additional data indicated that IL-8 transcription is dependent on ERK1/2 and p38 signaling and activation of the transcription factors NF-κB and AP-1 (Lee et al., 2012). However, the receptors involved in recognition of parasite antigens were not identified and the role of macrophage responses in contributing to the outcomes of infection remain unclear.

6.3 CD8$^+$ T Cells and disaccharidase deficiency

As we mentioned during discussion of the role of the microbiome in giardiasis, CD8$^+$ T cells have been implicated in mediating some of the epithelial damage observed in giardiasis. Specifically, upon adoptive transfer of either total mesenteric lymph node cells or purified CD8$^+$ T cells from mice infected with *G. muris* to athymic mice, shortening of the microvilli, loss of sucrase activity, and increase of the crypt/villus ratio are observed in the mucosa (Scott et al., 2004). The same effects are not observed in an adoptive transfer of CD4$^+$ T cells from infected mice (Scott et al., 2004). These observations were confirmed by analysis of mice with a deletion in the gene for β_2-microglobulin, a component of all class I MHC molecules. These mice lack class I MHC molecules, do not develop CD8$^+$ T cell populations and do not exhibit sucrase defects following *Giardia* infection, although they eliminate the infections as well as wild-type mice (Solaymani-Mohammadi and Singer, 2011).

Given that *Giardia* is an extracellular pathogen, it is unclear if or how CD8$^+$ T cells, which normally respond to viral antigens or other peptides found in host cell cytosol, would become activated. Keselman used flow cytometry to demonstrate that CD8$^+$ T cells in the lamina propria of *Giardia* infected mice exhibit an activated phenotype, i.e. high expression of CD44 and CD69. Interestingly, antibiotic treatment of mice ameliorated the sucrase deficiency normally seen following *Giardia* infection. It also prevented the increase in $CD8^+$ T cells with an activated phenotype (Keselman et al., 2016). In contrast, antibiotic treatment did not seem to have an effect on the increased accumulation of $CD4^+$ T cells in the lamina propria following infection (Keselman et al., 2016). Activation of certain intraepithelial lymphocyte populations was also observed following *Giardia* infection in this study, although antibiotic treatment did not seem to affect this response. These data suggest that intestinal microbiota somehow contribute to activation of $CD8^+$ T cells and the reduction in disaccharidase activity that is often observed in giardiasis.

Mucosal integrity can be severely affected by a *Giardia* infection, especially if coupled with malnourishment. Shukla et al. measured sucrase, lactase, and maltase activity, as well as alkaline phosphatase in wildtype and malnourished mice infected with *Giardia duodenalis* (Shukla et al., 2013). *Giardia* decreased disaccharide activity and alkaline phosphatase at 4, 9, and 10 days of infection (Shukla et al., 2013). Malnutrition and probiotic treatment at different time points modified the effect of the parasite on disaccharide activity, although the specifics varied based on the disaccharidase being analyzed (Shukla et al., 2013). Nevertheless, these data are consistent with the model that intestinal microbiota are key players in the development of the disaccharidase deficiency phenotype and that they act by modulating the activation of $CD8^+$ T cells. The exact role of the microbiota in activation of these cells remains to be determined.

6.4 Mast cells and irritable bowel syndrome

Giardiasis has been linked to a number of long-term sequelae, including chronic fatigue and irritable bowel syndromes. Several studies followed a population in Norway after a *Giardia* infection outbreak there in 2004. Hanevik et al. considered a group of patients for post-infectious chronic fatigue syndrome (PI-CFS), post-infectious functional gastrointestinal disorders (PI-FGID), as well as a potential co-morbidity relationship between the two (Hanevik et al., 2012). Five years post-infection the population of $CD8^+$ cells in PI-FGID-reporting patients was increased, while PI-CFS-reporting patients had a lower count of natural killer cells (Hanevik et al., 2012). Later work in the same population specifically focused on PBMCs from PI-CFS patients stimulated with antigens from *Giardia* assemblage A or assemblage B parasites. No statistical differences were seen comparing activation of $CD4^+$ T cell responses between patients with PI-CFS and those who had been infected with *Giardia* but did not develop CFS (Hanevik et al., 2017). Similarly, the amount of cytokines produced including IL-4, IL-6, IL-10, IFN-γ, TNF-α, and IL-2 were also similar (Hanevik et al., 2017). There was significantly more sCD40L in supernatants of stimulated PBMCs obtained from PI-CFS patients, although the authors concluded that further studies will be needed to determine if this is specifically a marker of post-*Giardia* infectious CFS (Hanevik et al., 2017).

In terms of irritable bowel syndrome (IBS), work in mice has shown that tight junctions in the jejunum are impaired during *Giardia* infection, specifically that occludin is cleaved on day 7 post-infection (peak of giardiasis) and day 35 post-infection (after resolution) (Chen et al., 2013). Permeability is also increased in jejunal tissues at both time points and in colon tissues at the later time point (Chen et al., 2013). Neutrophil counts, as well as myeloperoxidase activity, in the mucosa are higher both at day 7 and day 35 after oral gavage with *G. duodenalis* (Chen et al., 2013). IFN-γ levels are also increased on day 7 and day 35, while TNF-α and IL-1β levels are only increased on day 35 (Chen et al., 2013). Overall, the authors hypothesized that a *Giardia* infection leads to disrupted epithelial integrity, followed by an immune response to the microbes in the intestine that are now able to traffic across the damaged layer (Chen et al., 2013).

Fisher et al set up an *in vitro* system to model the interactions between *G. duodenalis*, the epithelial layer, and macrophages residing under the epithelium. The purpose of this model was to allow for study of prolonged giardiasis *in vitro* (Fisher et al., 2013). Similar to earlier work using either a different cell line or patient biopsies (Chin et al., 2002; Troeger et al., 2007), they showed that *Giardia* led to an increase in the activation of caspase-3 in epithelial cells, indicating apoptosis of these cells (Fisher et al., 2013). Furthermore, when culturing CaCo2 cells and macrophages together, the authors saw an increase in production of the chemokines GRO and IL-8, both of which are involved in neutrophil recruitment. Interestingly, this response was diminished when *Giardia* was cultured with the CaCo2 cells and macrophages (Fisher et al., 2013), consistent with results described above where parasite proteases can degrade IL-8.

In addition to acute symptomatic infections, *Giardia* often causes subclinical infections which can become chronic or recurrent. It is thought that chronic and recurrent *Giardia* infections contribute to growth faltering in children. Although studies have often been contradictory and inconclusive (Bartelt and Sartor, 2015), recent data from the very large MAL-ED cohort study suggests that *Giardia* is one of the four main contributors to stunting in children (Bartelt and Sartor, 2015; Rogawski et al., 2017, 2018). Bartelt et al. (2017) developed a chronic giardiasis mouse model utilizing H3 *G. duodenalis* cysts in under-nourished mice to investigate the interaction of *Giardia* infection and malnutrition. Similar parasite counts were observed at 8 days post infection and at 64 days post infection in the duodenum, indicating a chronic infection (Bartelt et al., 2013). Additionally, increased crypt depth and eosinophil counts in both the villi and crypts were observed on day 64 (Bartelt et al., 2013). Mice with *Giardia* had reduced weight gain compared to uninfected mice on the low-protein diet; additionally, villus height was also shown to decrease with malnourishment prior to infection (Bartelt et al., 2013). In varying the length of malnourishment prior to infection, the authors discovered that a 15-day low-protein diet expedited weight loss compared to an 8-day diet (Bartelt et al., 2013). Furthermore, while in nourished infected mice, there was an influx of neutrophils and an increase in IL-4 and IL-5 mRNA, these responses were decreased in malnourished infected mice (Bartelt et al., 2013). These data indicate that nutrition and infection interact with immune responses in complicated ways and provide a valuable model for environmental enteropathy in humans.

7. Remaining questions

While there has been significant progress in several areas, there remain numerous areas important for further study. In terms of the innate response to *Giardia*, it remains unclear which pattern recognition receptors recognize antigens from *Giardia* and contribute to the activation of macrophages and dendritic cells. Importantly, we do not know which innate cells provide the signals that help drive differentiation of the IL-17 producing $CD4^+$ T cells that are required for control of the infection. While several responses downstream of IL-17 have been investigated, it remains unclear which effector mechanisms are most important for control of the infection. Similarly, it is unclear how the $CD8^+$ T cell response that leads to shortening of the microvilli and reduced levels of disaccharidases in the mucosa are activated. If these $CD8^+$ T cells target parasite antigens, it is unclear how peptides from an extracellular pathogen would be presented in class I MHC molecules that normally present antigens from the host cell cytosol. Finally, the contribution of immune responses to the development of acute symptoms of giardiasis in humans has not been thoroughly studied, nor is the role of immune responses in long-term sequelae (e.g., stunting, irritable bowel syndrome or chronic fatigue syndrome) of the infection understood.

Acknowledgment

Work in the Singer lab is supported by grant AI109591 from the National Institutes of Health.

References

Abreu, M.T., 2010. Toll-like receptor signalling in the intestinal epithelium: how bacterial recognition shapes intestinal function. Nat. Rev. Immunol. 10, 131–144.

Adam, R.D., 2001. Biology of Giardia lamblia. Clin. Microbiol. Rev. 14, 447–475.

Aley, S.B., Zimmerman, M., Hetsko, M., Selsted, M.E., Gillin, F.D., 1994. Killing of Giardia lamblia by cryptdins and cationic neutrophil peptides. Infect. Immun. 62, 5397–5403.

Allain, T., Chaouch, S., Thomas, M., Travers, M.A., Valle, I., Langella, P., Grellier, P., Polack, B., Florent, I., Bermúdez-Humarán, L.G., 2018. Bile salt hydrolase activities: a novel target to screen anti-*Giardia* lactobacilli? Front. Microbiol. 9, 89.

Amat, C.B., Motta, J.P., Fekete, E., Moreau, F., Chadee, K., Buret, A.G., 2017. Cysteine protease-dependent mucous disruptions and differential mucin gene expression in Giardia duodenalis infection. Am. J. Pathol. 187, 2486–2498.

Andersen, Y.S., Gillin, F.D., Eckmann, L., 2006. Adaptive immunity-dependent intestinal hypermotility contributes to host defense against Giardia spp. Infect. Immun. 74, 2473–2476.

Babaei, Z., Malihi, N., Zia-Ali, N., Sharifi, I., Mohammadi, M.A., Kagnoff, M.F., Eckmann, L., Singer, S.M., Solaymani-Mohammadi, S., 2016. Adaptive immune response in symptomatic and asymptomatic enteric protozoal infection: evidence for a determining role of parasite genetic heterogeneity in host immunity to human giardiasis. Microbes Infect. 18, 687–695.

Barash, N.R., Maloney, J.G., Singer, S.M., Dawson, S.C., 2017. Giardia alters commensal microbial diversity throughout the murine gut. Infect. Immun. 85, e00948.

Bartelt, L.A., Sartor, R.B., 2015. Advances in understanding Giardia: determinants and mechanisms of chronic sequelae. F1000Prime Rep. 7, 62.

Bartelt, L.A., Roche, J., Kolling, G., Bolick, D., Noronha, F., Naylor, C., Hoffman, P., Warren, C., Singer, S., Guerrant, R., 2013. Persistent G. lamblia impairs growth in a murine malnutrition model. J. Clin. Invest. 123, 2672–2684.

Bartelt, L.A., Bolick, D.T., Mayneris-Perxachs, J., Kolling, G.L., Medlock, G.L., Zaenker, E.I., Donowitz, J., Thomas-Beckett, R.V., Rogala, A., Carroll, I.M., et al., 2017. Cross-modulation of pathogen-specific pathways enhances malnutrition during enteric co-infection with Giardia lamblia and enteroaggregative *Escherichia coli*. PLoS Pathog. 13, e1006471.

Beatty, J.K., Akierman, S.V., Motta, J.P., Muise, S., Workentine, M.L., Harrison, J.J., Bhargava, A., Beck, P.L., Rioux, K.P., McKnight, G.W., et al., 2017. Giardia duodenalis induces pathogenic dysbiosis of human intestinal microbiota biofilms. Int. J. Parasitol. 47, 311–326.

Benyacoub, J., Perez, P.F., Rochat, F., Saudan, K.Y., Reuteler, G., Antille, N., Humen, M., De Antoni, G.L., Cavadini, C., Blum, S., Schiffrin, E.J., 2005. Enterococcus faecium SF68 enhances the immune response to Giardia intestinalis in mice. J. Nutr. 135, 1171–1176.

Bhargava, A., Cotton, J.A., Dixon, B.R., Gedamu, L., Yates, R.M., Buret, A.G., 2015. Giardia duodenalis surface cysteine proteases induce cleavage of the intestinal epithelial cytoskeletal protein villin via myosin light chain kinase. PLoS One 10, e0136102.

Bienz, M., Dai, W.J., Welle, M., Gottstein, B., Muller, N., 2003. Interleukin-6-deficient mice are highly susceptible to Giardia lamblia infection but exhibit normal intestinal immunoglobulin a responses against the parasite. Infect. Immun. 71, 1569–1573.

Byrd, L.G., Conrad, J.T., Nash, T.E., 1994. Giardia lamblia infections in adult mice. Infect. Immun. 62, 3583–3585.
Cabrera-Licona, A., Solano-González, E., Fonseca-Liñán, R., Bazán-Tejeda, M.L., Argüello-García, R., Bermúdez-Cruz, R.M., Ortega-Pierres, G., 2017. Expression and secretion of the Giardia duodenalis variant surface protein 9B10A by transfected trophozoites causes damage to epithelial cell monolayers mediated by protease activity. Exp. Parasitol. 179, 49–64.
Cao, A.T., Yao, S., Gong, B., Elson, C.O., Cong, Y., 2012. Th17 cells upregulate polymeric Ig receptor and intestinal IgA and contribute to intestinal homeostasis. J. Immunol. 189, 4666–4673.
Chen, T.L., Chen, S., Wu, H.W., Lee, T.C., Lu, Y.Z., Wu, L.L., Ni, Y.H., Sun, C.H., Yu, W.H., Buret, A.G., Yu, L.C., 2013. Persistent gut barrier damage and commensal bacterial influx following eradication of Giardia infection in mice. Gut Pathog. 5, 26.
Chin, A.C., Teoh, D.A., Scott, K.G., Meddings, J.B., Macnaughton, W.K., Buret, A.G., 2002. Strain-dependent induction of enterocyte apoptosis by Giardia lamblia disrupts epithelial barrier function in a caspase-3-dependent manner. Infect. Immun. 70, 3673–3680.
Cotton, J.A., Bhargava, A., Ferraz, J.G., Yates, R.M., Beck, P.L., Buret, A.G., 2014a. Giardia duodenalis cathepsin B proteases degrade intestinal epithelial interleukin-8 and attenuate interleukin-8-induced neutrophil chemotaxis. Infect. Immun. 82, 2772–2787.
Cotton, J.A., Motta, J.P., Schenck, L.P., Hirota, S.A., Beck, P.L., Buret, A.G., 2014b. Giardia duodenalis infection reduces granulocyte infiltration in an in vivo model of bacterial toxin-induced colitis and attenuates inflammation in human intestinal tissue. PLoS One 9, e109087.
Dann, S.M., Manthey, C.F., Le, C., Miyamoto, Y., Gima, L., Abrahim, A., Cao, A.T., Hanson, E.M., Kolls, J.K., Raz, E., et al., 2015. IL-17A promotes protective IgA responses and expression of other potential effectors against the lumen-dwelling enteric parasite Giardia. Exp. Parasitol. 156, 68–78.
Dann, S.M., Le, C.H.Y., Hanson, E.M., Ross, M.C., Eckmann, L., 2018. Infection of the small intestine induces chronic colitis in genetically susceptible hosts. J. Immunol. 201, 548–559.
Davids, B.J., Palm, J.E., Housley, M.P., Smith, J.R., Andersen, Y.S., Martin, M.G., Hendrickson, B.A., Johansen, F.E., Svärd, S.G., Gillin, F.D., Eckmann, L., 2006. Polymeric immunoglobulin receptor in intestinal immune defense against the lumen-dwelling protozoan parasite Giardia. J. Immunol. 177, 6281–6290.
de Carvalho, T.B., David, E.B., Coradi, S.T., Guimaraes, S., 2008. Protease activity in extracellular products secreted in vitro by trophozoites of Giardia duodenalis. Parasitol. Res. 104, 185–190.
Dreesen, L., Rinaldi, M., Chiers, K., Li, R., Geurden, T., Van den Broeck, W., Goddeeris, B., Vercruysse, J., Claerebout, E., Geldhof, P., 2012. Microarray analysis of the intestinal host response in Giardia duodenalis assemblage E infected calves. PLoS One 7, e40985.
Dreesen, L., De Bosscher, K., Grit, G., Staels, B., Lubberts, E., Bauge, E., Geldhof, P., 2014. Giardia muris infection in mice is associated with a protective interleukin 17A response and induction of peroxisome proliferator-activated receptor alpha. Infect. Immun. 82, 3333–3340.
Dubourg, A., Xia, D., Winpenny, J.P., Al Naimi, S., Bouzid, M., Sexton, D.W., Wastling, J.M., Hunter, P.R., Tyler, K.M., 2018. Giardia secretome highlights secreted tenascins as a key component of pathogenesis. Gigascience 7, 1–13.
Eckmann, L., Laurent, F., Langford, T.D., Hetsko, M.L., Smith, J.R., Kagnoff, M.F., Gillin, F.D., 2000. Nitric oxide production by human intestinal epithelial cells and competition for arginine as potential determinants of host defense against the lumen-dwelling pathogen Giardia lamblia. J. Immunol. 164, 1478–1487.

El-Gebaly, N.S., Halawa, E.F., Moussa, H.M., Rabia, I., Abu-Zekry, M., 2012. Saliva and sera IgA and IgG in Egyptian Giardia-infected children. Parasitol. Res. 111, 571–575.

Evans-Osses, I., Ansa-Addo, E.A., Inal, J.M., Ramirez, M.I., 2010. Involvement of lectin pathway activation in the complement killing of Giardia intestinalis. Biochem. Biophys. Res. Commun. 395, 382–386.

Feng, X.M., Zheng, W.Y., Zhang, H.M., Shi, W.Y., Li, Y., Cui, B.J., Wang, H.Y., 2016. Vaccination with bivalent DNA vaccine of α1-Giardin and CWP2 delivered by attenuated Salmonella typhimurium reduces Trophozoites and cysts in the feces of mice infected with Giardia lamblia. PLoS One 11, e0157872.

Fink, M.Y., Singer, S.M., 2017. The intersection of immune responses, microbiota, and pathogenesis in giardiasis. Trends Parasitol. 33, 901–913.

Fisher, B.S., Estrano, C.E., Cole, J.A., 2013. Modeling long-term host cell-Giardia lamblia interactions in an in vitro co-culture system. PLoS One 8, e81104.

Frontera, L.S., Moyano, S., Quassollo, G., Lanfredi-Rangel, A., Rópolo, A.S., Touz, M.C., 2018. Lactoferrin and lactoferricin endocytosis halt Giardia cell growth and prevent infective cyst production. Sci. Rep. 8, 18020.

Gerbaba, T.K., Gupta, P., Rioux, K., Hansen, D., Buret, A.G., 2015. Giardia duodenalis-induced alterations of commensal bacteria kill Caenorhabditis elegans: a new model to study microbial-microbial interactions in the gut. Am. J. Physiol. Gastrointest. Liver Physiol. 308, G550–G561.

Goyal, N., Shukla, G., 2013. Probiotic lactobacillus rhamnosus GG modulates the mucosal immune response in Giardia intestinalis-infected BALB/c mice. Dig. Dis. Sci. 58, 1218–1225.

Goyal, N., Rishi, P., Shukla, G., 2013. Lactobacillus rhamnosus GG antagonizes Giardia intestinalis induced oxidative stress and intestinal disaccharidases: an experimental study. World J. Microbiol. Biotechnol. 29, 1049–1057.

Hagel, I., Cabrera, M., Puccio, F., Santaella, C., Buvat, E., Infante, B., Zabala, M., Cordero, R., Di Prisco, M.C., 2011. Co-infection with Ascaris lumbricoides modulates protective immune responses against Giardia duodenalis in school Venezuelan rural children. Acta Trop. 117, 189–195.

Hanevik, K., Kristoffersen, E.K., Sørnes, S., Mørch, K., Næss, H., Rivenes, A.C., Bødtker, J.E., Hausken, T., Langeland, N., 2012. Immunophenotyping in post-giardiasis functional gastrointestinal disease and chronic fatigue syndrome. BMC Infect. Dis. 12, 258.

Hanevik, K., Kristoffersen, E., Mørch, K., Rye, K.P., Sørnes, S., Svärd, S., Bruserud, Ø., Langeland, N., 2017. Giardia-specific cellular immune responses in post-giardiasis chronic fatigue syndrome. BMC Immunol. 18, 5.

Hill, D.R., Burge, J.J., Pearson, R.D., 1984. Susceptibility of Giardia lamblia trophozoites to the lethal effect of human serum. J. Immunol. 132, 2046–2052.

Hjøllo, T., Bratland, E., Steinsland, H., Radunovic, M., Langeland, N., Hanevik, K., 2018. Longitudinal cohort study of serum antibody responses towards Giardia lamblia variant-specific surface proteins in a non-endemic area. Exp. Parasitol. 191, 66–72.

Humen, M.A., De Antoni, G.L., Benyacoub, J., Costas, M.E., Cardozo, M.I., Kozubsky, L., Saudan, K.Y., Boenzli-Bruand, A., Blum, S., Schiffrin, E.J., Perez, P.F., 2005. Lactobacillus johnsonii La1 antagonizes Giardia intestinalis in vivo. Infect. Immun. 73, 1265–1269.

Jiménez, J.C., Uzcanga, G., Zambrano, A., Di Prisco, M.C., Lynch, N.R., 2000. Identification and partial characterization of excretory/secretory products with proteolytic activity in Giardia intestinalis. J. Parasitol. 86, 859–862.

Jimenez, J.C., Fontaine, J., Creusy, C., Fleurisse, L., Grzych, J.M., Capron, M., Dei-Cas, E., 2014. Antibody and cytokine responses to Giardia excretory/secretory proteins in Giardia intestinalis-infected BALB/c mice. Parasitol. Res. 113, 2709–2718.

Kamda, J.D., Singer, S.M., 2009. Phosphoinositide 3-kinase-dependent inhibition of dendritic cell interleukin-12 production by Giardia lamblia. Infect. Immun. 77, 685–693.

Kamda, J.D., Nash, T.E., Singer, S.M., 2012. Giardia duodenalis: dendritic cell defects in IL-6 deficient mice contribute to susceptibility to intestinal infection. Exp. Parasitol. 130, 288–291.

Keselman, A., Li, E., Maloney, J., Singer, S.M., 2016. The microbiota contributes to CD8+ T cell activation and nutrient malabsorption following intestinal infection with Giardia duodenalis. Infect. Immun. 84, 2853–2860.

Lee, H.Y., Hyung, S., Lee, N.Y., Yong, T.S., Han, S.H., Park, S.J., 2012. Excretory-secretory products of Giardia lamblia induce interleukin-8 production in human colonic cells via activation of p38, ERK1/2, NF-κB and AP-1. Parasite Immunol. 34, 183–198.

Lee, H.Y., Kim, J., Noh, H.J., Kim, H.P., Park, S.J., 2014. Giardia lamblia binding immunoglobulin protein triggers maturation of dendritic cells via activation of TLR4-MyD88-p38 and ERK1/2 MAPKs. Parasite Immunol. 36, 627–646.

Li, E., Zhou, P., Petrin, Z., Singer, S.M., 2004. Mast cell-dependent control of Giardia lamblia infections in mice. Infect. Immun. 72, 6642–6649.

Li, E., Zhou, P., Singer, S.M., 2006. Neuronal nitric oxide synthase is necessary for elimination of Giardia lamblia infections in mice. J. Immunol. 176, 516–521.

Li, E., Zhao, A., Shea-Donohue, T., Singer, S.M., 2007. Mast cell mediated changes in smooth muscle contractility during mouse giardiasis. Infect. Immun. 75, 4514–4518.

Li, E., Liu, M., Singer, S.M., 2014. Resistance to reinfection in mice as a vaccine model for giardiasis. Hum. Vaccin. Immunother. 10, 1536–1543.

Li, E., Tako, E.A., Singer, S.M., 2016. Complement activation by Giardia duodenalis parasites through the Lectin pathway contributes to mast cell responses and parasite control. Infect. Immun. 84, 1092–1099.

Li, X., Zhang, X., Gong, P., Xia, F., Li, L., Yang, Z., Li, J., 2017. TLR2−/− mice display decreased severity of giardiasis via enhanced proinflammatory cytokines production dependent on AKT signal pathway. Front. Immunol. 8, 1186.

Li, J., Casanova, J.L., Puel, A., 2018a. Mucocutaneous IL-17 immunity in mice and humans: host defense vs. excessive inflammation. Mucosal Immunol. 11, 581–589.

Li, L., Li, X., Li, G., Gong, P., Zhang, X., Yang, Z., Yang, J., Li, J., 2018b. Mouse macrophages capture and kill Giardia lamblia by means of releasing extracellular trap. Dev. Comp. Immunol. 88, 206–212.

Liu, J., Ma'ayeh, S., Peirasmaki, D., Lundström-Stadelmann, B., Hellman, L., Svärd, S.G., 2018. Secreted Giardia intestinalis cysteine proteases disrupt intestinal epithelial cell junctional complexes and degrade chemokines. Virulence 9, 879–894.

Liu, J., Fu, Z., Hellman, L., Svärd, S.G., 2019. Cleavage specificity of recombinant Giardia intestinalis cysteine proteases: degradation of immunoglobulins and defensins. Mol. Biochem. Parasitol. 227, 29–38.

Lopez-Romero, G., Garzon, T., Rascon, R., Valdez, A., Quintero, J., Arvizu-Flores, A.A., Garibay-Escobar, A., Rascon, L., Astiazarán-García, H., Velazquez, C., 2017. Characterization of BIP protein of G. lamblia as a potential immunogen in a mouse infection model. Immunobiology 222, 884–891.

Ma'ayeh, S.Y., Liu, J., Peirasmaki, D., Hörnaeus, K., Bergström Lind, S., Grabherr, M., Bergquist, J., Svärd, S.G., 2017. Characterization of the Giardia intestinalis secretome during interaction with human intestinal epithelial cells: the impact on host cells. PLoS Negl. Trop. Dis. 11, e0006120.

Ma'ayeh, S.Y., Knörr, L., Sköld, K., Granham, A., Ansell, B.R.E., Jex, A.R., Svärd, S.G., 2018. Responses of the differentiated intestinal epithelial cell line Caco-2 to infection with the. Front. Cell. Infect. Microbiol. 8, 244.

Maloney, J., Keselman, A., Li, E., Singer, S.M., 2015. Macrophages expressing arginase 1 and nitric oxide synthase 2 accumulate in the small intestine during Giardia lamblia infection. Microbes Infect. 17, 462–467.

Manko, A., Motta, J.P., Cotton, J.A., Feener, T., Oyeyemi, A., Vallance, B.A., Wallace, J.L., Buret, A.G., 2017. Giardia co-infection promotes the secretion of antimicrobial peptides beta-defensin 2 and trefoil factor 3 and attenuates attaching and effacing bacteria-induced intestinal disease. PLoS One 12, e0178647.

Nash, T.E., Keister, D.B., 1985. Differences in excretory-secretory products and surface antigens among 19 isolates of Giardia. J. Infect. Dis. 152, 1166–1171.

Nash, T.E., Gillin, F.D., Smith, P.D., 1983. Excretory-secretory products of Giardia lamblia. J. Immunol. 131, 2004–2010.

Obendorf, J., Renner Viveros, P., Fehlings, M., Klotz, C., Aebischer, T., Ignatius, R., 2013. Increased expression of CD25, CD83, and CD86, and secretion of IL-12, IL-23, and IL-10 by human dendritic cells incubated in the presence of toll-like receptor 2 ligands and Giardia duodenalis. Parasit. Vectors 6, 317.

Ortega-Pierres, G., Argüello-García, R., Laredo-Cisneros, M.S., Fonseca-Linán, R., Gómez-Mondragón, M., Inzunza-Arroyo, R., Flores-Benítez, D., Raya-Sandino, A., Chavez-Munguía, B., Ventura-Gallegos, J.L., et al., 2018. Giardipain-1, a protease secreted by Giardia duodenalis trophozoites, causes junctional, barrier and apoptotic damage in epithelial cell monolayers. Int. J. Parasitol. 48, 621–639.

Paerewijck, O., Maertens, B., Dreesen, L., Van Meulder, F., Peelaers, I., Ratman, D., Li, R.W., Lubberts, E., De Bosscher, K., Geldhof, P., 2017. Interleukin-17 receptor A (IL-17RA) as a central regulator of the protective immune response against Giardia. Sci. Rep. 7, 8520.

Perez, P.F., Minnaard, J., Rouvet, M., Knabenhans, C., Brassart, D., De Antoni, G.L., Schiffrin, E.J., 2001. Inhibition of Giardia intestinalis by extracellular factors from lactobacilli: an in vitro study. Appl. Environ. Microbiol. 67, 5037–5042.

Prucca, C.G., Slavin, I., Quiroga, R., Elias, E.V., Rivero, F.D., Saura, A., Carranza, P.G., Lujan, H.D., 2008. Antigenic variation in Giardia lamblia is regulated by RNA interference. Nature 456, 750–754.

Prucca, C.G., Rivero, F.D., Lujan, H.D., 2011. Regulation of antigenic variation in Giardia lamblia. Annu. Rev. Microbiol. 65, 611–630.

Quintero, J., Figueroa, D.C., Barcelo, R., Breci, L., Astiazaran-Garcia, H., Rascon, L., Robles-Zepeda, R., Garibay-Escobar, A., Velazquez-Contreras, E., Avila, G.L., et al., 2013. Identification of an immunogenic protein of Giardia lamblia using monoclonal antibodies generated from infected mice. Mem. Inst. Oswaldo Cruz 108, 616–622.

Quintero, J., Valdez, A., Samaniego, B., Lopez-Romero, G., Astiazaran-Garcia, H., Rascon, L., Breci, L., Garibay-Escobar, A., Robles-Zepeda, R., Velazquez, C., 2017. Isolation and partial characterization of an immunogenic antigen of Giardia lamblia. Parasitol. Int. 66, 324–330.

Ratner, D.M., Cui, J., Steffen, M., Moore, L.L., Robbins, P.W., Samuelson, J., 2008. Changes in the N-glycome, glycoproteins with Asn-linked glycans, of Giardia lamblia with differentiation from trophozoites to cysts. Eukaryot. Cell 7, 1930–1940.

Rivero, F.D., Saura, A., Prucca, C.G., Carranza, P.G., Torri, A., Lujan, H.D., 2010. Disruption of antigenic variation is crucial for effective parasite vaccine. Nat. Med. 16, 551–557. 551p following 557.

Rodriguez-Fuentes, G.B., Cedillo-Rivera, R., Fonseca-Linan, R., Arguello-Garcia, R., Munoz, O., Ortega-Pierres, G., Yepez-Mulia, L., 2006. Giardia duodenalis: analysis of secreted proteases upon trophozoite-epithelial cell interaction in vitro. Mem. Inst. Oswaldo Cruz 101, 693–696.

Rogawski, E.T., Bartelt, L.A., Platts-Mills, J.A., Seidman, J.C., Samie, A., Havt, A., Babji, S., Trigoso, D.R., Qureshi, S., Shakoor, S., et al., 2017. Determinants and impact of Giardia infection in the first 2 years of life in the MAL-ED birth cohort. J. Pediatric. Infect. Dis. Soc. 6, 153–160.

Rogawski, E.T., Liu, J., Platts-Mills, J.A., Kabir, F., Lertsethtakarn, P., Siguas, M., Khan, S.S., Praharaj, I., Murei, A., Nshama, R., et al., 2018. Use of quantitative molecular diagnostic methods to investigate the effect of enteropathogen infections on linear growth in children in low-resource settings: longitudinal analysis of results from the MAL-ED cohort study. Lancet Glob. Health 6, e1319–e1328.

Roxstrom-Lindquist, K., Ringqvist, E., Palm, D., Svard, S., 2005. Giardia lamblia-induced changes in gene expression in differentiated Caco-2 human intestinal epithelial cells. Infect. Immun. 73, 8204–8208.

Saghaug, C.S., Sørnes, S., Peirasmaki, D., Svärd, S., Langeland, N., Hanevik, K., 2016. Human memory CD4+ T cell immune responses against Giardia lamblia. Clin. Vaccine Immunol. 23, 11–18.

Samra, H.K., Ganguly, N.K., Garg, U.C., Goyal, J., Mahajan, R.C., 1988. Effect of excretory-secretory products of Giardia lamblia on glucose and phenylalanine transport in the small intestine of Swiss albino mice. Biochem. Int. 17, 801–812.

Scott, K.G., Meddings, J.B., Kirk, D.R., Lees-Miller, S.P., Buret, A.G., 2002. Intestinal infection with Giardia spp. reduces epithelial barrier function in a myosin light chain kinase-dependent fashion. Gastroenterology 123, 1179–1190.

Scott, K.G., Yu, L.C., Buret, A.G., 2004. Role of CD8+ and CD4+ T lymphocytes in jejunal mucosal injury during murine giardiasis. Infect. Immun. 72, 3536–3542.

Serradell, M.C., Saura, A., Rupil, L.L., Gargantini, P.R., Faya, M.I., Furlan, P.J., Lujan, H.D., 2016. Vaccination of domestic animals with a novel oral vaccine prevents. NPJ Vaccines 1, 16018.

Serradell, M.C., Gargantini, P.R., Saura, A., Oms, S.R., Rupil, L.L., Berod, L., Sparwasser, T., Luján, H.D., 2018. Cytokines, antibodies, and histopathological profiles during Giardia infection and variant-specific surface protein-based vaccination. Infect. Immun. 86, e00773.

Serradell, M.C., Rupil, L.L., Martino, R.A., Prucca, C.G., Carranza, P.G., Saura, A., Fernandez, E.A., Gargantini, P.R., Tenaglia, A.H., Petiti, J.P., Tonelli, R.R., Reinoso-Vizcaino, N., Echenique, J., Berod, L., Piaggio, E., Bellier, B., Sparwasser, T., Klatzman, D., Lujan, H.D., 2019. Efficient oral vaccination by bioengineering virus-like particles with protozoan surface proteins. Nat. Commun. 10, 361–375.

Shukla, G., Devi, P., Sehgal, R., 2008. Effect of Lactobacillus casei as a probiotic on modulation of giardiasis. Dig. Dis. Sci. 53, 2671–2679.

Shukla, G., Singh, S., Verma, A., 2013. Oral Administration of the Probiotic Lactobacillus casei ameliorates gut morphology and physiology in malnourished-Giardia intestinalis-infected BALB/c mice. ISRN Parasitol. 2013, 762638.

Shukla, G., Kamboj, S., Sharma, B., 2019. Comparative analysis of Antigiardial potential of heat inactivated and probiotic protein of probiotic lactobacillus rhamnosus GG in murine giardiasis. Probiotics Antimicrob. Proteins, in press.

Singer, S.M., Nash, T.E., 2000a. The role of Normal Flora in Giardia lamblia infections in mice. J. Infect. Dis. 181, 1510–1512.

Singer, S.M., Nash, T.E., 2000b. T-cell-dependent control of acute Giardia lamblia infections in mice. Infect. Immun. 68, 170–175.

Solaymani-Mohammadi, S., Singer, S.M., 2010. Giardia duodenalis: the double-edged sword of immune responses in giardiasis. Exp. Parasitol. 126, 292–297.

Solaymani-Mohammadi, S., Singer, S.M., 2011. Host immunity and pathogen strain contribute to intestinal disaccharidase impairment following gut infection. J. Immunol. 187, 3769–3775.

Stadelmann, B., Merino, M.C., Persson, L., Svard, S.G., 2012. Arginine consumption by the intestinal parasite Giardia intestinalis reduces proliferation of intestinal epithelial cells. PLoS One 7, e45325.

Summan, A., Nejsum, P., Williams, A.R., 2018. Modulation of human dendritic cell activity by Giardia and helminth antigens. Parasite Immunol. 40, e12525.

Tako, E.A., Hassimi, M.F., Li, E., Singer, S.M., 2013. Transcriptomic analysis of the host response to Giardia duodenalis infection reveals redundant mechanisms for parasite control. MBio 4, e00660–00613.

Toro-Londono, M.A., Bedoya-Urrego, K., Garcia-Montoya, G.M., Galvan-Diaz, A.L., Alzate, J.F., 2019. Intestinal parasitic infection alters bacterial gut microbiota in children. PeerJ 7, e6200.

Torres, M.F., Uetanabaro, A.P., Costa, A.F., Alves, C.A., Farias, L.M., Bambirra, E.A., Penna, F.J., Vieira, E.C., Nicoli, J.R., 2000. Influence of bacteria from the duodenal microbiota of patients with symptomatic giardiasis on the pathogenicity of Giardia duodenalis in gnotoxenic mice. J. Med. Microbiol. 49, 209–215.

Travers, M.A., Sow, C., Zirah, S., Deregnaucourt, C., Chaouch, S., Queiroz, R.M., Charneau, S., Allain, T., Florent, I., Grellier, P., 2016. Deconjugated bile salts produced by extracellular bile-salt hydrolase-like activities from the probiotic lactobacillus johnsonii La1 inhibit Giardia duodenalis in vitro growth. Front. Microbiol. 7, 1453.

Troeger, H., Epple, H.J., Schneider, T., Wahnschaffe, U., Ullrich, R., Burchard, G.D., Jelinek, T., Zeitz, M., Fromm, M., Schulzke, J.D., 2007. Effect of chronic Giardia lamblia infection on epithelial transport and barrier function in human duodenum. Gut 56, 328–335.

Ward, H.D., Alroy, J., Lev, B.I., Keusch, G.T., Pereira, M.E., 1988. Biology of Giardia lamblia. Detection of N-acetyl-D-glucosamine as the only surface saccharide moiety and identification of two distinct subsets of trophozoites by lectin binding. J. Exp. Med. 167, 73–88.

Weatherhead, J., Cortés, A.A., Sandoval, C., Vaca, M., Chico, M., Loor, S., Cooper, P.J., Mejia, R., 2017. Comparison of cytokine responses in Ecuadorian children infected with. Am. J. Trop. Med. Hyg. 96, 1394–1399.

Weaver, C.T., Harrington, L.E., Mangan, P.R., Gavrieli, M., Murphy, K.M., 2006. Th17: an effector CD4 T cell lineage with regulatory T cell ties. Immunity 24, 677–688.

Zarebavani, M., Dargahi, D., Einollahi, N., Dashti, N., Mohebali, M., Rezaeian, M., 2012. Serum levels of zinc, copper, vitamin B12, folate and immunoglobulins in individuals with giardiasis. Iran. J. Public Health 41, 47–53.

Zhou, P., Li, E., Zhu, N., Robertson, J., Nash, T., Singer, S.M., 2003. Role of interleukin-6 in the control of acute and chronic Giardia lamblia infections in mice. Infect. Immun. 71, 1566–1568.

Zhou, P., Li, E., Shea-Donohue, T., Singer, S.M., 2007. Tumour necrosis factor alpha contributes to protection against Giardia lamblia infection in mice. Parasite Immunol. 29, 367–374.

CHAPTER SIX

Molecular epidemiology of giardiasis from a veterinary perspective

Una Ryan*, Alireza Zahedi
College of Science, Health, Education and Engineering, Murdoch University, Perth, WA, Australia
*Corresponding author: e-mail address: una.ryan@murdoch.edu.au

Contents

Abstract

A total of eight *Giardia* species are accepted. These include: *Giardia duodenalis* (syn. *Giardia intestinalis* and *Giardia lamblia*), which infects humans and animals, *Giardia agilis*, *Giardia ardeae*, *Giardia psittaci*, *Giardia muris*, *Giardia microti*, *Giardia peramelis* and *G. cricetidarum,* which infect non-human hosts including amphibians, birds, rodents and marsupials. *Giardia duodenalis* is a species complex consisting of eight assemblages (A-H), with assemblages A and B the dominant assemblages in humans. Molecular studies to date on the zoonotic potential of *Giardia* in animals are problematic and are hampered by lack of concordance between loci. Livestock (cattle, sheep, goats and pigs) are predominantly infected with *G. duodenalis* assemblage E, which has recently been shown to be zoonotic, followed by assemblage A. In cats and dogs, assemblages A, B, C, D and F are commonly reported but relatively few studies have conducted molecular typing of humans and their pets and the results are contradictory with some studies support zoonotic transmission but the majority of studies suggesting

Advances in Parasitology, Volume 106
ISSN 0065-308X
https://doi.org/10.1016/bs.apar.2019.07.002

separate transmission cycles. *Giardia* also infects a broad range of wildlife hosts and although much less well studied, host-adapted species as well as *G. duodenalis* assemblages (A-H) have been identified. Fish and other aquatic wildlife represent a source of infection for humans with *Giardia* via water contamination and/or consumption of undercooked fish and interestingly, assemblage B and A predominated in the two molecular studies conducted to date. Our current knowledge of the transmission dynamics of *Giardia* is still poor and the development of more discriminatory typing tools such as whole genome sequencing (WGS) of *Giardia* isolates is therefore essential.

1. Introduction

The protozoan parasite *Giardia*, is a very common enteric parasite of humans and animals with a global distribution and 250–300 million symptomatic human infections reported annually and is responsible for numerous waterborne outbreaks (Einarsson et al., 2016; Feng and Xiao, 2011; Karanis et al., 2007). Clinical signs of giardiasis in animals range from asymptomatic to diarrhoea and failure to thrive (Feng and Xiao, 2011; Siwila, 2017). The pathogenesis in humans and animals is not well understood but is due to both parasite and host factors including parasite virulence, host immunity and the prevalence of cysts in the environment (Geurden et al., 2010a).

Currently eight *Giardia* species are accepted as valid. These include: *Giardia duodenalis* (syn. *Giardia intestinalis* and *Giardia lamblia*), *Giardia agilis*, *Giardia ardeae*, *Giardia psittaci*, *Giardia muris*, *Giardia microti Giardia peramelis* and *G. cricetidarum* (Monis et al., 2009; Ryan and Cacciò, 2013; Hillman et al., 2016; Lyu et al., 2018) (Table 1). Of these, *G. duodenalis* has the broadest host range infecting humans and a wide variety of animals, whereas the remaining species predominantly infect amphibians, rodents, birds and marsupials (Chilvers et al., 2010). *Giardia duodenalis* is a species complex consisting of eight assemblages; assemblages A and B, which commonly infect humans and other mammals, assemblages C and D in dogs and other canids, assemblage E in hoofed animals, assemblage F in cats, assemblage G in rodents and assemblage H in pinnipeds (Cacciò et al., 2018; Table 1). Until recently, assemblages C-H were considered host specific, but sporadic cases of assemblages C, D, E and F have been reported in humans (Broglia et al., 2013; Gelanew et al., 2007; Liu et al., 2014; Scalia et al., 2016; Štrkolcová et al., 2015; Zahedi et al., 2017) and therefore these assemblages should be considered potentially zoonotic. However, it should be noted that these reports have been based on the detection of *Giardia* DNA and not demonstration

Table 1 Recognised *Giardia* species and assemblages.

***Giardia* spp./ assemblages**	**Author(s)**	**Major hosts**	**Reports in humans**
G. duodenalis	Filice (1952)	Mammals	Commonly reported
Assemblage A		Wide range of mammals (including humans)	Commonly reported
Assemblage B		Wide range of mammals (including humans)	Commonly reported
Assemblage C	Hopkins et al. (1997), Monis et al. (1998)	Canids	Reports in humans in China and Slovakia
Assemblage D	Hopkins et al. (1997), Monis et al. (1998)	Canids	Single report in German travellers
Assemblage E	Ey et al. (1997)	Hoofed animals	Several reports
Assemblage F	Monis et al. (1999)	Felines	Single report in humans in Ethiopia
Assemblage G	Monis et al. (1999)	Rodents	None reported
Assemblage H	Lasek-Nesselquist et al. (2010)	Pinnipeds	None reported
G. agilis	Kunstler (1882)	Amphibians	None reported
G. microti	Filice (1952)	Rodents	None reported
G. muris	Filice (1952)	Rodents	None reported
G. ardeae	Filice (1952)	Birds	None reported
G. psittaci	Erlandsen and Bemrick (1987)	Birds	None reported
G. peramelis	Hillman et al. (2016)	Southern brown bandicoots (*Isoodon obesulus*)	None reported
G. cricetidarum	Lyu et al. (2018)	Hamsters (*Phodopus sungorus*)	None reported

of an actual infection. Assemblages A and B can be subtyped into sub-assemblages (e.g. AI, AII, AIII, BIII and BIV) using multilocus typing to facilitate transmission studies (Cacciò et al., 2018). Sub-assemblages AI and AII infect humans and animals (with AII more commonly identified in humans), whereas sub-assemblage AIII appears to predominantly infect wild hoofed animals (Cacciò et al., 2008; Lebbad et al., 2010).

The reported prevalences of *Giardia* in animals varies with the diagnostic methods used, the number of faecal samples screened per individual, the age and immune status of the animals screened and the geographic area studied, with microscopy performing poorly compared to other detection methods in most studies (Ballweber et al., 2010; Bouzid et al., 2015). Animal hosts can become infected through the ingestion of infectious cysts from contaminated environments. The maximum cyst excretion can be as high as 1.7×10^6, 4.7×10^9, 2.1×10^4 and 2.25×10^5 cysts per gram of faeces for cattle, sheep, pigs and dogs respectively (Mark-Carew et al., 2010; Petersen et al., 2015; Rehbein et al., 2019; Yang et al., 2014), with peaks in young animals, due to the slow development of immunity by the host (O'Handley et al., 2003). Young animals should therefore be considered as the major source of transmission however, adult hosts are also a source of infection with periparturient rises in cyst excretion reported in sheep, goats, pigs and cattle (Castro-Hermida et al., 2005; Wade et al., 2000; Xiao and Herd, 1994).

As *G. duodenalis* assemblages are morphologically identical, molecular tools are required to identify them. The most commonly used loci for typing *Giardia* are 18S rRNA, glutamate dehydrogenase (*gdh*), elongation factor 1-alfa (*el1-α*), triose-phosphate isomerase (*tpi*) and β-giardin (*bg*) (Ryan and Cacciò, 2013). Molecular studies conducted to date however, are problematic as some studies have only used one locus, which frequently does not detect mixed infections or provide sufficient information to determine possible zoonotic transmission and/or have relied on restriction fragment polymorphism analysis rather than sequencing. Also, sequence analysis of the 18S rRNA and/or the elongation factor alpha gene is problematic as these loci cannot accurately discriminate within assemblages A or B and are therefore not useful for transmission studies (Traub et al., 2004). The 18S locus is particularly problematic as many studies which rely on typing at the 18S locus use a very small amplicon (292 bp) (based on primers by Hopkins et al., 1997), with very few genetic differences between the assemblages. Even when multiple loci have been used, there is frequently a lack of concordance between loci due to either mixed infections or allelic sequence heterogeneity (Cacciò et al., 2008; Ryan and Cacciò, 2013). The 18S locus is most commonly associated with discordant typing results when compared with other loci, largely due to the limited number of distinguishing single nucleotide polymorphisms between assemblages at this locus.

2. *Giardia* in livestock

Giardia duodenalis is one of the most commonly identified protozoan parasites in livestock, particularly sheep, cattle and goats. Infections are frequently asymptomatic but can cause diarrhoea and can impair the growth and development of calves (Geurden et al., 2010a,b). In sheep and goats, *Giardia* can cause severe diarrhoea, depression, weight loss and mortality (Bomfim et al., 2005; O'Handley and Olson, 2006; Geurden et al., 2008) and have been associated with poor feed efficiency and decreased weight gain (Geurden et al., 2010a). In pigs, *Giardia* has been associated with diarrhoea (Armson et al., 2009), however high rates of infection have also been reported in asymptomatic pigs (Akinkuotu et al., 2019). Treatment options are limited in livestock. In calves, repeat fenbendazole treatments reduced the number of infective cysts shed by calves and improved weight gain, but calves rapidly became re-infected (Geurden et al., 2010b; O'Handley et al., 2000). In experimentally infected calves, paromomycin reduced *Giardia* cyst excretion, when administered at 50 and 75 mg/kg/day during five consecutive days (Geurden et al., 2006). Control programs which combine both treatment and reducing cyst contamination of the environment are essential to minimise the risk of reinfection. Flies have also been shown to be transport vehicles for *Giardia* on farms, with 5% of batches of flies at a dairy farm in China identified as positive for *Giardia* (Zhao et al., 2014).

Assemblage E is the dominant assemblage reported in livestock in most studies. As discussed above, this assemblage was previously thought to be host-specific but has been reported in humans in several studies (Abdel-Moein and Saeed, 2016; Fantinatti et al., 2016; Foronda et al., 2008; Helmy et al., 2014; Scalia et al., 2016; Zahedi et al., 2017) and at a whole genome level, assemblages A and E are more similar to each than to assemblage B (Franzén et al., 2009; Jerlström-Hultqvist et al., 2010).

2.1 *Giardia* in cattle and other bovids

Giardia has a worldwide distribution in cattle. The prevalence of *G. duodenalis* in cattle varies in different studies with prevalences ranging from 1.09% to 74.2% (Feng and Xiao, 2011; Feng et al., 2019) (Table 2), but are generally much higher in calves and in dairy cattle compared to beef cattle (Abeywardena et al., 2015; Bartley et al., 2018; Feng and Xiao, 2011;

Table 2 Reports of *Giardia duodenalis* prevalence and assemblages in livestock since 2012.[a]

Animal	Location	No of samples	Prevalence (%)	No of samples typed	Assemblages				References
					A	B	E	Other	
Buffalo	Australia	476	13	13	10	0	3	0	Abeywardena et al. (2013a)
Buffalo	Sri Lanka	297	0.7	2	0	0	2	0	Abeywardena et al. (2014)
Cattle	Australia	175	36.6	29	0	9	20	0	Asher et al. (2016)
Cattle	Australia	474	29.5	140	10	0	130	0	Abeywardena et al. (2013b)
Cattle	Bangladesh	623	22	60	10	3	47	0	Ehsan et al. (2015)
Cattle	Brazil	256	11.7	9	0	0	9	0	Fava et al. (2013)
Cattle	Canada	739	42	25	2	0	23	0	Budu-Amoako et al. (2012)
Cattle	China	388	74.2	288	1	0	282	Mixed A and E (n=5)	Feng et al. (2019)
Cattle	China	1440	2.2	31	2	0	29	0	Cui et al. (2018)
Cattle	China	389	10	39	0	0	39	0	Jian et al. (2018)
Cattle	China	339	22.6	77	0	0	77	0	Fan et al. (2017)
Cattle	China	1040	4.7	49	0	0	47	Mixed A and E (n=2)	Hu et al. (2017)
Cattle	China	818	60.1	492	5	1	482	Mixed A and E (n=4)	Wang et al. (2017a)
Cattle	China	822	1.09	9	0	0	9	0	Li et al. (2016a)
Cattle	China	371	18.9	70	8	0	62	0	Wang et al. (2016a)
Cattle	China	2945	3.6	107	1	0	106	0	Zhang et al. (2016b)

Cattle	China	655	7.9	52	1	0	50	Mixed A and E (n=1)	Liu et al. (2015)
Cattle	China	1366	2.1	29	0	4	25	0	Huang et al. (2014)
Cattle	China	1777	7.2	79	58	0	21	Mixed A and E (n=2)	Wang et al. (2014)
Cattle	Egypt	248	13.3	33	1	0	32	0	Naguib et al. (2018)
Cattle	Ethiopia	449	9.6	43	2	0	41	0	Wegayehu et al. (2016)
Cattle	Germany	536	51.2	110	8	0	101	Mixed A and E (n=1)	Gillhuber et al. (2013)
Cattle	Ghana	328	8.5	14	0	0	14	9	Squire et al. (2017)
Cattle	Iran	246	9.3	23	4	0	19	0	Malekifard and Ahmadpour (2018)
Cattle	Korea	590	13.1	15	0	0	15	0	Lee et al. (2016)
Cattle	Korea	90	10	7	2	0	5	0	Lee et al. (2018)
Cattle	Malaysia	240	12.5	25	0	0	25	0	Muhid et al. (2012)
Cattle	New Zealand	180	6.1	11	2	0	9	0	Abeywardena et al. (2012)
Cattle	Poland	86	18.6	5	1	0	4	0	Stojecki et al. (2015a)
Cattle	Sicily	149	35.6	27	5	0	22	0	Di Piazza et al. (2013)
Cattle	Scotland	388	32.5	66	3	12	51	0	Bartley et al. (2018)
Cattle	Spain	362	12.4	19	0	0	15	F (n=4)	Cardona et al. (2015)
Cattle	Sri Lanka	340	41.5	141	4	0	137	0	Abeywardena et al. (2014)
Cattle	Thailand	900	6	54	12	0	42	0	Inpankaew et al. (2015)

Continued

Table 2 Reports of *Giardia duodenalis* prevalence and assemblages in livestock since 2012.[a]—cont'd

Animal	Location	No of samples	Prevalence (%)	No of samples typed	Assemblages				References
					A	B	E	Other	
Cattle	Uganda	45	4.4	1	0	0	1	0	Nolan et al. (2017)
Cattle	UK	283	32.9	63	16	0	33	C (2), D (4), Mixed A and C (n=1) Mixed A and D (n=1) Mixed A and E (n=6)	Minetti et al. (2014)
Cattle	US	2109	23.9	131	29	0	102	0	Mark-Carew et al. (2012)
Cattle	US	819	33.5	274	10	0	260	Mixed A and E (n=4)	Santin et al. (2012)
Cattle	Vietnam	412	13.8	25	0	0	25	0	Nguyen et al. (2016)
Yaks	China	297	5.4	10	0	0	10	0	Wang et al. (2017a)
Yaks	China	344	5.2	18	0	9	9	0	Wang et al. (2018)
Yaks	China	605	10.4	63	2	0	60	Mixed A and E (n=1)	Jin et al. (2017)
Yaks	China	208	1.9	4	0	0	4	0	Song et al. (2016)
Yaks	China	545	6	16	0	0	16	0	Qi et al. (2015a)
Sheep	Australia	3412	20.2	473	106	0	359	Mixed A and E (n=8)	Yang et al. (2014)
Sheep	Australia								
Sheep	Brazil	100	34	34	0	0	34	0	Paz e Silva et al. (2014)
Sheep	Brazil	105	24.8	14	0	0	14	0	Fava et al. (2013)
Tibetan Sheep	China	177	1.7	3	0	0	3	0	Wu et al. (2018)

Tibetan Sheep	China	495	13.1	75	10	0	51	Mixed A and E (n=4)	Jin et al. (2017)
Sheep	China	716	4.3	36	5	0	31	Mixed E and A (3)	Wang et al. (2016b)
Sheep	China	375	4.3	13	13	0	0	0	Ye et al. (2015)
Sheep	China	539	5.6	25	4	2	19	0	Zhang et al. (2012a)
Sheep	Ethiopia	389	2.6	10	0	0	10	0	Wegayehu et al. (2017)
Sheep	Ghana	217	12.9	12	0	0	12	0	Squire et al. (2017)
Sheep	Greece	429	37.3	39	1	0	35	Mixed A and E (n=3)	Tzanidakis et al. (2014)
Sheep	Iran	86	19.8	14	0	0	14	0	Jafari et al. (2014)
Sheep	Poland	81	21	14	6	0	8	0	Stojecki et al. (2015a)
Sheep	Spain	120	89.2	107	59	0	21	Mixed A and E (n=27)	Gómez-Muñoz et al. (2012)
Sheep	UK	64	43.7	24	4	0	19	C (1)	Minetti et al. (2014)
Goats	Australia	500	7.6	26	0	0	26	0	Al-Habsi et al. (2017)
Goats	China	907	4.2	38	0	0	38	0	Xie et al. (2018)
Goats	China	1311	7.1	93	4	3	84	Mixed A and E (n=2)	Yin et al. (2018)
Goats	China	342	14.9	51	0	0	51	0	Zhong et al. (2018a,b,c)
Goats	China	139	2.9	4	0	0	4	0	Zhang et al. (2012a)
Goats	China	315	12.7	80	4	0	76	0	Peng et al. (2016)
Goats	China	342	4.7	16	0	0	16	0	Zhong et al. (2018a,b,c)
Goats	China	629	12.7	80	4		76	0	Peng et al. (2016)

Continued

Table 2 Reports of *Giardia duodenalis* prevalence and assemblages in livestock since 2012.[a]—cont'd

Animal	Location	No of samples	Prevalence (%)	No of samples typed	Assemblages				References
					A	B	E	Other	
Goats	China	506	6.3	23	0	0	23	0	
Goats	Ghana	285	12.3	3	0	0	3	0	Squire et al. (2017)
Goats	Greece	255	40.4	30	1	0	26	Mixed A and E (n=3)	Tzanidakis et al. (2014)
Goats	India	207	33.8	28	10	9	8	D (1)	Utaaker et al. (2017)
Goats	Iran	94	15.9	5	0	0	5	0	Jafari et al. (2014)
Goat- antelope (Chamois)	Italy	157	4.4	7	4	0	3	0	De Liberato et al. (2015)
Goat	Malaysia	310	6.8	16	3	1	12	0	Lim et al. (2013)
Goats	Tanzania	41	21.9	9	1	2	6	0	Di Cristanziano et al. (2014)
Pigs	Nigeria	209	25.4	55	0	14	37	Mixed B and E (n=4)	Akinkuotu et al. (2019)
Pigs (wild boar)	China	357	3.1	11	2	0	9	0	Li et al. (2017a)
Pigs	China	560	8.0	45	9	0	36	0	Wang et al. (2017b)
Pigs	Denmark	856	14.0	13	2	0	11	0	Petersen et al. (2015)
Pigs	Poland	84	29.8	5	0	1	4	0	Stojecki et al. (2015a)
Pigs (feral)	US	370	4.3	16	6	0	10	0	Rodriguez-Rivera et al. (2016)

[a]Data prior to 2012 is detailed in the review by Feng and Xiao (2011).

Mahato et al., 2018). Numerous studies worldwide have reported that assemblage E is the most common assemblage detected in cattle (Table 2), followed by assemblage A (sub-assemblages AI and AII) and more rarely assemblage B (BIII and BIV). One study also reported assemblages C, D and F in cattle in England and Wales (Minetti et al., 2014) and assemblage F was also reported in asymptomatic cattle in Spain (Cardona et al., 2015). However, in the study by Minetti et al. (2014), samples were only typed at the 18S locus. In another recent study in cattle in the UK (n=388), assemblage B was the second most common assemblage detected in cattle (after assemblage E) at the β-giardin locus and was reported at a prevalence of 18.2% compared to only 4.6% for assemblage A (Bartley et al., 2018). In that study, assemblage B sequences from cattle were 100% identical to assemblages B sequences from humans in Spain, suggest that cattle can be a reservoir for assemblage with consequent public health implications (Bartley et al., 2018). Few studies have specifically examined *Giardia* assemblages in cattle handlers and their calves and the data to date is equivocal. For example, a study in India, which used RFLP and sequence analysis of the β-giardin gene, detected assemblages A1 and AII (n=6) and B (n=8) in farm workers and A1 (n=5), E (n=15) and mixed A and E (n=3) in cattle (Khan et al., 2011). The AI β-giardin gene sequences from humans and cattle were 100% identical to each other, suggesting possible zoonotic transmission. In a more recent study in Bangladesh however, assemblages AII and BIII were identified in cattle handlers and assemblage E and AI in the calves, suggesting that zoonotic transmission was not occurring in that setting (Ehsan et al., 2015).

Very high levels of genetic diversity within assemblage E have been reported in some studies (Feng et al., 2019; Wang et al., 2017a; Zhang et al., 2016a), the reasons for which are unknown, but intra-assemblage genetic recombination has been suggested as a possible cause (Aguiar et al., 2016; Cacciò et al., 2008). With the exception of yaks (*Bos grunniens*) and water buffalo (*Bubalus bubalis*), relatively little is known about *Giardia* in other bovids (Abeywardena et al., 2015), with assemblages A (AII), E and B reported in yaks (Table 2) and assemblages E and A in water buffalo (Table 2).

2.2 *Giardia* in sheep

The prevalence of *Giardia* in sheep ranges from 1.5% to 89.2%, with lambs seven times more likely to be positive for *G. duodenalis* than adult sheep (Feng and Xiao, 2011; Ryan et al., 2005; Table 2). In addition to clinical signs, giardiasis in sheep also has production effects, with *Giardia* shedding pre-slaughter associated with reduced hot standard carcase weight (HSCW) (weight within 2 h of slaughter of a carcase with standard trim, all fats out) and dressing percentage (carcase weight expressed as a percentage of live weight) (Jacobson et al., 2016; Sweeny et al., 2012).

Assemblages E and A (AI and AII) are commonly reported in sheep (Table 2) with assemblage B rarely reported. In one study in Italy however, an outbreak of giardiasis in sheep which resulted in loose faeces, decreased weight gain and impairment in feed efficiency was attributed to *G. duodenalis* assemblage B (in the absence of viral, bacterial or parasitic pathogens in faeces or tissue samples) (Aliosio et al., 2006). In that study, the infection cleared after treatment with fenbendazole (10 mg/kg for 3 consecutive days). As with cattle, high levels of genetic diversity within assemblage E have been reported in sheep (Jin et al., 2017; Wegayehu et al., 2017; Xie et al., 2018).

2.3 *Giardia* in goats

Giardia is less well studied in goats with prevalences ranging from 4% to 43.5% reported (Feng and Xiao, 2011; Table 2). *G. duodenalis* assemblages A (AI, AII), B and E have been reported in goats with assemblage E most commonly reported (Table 2). There has been one report of assemblage D in goats, which was speculated to be due to mechanical transmission from goats ingesting canine faeces (Utaaker et al., 2017).

2.4 *Giardia* in pigs

Giardia duodenalis has been reported in pigs worldwide with prevalences ranging from 3.5% to 31.1% (Feng and Xiao, 2011; Langkjaer et al., 2007; Sprong et al., 2009; Table 2). Assemblages A, B (BIII, BIV), D and E have been reported. As with other livestock, assemblage E predominates, followed by assemblage A (Table 2; Feng and Xiao, 2011). One study reported that the presence of assemblage E in pigs was significantly associated with soft to diarrhoeic stool ($P < 0.05$), whereas assemblage A was not (Armson et al., 2009). In a recent study, a high prevalence of assemblage B was reported in pigs in Nigeria (Akinkuotu et al., 2019).

3. *Giardia* in companion animals

Giardia infections in dogs are mostly asymptomatic although clinical signs can occur ranging from slight abdominal discomfort to severe abdominal pain, cramping and soft to watery diarrhoea (Tangtrongsup and Scorza, 2010).

In cats, as with dogs, infections are mostly asymptomatic but clinical signs include acute diarrhoea and weight loss (Janeczko and Griffin, 2010). The prevalence of *Giardia* in cats and dogs varies widely from 1.1% to 45.9% (Table 3; Ballweber et al., 2010; Bouzid et al., 2015; Esch and Petersen, 2013; Feng and Xiao, 2011; Lucio-Forster et al., 2010; Ramírez-Ocampo et al., 2017), with the highest prevalence in younger animals and in kennel or shelter populations (Ballweber et al., 2010).

Dogs and cats have close personal relationships which favours increased transmission of *Giardia*. This potential for zoonotic transmission of *Giardia* from companion animals to humans has been widely used a rationale for treatment and febantel has been registered for dogs, fenbendazole for dogs and cats and nitazoxanide which is used to treat *Giardia* in humans, has been shown to reduce *Giardia* cyst shedding in dogs (Moron-Soto et al., 2017). A veterinary vaccine called GiardiaVax, which consists of killed trophozoites isolated from a sheep (unknown assemblage) for nonchronically infected dogs and cats has been licensed (Geurden et al., 2014; Olson et al., 2000). However, the efficacy of the vaccine is variable with some studies reporting it as ineffective (Anderson et al., 2004) and it has been withdrawn from use in several countries (Geurden et al., 2014). More recently, an oral vaccine formulation based on trophozoite variant-specific surface proteins (VSPs) was tested on gerbils, dogs and cats and it was reported that the reduced clinical signs in infected animals and prevented new infections (Serradell et al., 2016). Also, in that study, the number of children infected with *Giardia* in a highly endemic area decreased after immunisation of dogs in the area with the vaccine, suggesting that it has transmission blocking potential (Serradell et al., 2016), however, further studies are required.

The molecular epidemiology of giardiasis in cats and dogs has been extensively reviewed (Ballweber et al., 2010; Bouzid et al., 2015; Esch and Petersen, 2013; Feng and Xiao, 2011; Lucio-Forster et al., 2010; Ramírez-Ocampo et al., 2017). However, the role of dogs and cats as a source of human giardiasis is still unclear, particularly as some studies only used one locus or relied on restriction fragment polymorphism analysis and where multiple loci have been used due to the lack of concordance between loci, particularly between the 18S rRNA and other loci (Table 3; cf. Ballweber et al., 2010; Lucio-Forster et al., 2010). Assemblages A (A1 and AII), B (BIII, BIV), C, D and F have been identified in dogs. Some studies, have reported a high prevalence of assemblage A (mostly AII) and or B in dogs (Adell-Aledón et al., 2018; Ballweber et al., 2010; Fantinatti et al., 2018; Gultekin et al., 2017; Lee et al., 2017; Lucio-Forster et al., 2010), with the same

Table 3 Molecular detection of *G. duodenalis* in companion animals from 2015 on.[a]

Animal	Location	No of samples	Prevalence (%)	No of samples typed	Assemblages				References
					A	B	C	Other	
Dogs	Australia	721	16.1	42	0	0	42	0	Ash et al., (2019)
Dogs	Brazil	97	19.6	19	0	0	0	D (n=19)	Fava et al. (2016)
Dogs	Brazil	32	6.3	2	0	1	1	0	Colli et al. (2015)
Dogs	China	485	12.8	21	0	0	5	D (n=15) (F (n=1)	Yu et al. (2018)
Dogs	China	159	11.3	22	0	0	13	D (n=9)	Zhang et al. (2017)
Dogs	China	940	14.3	51	0	0	19	D (n=32)	Qi et al. (2016)
Dogs	China	267	13	13	0	0	7	E (n=5)	Li et al. (2015a)
Dogs	China	205	13.2	27	25	0	2	0	Li et al. (2013)
Dogs	Germany	31	42	6	2	0	1	Mixed A and B (n=1), D (n=2)	Rehbein et al. (2019)
Dogs	Germany	376	12.2	33	0	0	7	D (n=25), F (n=1)	Sommer et al. (2018)
Dogs	Germany	NR	NR	60	8	0	0	C (n=15), D (n=20), F (n=2), Mixed C and D (n=13), mixed B and D (n=2)	Pallant et al. (2015) (data based on *bg* locus)
Dogs	Greece	879	25.2	95	2	0	47	D (n=25), Mixed C and D (n=15), A with C or D (n=5), and C (n=1)	Kostopoulou et al. (2017)
Dogs	Italy	262	21.4	25	0	0	6	D (n=19)	Liberato et al. (2018)

Dogs	Italy	705	28.9	21	0	1	9	D (n = 11)	Simonato et al. (2017)
Dogs	Italy	502	8.2	20	0	0	15	D (n = 2), Mixed C and D (n = 3)	Paoletti et al. (2015)
Dogs	Italy	318	15.1	79	0	1	49	D (n = 29)	Simonato et al. (2015)
Dogs	Jamaica	225	19.6	44	43	0	0	Mixed A and B (n = 1)	Lee et al. (2017)
Dogs	Mexico	21	23.8	5	5	0	0	0	García-Cervantes et al. (2017)
Dogs	Poland	128	21.1	22	0	1	18	D (n = 2), Mixed C and D (n = 1)	Piekarska et al. (2016)
Dogs	Poland	36	19.4	2	1	0	1	0	Stojecki et al. (2015a)
Dogs	South Korea	202	33.2	3	2	0	1	0	Shin et al. (2015)
Dogs	Spain	348	36.5	35	5	8	2	D (n = 13), Mixed A and B (n = 4) Mixed A and D (n = 1), Mixed A, B and D (n = 1)	Adell-Aledón et al. (2018)
Dogs	Spain	55	29	0	0	0	3	0	de Lucio et al. (2017)
Dogs	Spain	194	33	19	7 (AII)	8	3	D (n = 1)	Gil et al. (2017)
Dogs	Spain	108	9.2	10	5 (A1)	3	2	0	Quadros et al. (2016)
Dogs	Thailand	109	45.9	21	0	0	8	D (n = 11), Mixed C and D (n = 2)	Tangtrongsup et al. (2017)
Dogs	Turkey	473	18.8	89	0	51	0	Mixed A and B (n = 38)	Gultekin et al. (2017)
Dogs	US	84	32	10	0	0	2	D (n = 4), Mixed C and D (n = 4)	Scorza and Lappin (2017)
Dogs	US	120	15	16	16	0	0	D (n = 1)	Munoz and Mayer (2016)

Continued

Table 3 Molecular detection of *G. duodenalis* in companion animals from 2015 on.[a]—cont'd

Animal	Location	No of samples	Prevalence (%)	No of samples typed	Assemblages				References
					A	B	C	Other	
Dogs	Vietnam	209	8.6	15	0	0	10	D (n=5)	Nguyen et al. (2018)
Cats	Australia	345	10.1	10	1	0	0	F (n=9)	Yang et al. (2015)
Cats	China	52	1.9	1	0	0	0	F (n=1)	Li et al. (2015a)
Cats	China	102	9.8	10	8	0	0	F (n=1), Mixed A and C (n=1)	Zheng et al. (2015)
Cats	Germany	145	5.5	4	0	0	0	F (n=4)	Sommer et al. (2018)
Cats	Germany	NR	NR	21	1	0	0	F (n=15), C (n=1), D (n=1), mixed A, D and F (n=3)	Pallant et al. (2015) (data based on bg locus)
Cats	Greece	264	20.5	14	6	1	1	F (n=2) Mixed F and A (n=4),	Kostopoulou et al. (2017)
Cats	Japan	342	18.7	41	5	0	1	F (n=28) Mixed F and A (n=4), Mixed F and C (n=2), Mixed C and D (n=1),	Ito et al. (2017)
Cats	Poland	33	15.1	1	0	0	0	F (n=4),	Piekarska et al. (2016)
Cats	Spain	34	5.9	3	2	0	0	F (n=2)	de Lucio et al. (2017)
Cats	Spain	65	9.2	1	1	0	0	F (n=1)	Gil et al. (2017)

[a]The prevalence in cats and dogs prior to 2015 has been extensively reviewed in Ballweber et al. (2010), Lucio-Forster et al. (2010), Esch and Petersen (2013), Bouzid et al. (2015), Feng and Xiao (2011) and Ramírez-Ocampo et al. (2017).

sub-assemblage (AII) dominant in both humans and dogs (but not from the same localities) (Lee et al., 2017). However, the majority of studies have reported that assemblage C and D is more common in dogs (Table 3; cf. Ballweber et al., 2010; Lucio-Forster et al., 2010). In cats, assemblages A (AI and AII), B (BIII and BIV), C, D, E and F have been reported, with assemblage F the most common, followed by assemblage A (Ramírez-Ocampo et al., 2017).

Relatively few studies have conducted molecular typing of humans and their pets. Of these, some studies, have identified assemblages A and or B in both humans and dogs (Inpankaew et al., 2007; Minvielle et al., 2008; Traub et al., 2004), however, the majority of studies have shown that molecular data does not support transmission of *Giardia* from pets to humans (Ballweber et al., 2010; Inpankaew et al., 2014; Lucio-Forster et al., 2010; Souza et al., 2007; van der Giessen et al., 2006). The most recent study was conducted in households with dogs and cats in Berlin/Brandenburg (Germany) and reported that while both a dog and a human from the same household were positive for assemblage B at the *tpi* locus, the sequences were only 98% similar (Rehbein et al., 2019). Another study in Spain, which examined faecal samples from 179 humans, 55 dogs, and 34 cats, identified assemblage BIV in a single human isolate and assemblage C and F in dogs and cats respectively (de Lucio et al., 2017). More multilocus typing studies need to be conducted on isolates longitudinally over consecutive days from humans and their pets from the same household to better understand the transmission dynamics of *Giardia* between humans and pets.

4. *Giardia* in wildlife

Giardia infects a broad range of wildlife hosts including mammals, amphibians, reptiles, birds and fish worldwide, causing asymptomatic or mild to severe gastrointestinal disease in their host species (Cacciò et al., 2018; Feng and Xiao, 2011; Ryan and Cacciò, 2013).

Unlike livestock, where the molecular epidemiology and transmission dynamics of *G. duodenalis* have been extensively studied, giardiasis in wildlife has only been investigated opportunistically and relatively little is known about the distribution, genetic diversity and zoonotic potential of *Giardia* spp. and assemblages in terrestrial and aquatic wildlife populations (Cacciò et al., 2018; Li et al., 2017a). Host-adapted species (*G. muris, G. microti, G. peramelis, G. agilis, G. cricetidarum, G. ardeae* and *G. psittaci* as well as *G. duodenalis* assemblages (Tables 4–6) have been identified.

Table 4 *G. duodenalis* assemblages/sub-assemblages identified with molecular tools in captive and wild animals.

Host species	Assemblages/ sub-assemblages	References
Aquatic mammals: Atlantic harbour seal (*Phoca vituline vitulina*), Grey seal (*Halichoerus grypus*), Pacific harbour seals (*Phoca vitulina richardsi*), harp seal (*Phoca groenlandica*), hooded seal (*Cystophora cristata*), ringed seals (*Phoca hispida*), bearded seals (*Erignathus barbatus*), harbour porpoise (*Phocoena phocoena*), striped dolphin (*Stenella coeruleoalba*), minke whale (*Balaenoptera acutorostrata*) and a Pygmy Sperm Whale (*Kogia breviceps*)	A (AI and AII), B, C, D, F and H	Dixon et al. (2008), Gaydos et al. (2008), Appelbee et al. (2010), Lasek-Nesselquist et al. (2010), Reboredo-Fernández et al. (2015a)
Anteater (*Tanamuda* sp.)	B	Solarczyk (2009)
Beech marten (*Martes foina*)	NA	Mateo et al. (2017)
Hoofed animals: Alpine chamois (*Rupicapra rupicapra rupicapra*), Apennine chamois (*Rupicapra pyrenaica ornata*), Caribou (*Rangifer tarandus*), Fallow Deer (*Dama dama*), Orest musk deer (*Moschus berezovskii*), Gazelle (*Gazella thomsonii*), Moose (*Alces alces*), Muskoxen (*Ovibos moschatus*), Père David's deer (*Elaphurus davidianus*), Red deer (*Cervus elaphus*), Reindeer (*Rangifer tarandus*), Roe deer (*Capreolus capreolus*), Sika deer (*Cervus nippon*), Samber deer (*Rusa unicolor*), Scimitar horned oryx (*Oryx dammah*), Water buffalo (*Bubalus bubalis*), White-tailed Deer (*Odocoileus virginianus*), Wild boar (*Sus scrofa*)	AI, AII, AIII, B, D and E	Trout et al. (2003), Lalle et al. (2005), (2007), Cacciò et al. (2007, 2008), Paziewska et al. (2007), Robertson et al. (2007), Solarczyk (2009), Johnson et al. (2010), Lebbad et al. (2010), Beck et al. (2011b), Majewska et al. (2012), Solarczyk et al. (2012), Solarczyk et al. (2014), De Liberato et al. (2015), Li et al. (2016a,b), Stojecki et al. (2015a), Stojecki et al. (2015b), Li et al. (2017a), Adriana et al. (2016), Koehler et al. (2016), Huang et al. (2018), Song et al. (2018)
Marsupials: Brush-tailed rock-wallaby (*Petrogale penicillata*), Common planigale (*Planigale maculata*), Quenda (*Isoodon obesulus*), Quokka (*Setonix brachyurus*), Red kangaroo (*Macropus rufus*), Spotted-tailed quoll (*Dasyurus maculatus*), Swamp wallaby (*Wallabia bicolor*), Tammar wallaby (*Macropus eugenii*), Tasmanian devil (*Sarcophilus harrisii*), Western grey kangaroo (*Macropus fuliginosus*), Yellow-footed rock-wallaby (*Petrogale xanthopus*)	A, BIV, C, D and E	McCarthy et al. (2008), Thompson et al. (2008), (2010), Ng et al. (2011), Vermeulen et al. (2015), Wait et al. (2017)

Non-Human Primates (*NHPs*): Assam macaque (*Macaca assamensis*), Barbary macaques (*Macaca sylvanus*), Black-capped squirrel monkey (*Saimiri boliviensis*), Black-headed spider monkey (*Ateles fusciceps*), Bornean orangutan (*Pongo pygmaeus*), Colobus monkey (*Colobus vellerosus*), Common chimpanzee (*Pan troglodytes*), Cottontop tamarin (*Saguinus oedipus*), Crab-eating macaque (*Macaca fascicularis*), Cynomolgus monkey (*Macaca fascicularis*), Diana monkey (*Cercopithecus diana*), Golden monkey (*Rhinopithecus roxellana*), Hamadryas baboon (*Papio hamadryas*), Howler Monkeys (*Alouatta clamitans*), Hussar monkey (*Erythrocebus patas*), Japanese macaque (*Macaca fuscata*), Javan lutung (*Trachypithecus auratus*), Leaf monkey (*Presbytis leucocephalus*), Long-tailed macaques (*Macaca fascicularis*), Mandrill (*Mandrillus sphinx*), Mantled guereza (*Colobus guereza*), Mayotte lemur (*Eulemur fulvus mayottensis*), Mona monkey (*Cercopithecus mona*), Mountain gorilla (*Gorilla beringei beringei*), Northern white-cheeked Gibbon (*Varecia variegata*), Olive baboon (*Papio cynocephalus anubis*), Pig-tailed macaque (*Macaca nemestrina*), Pygmy marmoset (*Cebuella pygmaea*), Red colobus (*Procolobus badius tephrosceles*), Red ruffed lemur (*Varecia rubra*), Rhesus macaque (*Macaca mulatta*), Ring-tailed lemur (*Lemur catta*), Southern Brown Squirrel monkey (*Saimiri sciureus*), Sunda slow loris (Nycticebus coucang), Vervet monkey (*Cercopithecus* sp.), White-Handed Gibbon (*Hylobates lar*), Wild western lowland gorillas (*Gorilla gorilla gorilla*), Yellow baboon (*Papio cynocephalus*)	AI, AII, AIII, BIII, BIV and E	Graczyk et al. (2002), Itagaki et al. (2005), Levecke et al. (2007, 2009), Cacciò et al. (2008), Kutz et al. (2008), Volotao et al. (2008), Johnston et al. (2010), Lebbad et al. (2010), Beck et al. (2011a), Berrilli et al. (2011), Martínez-Díaz et al. (2011), Li et al. (2011), Zhao et al. (2011), Ye et al. (2012), Li et al. (2013), Sak et al. (2013), Hogan et al. (2014), Karim et al. (2014), Ye et al. (2014), Du et al. (2015), Karim et al. (2015), Li et al. (2015a,b), Sricharern et al. (2016), Debenham et al. (2017), Li et al. (2017b), Mynářová et al. (2017), Saleh et al. (2017), Zhong et al. (2017)
Rabbits: European rabbit (*Oryctolagus cuniculus*)	A, BI, BII, BIII, BIV, BV, BVI and E	Zhang et al., 2012b), Liu et al. (2014), Pantchev et al. (2014), Qi et al. (2015c), Koehler et al. (2016), Jiang et al. (2018)

Continued

Table 4 *G. duodenalis* assemblages/sub-assemblages identified with molecular tools in captive and wild animals.—cont'd

Host species	Assemblages/ sub-assemblages	References
Rodents: *Apodemus* spp. Ash-grey mouse (*Pseudomys albocinereus*), Asian house rats (*Rattus tanezumi*), Bamboo rat (*Rhizomyini*), Bank vole (*Myodes glareolus*), Beaver (genus Castor), Brown rats (*Rattus norvegicus*), Bush rat (*Rattus fuscipes*), Chinchillas (*Chinchilla lanigera*), Chipmunks (*Eutamias asiaticus*), Desmarest's hutia (*Capromys pilorides*), Deer Mice (*Peromyscus maniculatus*), Eurasian field mice (*Apodemus* sp.), House mice (*Mus musculus*), Muskrat (*Ondatra zibethicus*), Patagonian mara (*Dolichotis patagonum*), Prevost's Squirrel (*Callosciurus prevosti*)	AI, BIII, BIV, C, D, E, F, GI and GII	Appelbee et al. (2002), Sulaiman et al. (2003), Lebbad et al. (2010), Thompson et al. (2010), Beck et al. (2011a), Levecke et al. (2011), Veronesi et al. (2012), Fernandez-Alvarez et al. (2014), Pantchev et al. (2014), Qi et al. (2015a), Zhao et al. (2015), Adriana et al. (2016), Kilonzo et al. (2017), Deng et al. (2018), Helmy et al. (2018), Gherman et al. (2018), Ma et al. (2018), Schug et al. (2018), Tan et al. (2019)
Reptiles: Bocage's wall lizard (*Podarcis bocagei*), Iberian rock lizard (*Iberolacerta monticola*)	A, B and E	Reboredo-Fernández et al. (2017)
Rock hyrax (*Procavia capensis*)	B	Beck et al. (2011a)
Sun bear (*Ursidae Helarctos malayanus*)	B	Beck et al. (2011a)
Wild felids: Cheetah (*Acinonyx jubatus*), Chinese leopard (*Panthera pardus orientalis*), Lynx (*Lynx lynx*), Siberian tiger (*Panthera tigris altaica)*, Snow leopard (*Uncia uncial*)	AI and F	Beck et al. (2011a), Soares et al. (2011), Li et al. (2015a,b)
Wild canids: African painted dog (*Lycaon pictus*), Coyote (*Canis latrans*), Fox (*Vulpes vulpes*), Jackals (*Canis aureus*), Jaguar (*Panthera onca*), Maned wolf (*Chrysocyon brachyurus*), Raccoon dog (*Nyctereutes procyonoides*), Wolf (*Canis lupus*)	AI, AII, AVIII, B, C, DI and DII	Hamnes et al. (2007), Thompson et al. (2009b), Ash et al. (2010), Beck et al. (2011a,b), Ng et al. (2011), Oates et al. (2012), Stojecki et al. (2015a, b), Adriana et al. (2016), Zhang et al. (2016a,b), Debenham et al. (2017), Hermosilla et al. (2017), Mateo et al. (2017)

NA: Not Available.

Modified from Ryan, U., Cacciò, S.M., 2013. Zoonotic potential of Giardia. Int. J. Parasitol. 43(12–13), 943–56.

Table 5 *Giardia duodenalis* in fish.

Fish species	Location	No of samples	Prevalence (%)	No of samples typed	Assemblages A	B	E	Other	References
Tilapia nilotica	Egypt	68	2.9	2	2	0	0	0	Ghoneim et al. (2012)
Mugil cephalus	Egypt	24	4.2	1	1	0	0	0	Ghoneim et al. (2012)
Cultured fish	Australia	227	8.4	17	6	6	2	Mixed A and E (n=1), Mixed A and B (n=3)	Yang et al. (2011)
Freshwater fish	Australia	227	0.4	1	0	1	0	0	Yang et al. (2011)
Marine fish	Australia	255	8.4	7	1	5	0	Mixed A and B (n=1)	Yang et al. (2011)

4.1 *Giardia* in terrestrial wildlife

The majority of *Giardia* spp. found in captive and free-ranging terrestrial wildlife are *G. duodenalis* assemblages (Table 4; Hillman et al., 2016; Lyu et al., 2018; Thompson et al., 2009a). Few studies have been conducted in Australian native wildlife (Thompson et al., 2010), marsupials appear to be predominantly infected with zoonotic assemblages of *G. duodenalis* (mainly assemblage A and B), rather than host-specific *Giardia* species such as *G. peramelis* (Wait et al., 2017). Two novel *Giardia* genotypes were recently identified in the Tasmanian devil (*Sarcophilus harrisii*); *Giardia* sp. TD type 1 (94.4% similar to isolates from GenBank: U60982) and *Giardia* sp. TD type 2 (86.9% similar to *G. duodenalis* assemblage A from humans in South India GenBank: JN616252) (Wait et al., 2017). To date, molecular studies have identified *G. duodenalis* in 31 marsupial species belonging to 9 families with a prevalence ranging between 1.3% and 24.1% (Adams et al., 2004; McCarthy et al., 2008; Ng et al., 2011; Thompson et al., 2010; Vermeulen et al., 2015; Wait et al., 2017). In addition to assemblages A and B, other *G. duodenalis* assemblages including C, D (mainly found in canines) and E (mainly found in pigs) have also been reported sporadically in marsupials (Ng et al., 2011; Thompson et al., 2010), which suggests potential transmission routs of *G. duodenalis* assemblages between humans, livestock, companion animals and wildlife (Vermeulen et al., 2015).

Non-human-primates (NHPs) have been implicated as major wildlife reservoirs for zoonotic assemblages of *G. duodenalis*. To date, zoonotic

Table 6 Molecular identification of *Giardia* in birds.

Host	Location	No of samples	Prevalence (%)	No of samples typed	*Giardia* species	References
Straw-necked ibis *Threskiornis spinicollis*	Australia	63	70	9	*G. ardeae*	McRoberts et al. (1996)
Cyanoramphus sp., *Neophema* sp., cockatiel (*Nymphicus hollandicus*), Platycercus sp., Grey-hooded parakeet (*Psilopsiagon aymara*), Rose-ringed parakeet (*Psittacula krameri*)	Brazil	499	5.2	12	*G. psittaci*	Ichikawa et al. (2019)
Toco toucon (*Ramphastos toco*)	Brazil	85	1.2	1	*G. duodenalis* (Assemblage A)	da Cunha et al. (2017)
Aquatic birds	Spain	265	8.3	2	*G. duodenalis* (Assemblage B—n=2)	Cano et al. (2016)
Mallard Duck (*Anas platyrhynchos*), Common magpie (*Pica pica*), Common buzzard (*Buteo buteo*), European nightjar (*Caprimulgus europaeus*) Common quail (*Coturnix coturnix*), Eurasian jay (*Garrulus glandarius*)	Spain	433	2.1	8	*G. duodenalis* (Assemblage A—n=3, assemblage B—n=3, assemblage D—n=1, assemblage F—n=1)	Reboredo-Fernández et al. (2015b)
Blue-fronted amazon (*Amazona aestiva*), a blue-and-yellow macaw (*Ara ararauna*), scarlet macaw (*Ara macao*), and a white-bellied parrot (*Pionites leucogaster*)	Italy	146	5.2	4	*G. duodenalis* (Assemblage A—n=4)	Papini et al. (2012)
Greylag goose (*Anser anser*), Domestic duck (*Anser platyrhyncha f. domestica*), Gadwall (*Anas Strepera*)	Hungary	132	9.8	4	*G. duodenalis* (Assemblage A—n=1, assemblage B–n=3)	Plutzer and Tomor (2009)

G. duodenalis assemblages A (I, II and III), B (BIII and BIV) and E (sporadic cases in captive NHPs) have been reported in both wild and captive NHPs including chimpanzees, gibbons, gorrillas, macaques, monkeys and lemurs with a worldwide distribution (Table 4) (Du et al., 2015; Sricharern et al., 2016; Ryan and Cacciò, 2013). The overall infection rate of *G. duodenalis* in NHPs is documented to be between 1.3% (China) and 50.0% (Croatia) with Assemblage B the predominant assemblage reported (Beck et al., 2011a; Berrilli et al., 2011; Du et al., 2015; Johnston et al., 2010; Karim et al., 2014, 2015; Li et al., 2015b; Sricharern et al., 2016; Ye et al., 2012; Zhong et al., 2017). The monoxenous life cycle of *G. duodenalis* and confined space in captive environment means that *Giardia* cysts spread more rapidly in captivity, which results in higher infection rates among captive NHPs compared to free-ranging NHPs (Li et al., 2017b; Zhong et al., 2017).

Predominantly infected by the host-adapted *G. duodenalis* assemblage G, rodents also harbour all other assemblages of *G. duodenalis* except assemblage H (Table 4) (Li et al., 2017b; Helmy et al., 2018). The presence of assemblages other than the rodent-specific assemblage G in rodents may be due to habitat sharing of wildlife with domestic animals and humans (Bajer, 2008; Bitto and Aldras, 2009; Feng and Xiao, 2011; Levecke et al., 2011; Meerburg et al., 2009; Perec-Matysiak et al., 2015). While some studies report a higher prevalence of zoonotic assemblages of *G. duodenalis* in rodents compared to rodent-specific *Giardia* species (*G. micoti* and *G. muris*), and hence argue a higher potential risk for zoonotic transmission from *Giardia*-infected wild rodents (Fayer et al., 2006), other studies claim that rodent-specific *Giardia* species are more prevalent than *G. duodenalis* zoonotic assemblages in wild rodents (Helmy et al., 2018).

G. duodenalis infections have also been molecularly confirmed in other wildlife species including pinnipeds rabbits, reptiles, wild canids, wild felids, beach martin (*Martes foina*), rock hyrax (*Procavia capensis*), sun bear (*Ursidae Helarctos malayanus*) and anteaters (*Tanamuda* sp.) from Australia, Canada, China, Croatia, Germany, Poland, Romania, Spain, Sweden and United States (Table 3) with prevalences ranging from 0.6% to 41% (Adriana et al., 2016; Beck et al., 2011a; Debenham et al., 2017; Hermosilla et al., 2017; Jiang et al., 2018; Koehler et al., 2016; Lasek-Nesselquist et al., 2010; Li et al., 2015a,b; Mateo et al., 2017; Qi et al., 2015c; Reboredo-Fernández et al., 2017; Soares et al., 2011; Solarczyk, 2009; Stojecki et al., 2015a,b; Zhang et al., 2016a,b). Assemblages A and B have been reported in the majority of these studies (Table 4), suggesting that wild animals may potentially act as a major reservoir for human infections. However, conclusive molecular evidence, linking *Giardia* species/assemblages in wildlife with giardiasis in human populations, is scant.

In addition to zoonotic and rodent-specific assemblages of *G. duodenalis* (A, B, C, D, E, F and G), rodents harbour host-adapted species of *Giardia*; *G. muris* and *G. microti* (Helmy et al., 2018; Thompson and Monis, 2012). To date, *G. microti* has been documented in rodents of various genera including muskrats (*Ondatra. zibethicus*), prairie voles (*Microtus ochrogaster*), Père David's vole (*Eothenomys melanogaster*) and yellow-necked mouse (*Apodemus flavicollis*) (Backhans et al., 2013; Lyu et al., 2018; van Keulen et al., 1998). In addition to rodents, *C. microti* has been also reported in other species including a dog (van Keulen et al., 1998), a leopard (*Panthera pardus japonensis*) and a cheetah (*Acinonyx jubatus*) (confirmed only at 18S locus) (Beck et al., 2011a), Red deer (*Cervus elaphus*) and Roe deer (*Capreolus capreolus*) (Beck et al., 2011b), and Bramandi fish (*Lates calcarifer*), which suggests that this species might not be as host-specific as previously thought (Yang et al., 2010).

The most recently described species of *Giardia* is *G. cricetidarum* in hamsters (*Phodopus sungorus*), is most similar to *G. muris* on the basis of the morphology of the trophozoites shape and molecular data (Lyu et al., 2018). *Giardia cricetidarum* produced a detectable infection in golden hamsters (*Mesocricetus auratus*), Campbell's dwarf hamster (*Phodopus campbelli*) and winter white dwarf hamsters (*Phodopus sungorus*) but transmission studies with *G. cricetidarum* failed to establish infections in brown rats (*Rattus norvegicus*), house mice (*Mus musculus*) and lagomorphs including the European rabbit (*Oryctolagus cuniculus*) and natural infections were also not detected in those hosts (Lyu et al., 2018). To date, there is no other reports of *G. cricetidarum* in other host species, suggesting that this species is a hamster-specific parasite; however further evidence is required to confirm this. Further research is required to determine the true distribution and abundance of different *Giardia* species and assemblages among rodents.

Giardia peramelis (previously known as the 'quenda genotype') was first reported in southern brown bandicoots (Quendas) (*Isoodon obesulus)* from Western Australia in 2004 (Adams et al., 2004), and since this initial report, it has been identified in quendas from other locations in Western Australia (Thompson et al., 2010), in the Northern Territory (Barbosa et al., 2017) and in a single calf sample in New South Wales (Ng et al., 2011). However, it was not officially described as a unique *Giardia* species until recently (Hillman et al., 2016). The absence of *G. peramelis* in other Australian marsupials surveyed for *Giardia* spp. (McCarthy et al., 2008; Ng et al., 2011; Thompson et al., 2008, 2010; Vermeulen et al., 2015) led to an assumption that *G. peramelis* was highly host-specific infecting quendas only, however a recent study by Barbosa et al. (2017) identified *G. peramelis* in Northern-brown bandicoot (*Isoodon macrourus*), Brush-tail rabbit-rat (*Conilurus penicillatus*) and Brush-tail possum (*Trichosurus vulpecula*) extending the host range of *G. peramelis*.

4.2 *Giardia* in aquatic wildlife

Water is an important transmission route for zoonotic *G. duodenalis* but very little is known about *Giardia* in aquatic wildlife. *Giardia duodenalis* assemblages A (AI and AII), B, C, D, F and H have been identified in Atlantic harbour seals (*Phoca vituline vitulina*), grey seals (*Halichoerus grypus*), Pacific harbour seals (*Phoca vitulina richardsi*), harp seals (*Phoca groenlandica*), hooded seal (*Cystophora cristata*), ringed seals (*Phoca hispida*), bearded seals (*Erignathus barbatus*), harbour porpoise (*Phocoena phocoena*), striped dolphin (*Stenella coeruleoalba*), minke whale (*Balaenoptera acutorostrata*) and a Pygmy Sperm Whale (*Kogia breviceps*) (Table 4), with prevalences as high as 80% in some studies (Dixon et al., 2008).

Giardia agilis is the *Giardia* species that mainly parasites amphibians but its epidemiology and host range is largely unknown. It is thought to be non-pathogenic and host-specific and it has not been reported in humans (Adam, 1991). Recently *G. agilis* was identified a Yunnan pond frog (*Babina pleuraden*) and Chaochiao frog (*Rana chaochiaoensis*) with 100% and 65% prevalence, respectively, extending its known host range (Lyu et al., 2018).

4.2.1 Giardia *in fish*

Outbreaks of human giardiasis are most frequently waterborne. Fish represent a source of infection for humans with *Giardia* via (1) contamination of both recreational water and drinking water with *Giardia* cysts shed by fish, (2) hand-oral contamination from handling or cleaning fish and (3) consumption of fish contaminated with cysts that is raw or undercooked fish. Regarding the latter, there have been several reports of giardiasis thought to have been acquired through the consumption of undercooked fish (Cheng and Shieh, 2000; Osterholm et al., 1981). Despite the potential for transmission, very little is known about *Giardia* in fish and the only two studies that conducted molecular characterisation reported prevalences ranging from 0.4% to 8.4% (Ghoneim et al., 2012; Yang et al., 2011; Table 5), with another study which conducted microscopy detected *Giardia* in the intestines of a single Oscar fish (Nematollahi et al., 2016). In the study by Yang et al. (2011), molecular analyses detected *G. microti* in one sample from a cultured Barramundi (*Lates calcarifer*), with the remaining isolates identified as *G. duodenalis*. Of these, assemblage B (BIII and BIV) was the most common, followed by Assemblage A (AII) and assemblage E was detected in three samples (Ghoneim et al., 2012; Yang et al., 2011). Evidence also suggest that fish are not mechanical vectors of *Giardia* but are actually infected are infected, as in the study by Yang et al. (2011), histological analysis identified *Giardia* cysts and trophozoites in 10 tissue samples with large numbers of *Giardia* trophozoites and cysts (>100 parasites per field of view) detected in several samples. This coupled with the fact that genetic analysis was conducted on scrapings of stomach and intestinal tissue, suggests that the fish were naturally infected with zoonotic *G. duodenalis* assemblages, which has important public health implications.

5. *Giardia* in birds

Giardia is common in wild and captive birds (Abe et al., 2012; Erlandsen et al., 1991; McRoberts et al., 1996; Reboredo-Fernández et al., 2015a,b) and although frequently asymptomatic, clinical signs include diarrhoea, failure to thrive and feather plucking (Filippich et al., 1998; McRoberts et al., 1996; Upcroft et al., 1997). Birds and particularly waterfowl have the potential to contaminate aquatic habitats with infectious *Giardia* cysts including drinking and recreational water sources and the prevalence of *Giardia* cysts has been shown to be significantly higher in free-ranging than in captive or domestic birds (Majewska et al., 2009). The feeding habits of some birds such as omnivores and scavengers can also increase their exposure to *Giardia* cysts. For example, *Giardia* cysts have been identified in the faeces of migratory Canada geese (*Branta canadensis*) (Graczyk et al., 1998), which are known to follow cattle and eat undigested plant material in cattle feces (Graczyk et al., 1998). As cattle can carry zoonotic *G. duodenalis* assemblages, it is possible that birds can disseminate human-infectious *G. duodenalis* assemblages in aquatic environments. Whether birds are capable of being infected with *G. duodenalis* or disseminate via mechanical transmission remains to be determined. However, a *G. duodenalis* isolate from a sulphur-crested cockatoo (*Cacatua galerita*) established a chronic infection in mice (Upcroft et al., 1997). Very few molecular studies have been conducted on birds and *G. psittaci* and *G. ardeae* are the avian species reported in birds (which are considered non-zoonotic) (Table 6; Abe et al., 2012), however *G. duodenalis* is more commonly reported with assemblages A, B (BIV), D and F detected, which poses a public health risk (Table 6).

6. Future studies

Over the last few decades, diagnostic tools to detect and differentiate between *G. duodenalis* assemblages have improved, however, our understanding of the zoonotic potential and transmission dynamics of *Giardia* infections in animals and humans is still poor and remains a major knowledge gap due mainly to (i) insufficient diversity in the most commonly used markers and (ii) lack of concordance between markers. The development of more discriminatory typing tools and whole genome sequencing (WGS) of *Giardia* isolates is therefore essential to better understand the zoonotic transmission of *Giardia* from animals to humans and also anthroponotic transmission. Isolates from assemblages A, B and E have been analysed by WGS (Adam et al., 2013; Ankarklev et al., 2015; Franzén et al., 2009; Jerlström-Hultqvist et al., 2010; Wielinga et al., 2015) and direct WGS of clinical stool samples and water samples is now possible (Hanevik et al., 2014; Prystajecky et al., 2015; Tsui et al., 2018).

Most recently, WGS has been used to examine the transmission of *Giardia* from wildlife into surface water in Canada using geographically and epidemiologically linked cultured isolates from surface drinking water, human, and animals (including beavers) (Tsui et al., 2018). The study identified assemblages AI, AII and B and provided genomic evidence supporting the role of beavers as the cause of two previous waterborne outbreaks and also identified the presence of mixed infections during an outbreak. The increased ability of WGS to detect mixed infections is important not only for transmission studies but also for understanding the pathogenesis and treatment of giardiasis, as recent evidence suggests that mixed infections enhance intestinal cell damage (Cotton et al., 2015).

One of the current limitations of WGS is that both faecal samples and water samples are complex mixtures of bacterial, host and environmental DNA which requires renders WGS analysis bioinformatically difficult to separate target DNA from background DNA. Newer techniques such as selective whole-genome amplification (SWGA) which preferentially amplifies the genomes of pathogens from complex mixtures of target and host DNA (Clarke et al., 2017), coupled with the decreasing cost of WGS and the relatively small size of the *Giardia* genome (~10 Mb) will result in WGS becoming a more widespread and frequently used higher resolution tool to clarify the transmission dynamics of *Giardia* in different regions of the world.

Prevention and control of zoonotic giardiasis requires a multi-faceted approach, particularly as human encroachment into wildlife-populated areas means more direct contact between humans and wildlife and also increases the likelihood of contamination of drinking water catchments with *Giardia* cysts due to run-off from streams. Unlike *Cryptosporidium* where host-adapted species and genotypes predominate in wildlife (Zahedi et al., 2016), zoonotic *G. duodenalis* assemblages are common in wildlife (Table 4). Therefore, continuous monitoring and molecular typing of protozoan parasites in source water should become routine. The use of agricultural effluents from livestock for crop cultivation can also result in contamination of water and food and needs to be more tightly regulated. Improved financial support and co-operation between urban planners, water utilities and regulatory authorities are essential for effective prevention and should include multi-barrier approaches such as adequate riparian zones, "best practice" water monitoring and treatment and routine monitoring of water filtration performance to minimise the public health risks of waterborne transmission of zoonotic *Giardia*.

References

Abdel-Moein, K.A., Saeed, H., 2016. The zoonotic potential of *Giardia intestinalis* assemblage E in rural settings. Parasitol. Res. 115, 2302–3197.

Abe, N., Makino, I., Kojima, A., 2012. Molecular characterization of *Giardia psittaci* by multilocus sequence analysis. Infect. Genet. Evol. 12, 1710–1716.

Abeywardena, H., Jex, A.R., Nolan, M.J., Haydon, S.R., Stevens, M.A., McAnulty, R.W., Gasser, R.B., 2012. Genetic characterisation of *Cryptosporidium* and *Giardia* from dairy calves: discovery of species/genotypes consistent with those found in humans. Infect. Genet. Evol. 12 (8), 1984–1993.

Abeywardena, H., Jex, A.R., von Samson-Himmelstjerna, G., Haydon, S.R., Stevens, M.A., Gasser, R.B., 2013a. First molecular characterisation of *Cryptosporidium* and *Giardia* from *Bubalus bubalis* (water buffalo) in Victoria, Australia. Infect. Genet. Evol. 20, 96–102.

Abeywardena, H., Jex, A.R., Firestone, S.M., McPhee, S., Driessen, N., Koehler, A.V., Haydon, S.R., von Samson-Himmelstjerna, G., Stevens, M.A., Gasser, R.B., 2013b. Assessing calves as carriers of *Cryptosporidium* and *Giardia* with zoonotic potential on dairy and beef farms within a water catchment area by mutation scanning. Electrophoresis 34 (15), 2259–2267.

Abeywardena, H., Jex, A.R., Koehler, A.V., Rajapakse, R.P., Udayawarna, K., Haydon, S.R., Stevens, M.A., Gasser, R.B., 2014. First molecular characterization of *Cryptosporidium* and *Giardia* from bovines (*Bos taurus* and *Bubalus bubalis*) in Sri Lanka: unexpected absence of *C. parvum* from pre-weaned calves. Parasit. Vectors 7, 75.

Abeywardena, H., Jex, A.R., Gasser, R.B., 2015. A perspective on cryptosporidium and giardia, with an emphasis on bovines and recent epidemiological findings. Adv. Parasitol. 88, 243–301.

Adam, R.D., 1991. The biology of *Giardia* spp. Clin. Microbiol. Rev. 55, 706–732.

Adam, R.D., Dahlstrom, E.W., Martens, C.A., Bruno, D.P., Barbian, K.D., Ricklefs, S.M., Hernandez, M.M., Narla, N.P., Patel, R.B., Porcella, S.F., Nash, T.E., 2013.

Genome sequencing of *Giardia lamblia* genotypes A2 and B isolates (DH and GS) and comparative analysis with the genomes of genotypes A1 and E (WB and Pig). Genome Biol. Evol. 5 (12), 2498–2511.

Adams, P.J., Monis, P.T., Elliot, A.D., Thompson, R.C., 2004. Cyst morphology and sequence analysis of the small subunit rDNA and ef1 alpha identifies a novel *Giardia* genotype in a quenda (*Isoodon obesulus*) from Western Australia. Infect. Genet. Evol. 4, 365–370.

Adell-Aledón, M., Köster, P.C., de Lucio, A., Puente, P., Hernández-de-Mingo, M., Sánchez-Thevenet, P., Dea-Ayuela, M.A., Carmena, D., 2018. Occurrence and molecular epidemiology of *Giardia duodenalis* infection in dog populations in eastern Spain. BMC Vet. Res. 14 (1), 26.

Adriana, G., Zsuzsa, K., Mirabela Oana, D., Mircea, G.C., Viorica, M., 2016. *Giardia duodenalis* genotypes in domestic and wild animals from Romania identified by PCR-RFLP targeting the *gdh* gene. Vet. Parasitol. 217, 71–75.

Aguiar, J.M., Silva, S.O., Santos, V.A., Taniwaki, S.A., Oliveira, T.M., Ferreira, H.L., Keid, L.B., Gregori, F., Soares, R.M., 2016. Evidence of heterozygosity and recombinant alleles in single cysts of *Giardia duodenalis*. Rev. Bras. Parasitol. Vet. 25, 187–195.

Akinkuotu, O.A., Takeet, M.I., Otesile, E.B., Olufemi, F., Greenwood, S.J., McClure, J.T., 2019. Prevalence and mulilocus genotypes of Giardia duodenalis infecting pigs in Ogun state, Nigeria. Infect. Genet. Evol. 70, 53–60. In Press.

Al-Habsi, K., Yang, R., Williams, A., Miller, D., Ryan, U., Jacobson, C., 2017. Zoonotic *Cryptosporidium* and *Giardia* shedding by captured rangeland goats. Vet. Parasitol. Reg. Stud. Rep. 7, 32–35.

Aliosio, F., Filippini, G., Antenucci, P., Lepri, E., Pezzotti, G., Cacciò, S. M., and Pozio, E., 2006. Severe weight loss in lambs infected with *Giardia duodenalis* assemblage B. Vet. Parasitol. 142, 154–158.

Anderson, K.A., Brooks, A.S., Morrison, A.L., Reid-Smith, R.J., Martin, S.W., Benn, D.M., Peregrine, A.S., 2004. Impact of *Giardia* vaccination on asymptomatic *Giardia* infections in dogs at a research facility. Can. Vet. J. 45 (11), 924–930.

Ankarklev, J., Franzén, O., Peirasmaki, D., Jerlström-Hultqvist, J., Lebbad, M., Andersson, J., Andersson, B., Svärd, S.G., 2015. Comparative genomic analyses of freshly isolated Giardia intestinalis assemblage A isolates. BMC Genomics 16, 697.

Appelbee, A., Thorlakson, C., Olson, M.E., 2002. Genotypic characterization of *Giardia* cysts isolated from wild beaver in southern Alberta, Canada. In: Olson, B.E., Olson, M.E., Wallis, P.M. (Eds.), *Giardia*: The Cosmopolitan Parasite. CAB International, Wallingford, United Kingdom, pp. 299–300.

Appelbee, A.J., Thompson, R.C., Measures, L.M., Olson, M.E., 2010. Giardia and cryptosporidium in harp and hooded seals from the Gulf of St. Lawrence, Canada. Vet. Parasitol. 173 (1–2), 19–23.

Armson, A., Yang, R., Thompson, J., Johnson, J., Reid, S., Ryan, U.M., 2009. *Giardia* genotypes in pigs in Western Australia: prevalence and association with diarrhea. Exp. Parasitol. 121 (4), 381–383.

Ash, A., Lymbery, A., Lemon, J., Vitali, S., Thompson, R.C., 2010. Molecular epidemiology of *Giardia duodenalis* in an endangered carnivore-the African painted dog. Vet. Parasitol. 174, 206–212.

Ash, A., Lymbery, A., Godfrey, S., Shiel, R., Paul, A., 2019. Substrate type and age are risk factors for gastrointestinal parasitism in greyhound kennels. Vet. Parasitol. 265, 7–14.

Asher, A.J., Hose, G., Power, M.L., 2016. Giardiasis in NSW: identification of *Giardia duodenalis* assemblages contributing to human and cattle cases, and an epidemiological assessment of sporadic human giardiasis. Infect. Genet. Evol. 44, 157–161.

Backhans, A., Jacobson, M., Hansson, I., Lebbad, M., Lambertz, S.T., Gammelgard, E., Saager, M., Akande, O., Fellström, C., 2013. Occurrence of pathogens in wild rodents caught on Swedish pig and chicken farms. Epidemiol. Infect. 141, 1885–1891.

Bajer, A., 2008. Between-year variation and spatial dynamics of *Cryptosporidium* spp. and *Giardia* spp. infections in naturally infected rodent populations. Parasitology 135, 1629–1649.

Ballweber, L.R., Xiao, L., Bowman, D.D., Kahn, G., Cama, V.A., 2010. Giardiasis in dogs and cats: update on epidemiology and public health significance. Trends Parasitol. 26 (4), 180–189.

Barbosa, A., Reiss, A., Jackson, B., Warren, K., Paparini, A., Gillespie, G., Stokeld, D., Irwin, P., Ryan, U., 2017. Prevalence, genetic diversity and potential clinical impact of blood-borne and enteric protozoan parasites in native mammals from northern Australia. Vet. Parasitol. 238, 94–105.

Bartley, P.M., Roehe, B.K., Thomson, S., Shaw, H.J., Peto, F., Innes, E.A., Katzer, F., 2018. Detection of potentially human infectious assemblages of *Giardia duodenalis* in fecal samples from beef and dairy cattle in Scotland. Parasitology 6, 1–8.

Beck, R., Sprong, H., Bata, I., Lucinger, S., Pozio, E., Cacciò, S.M., 2011a. Prevalence and molecular typing of *Giardia* spp. in captive mammals at the zoo of Zagreb, Croatia. Vet. Parasitol. 175, 40–46.

Beck, R., Sprong, H., Lucinger, S., Pozio, E., Cacciò, S.M., 2011b. A large survey of Croatian wild mammals for *Giardia duodenalis* reveals a low prevalence and limited zoonotic potential. Vector Borne Zoonotic Dis. 11, 1049–1055.

Berrilli, F., Prisco, C., Friedrich, K.G., Di Cerbo, P., Di Cave, D., De Liberato, C., 2011. *Giardia duodenalis* assemblages and *Entamoeba* species infecting non-human primates in an Italian zoological garden: zoonotic potential and management traits. Parasit. Vectors 4, 199.

Bitto, A., Aldras, A., 2009. Prevalence of *Giardia* and *Cryptosporidium* in muskrats in northeastern Pennsylvania and New Jersey. J. Environ. Health 71, 20–26.

Bomfim, T.C., Huber, F., Gomes, R.S., Alves, L.L., 2005. Natural infection by *Giardia* sp. and *Cryptosporidium* sp. in dairy goats, associated with possible risk factors of the studied properties. Vet. Parasitol. 134 (1–2), 9–13.

Bouzid, M., Halai, K., Jeffreys, D., Hunter, P.R., 2015. The prevalence of *Giardia* infection in dogs and cats, a systematic review and meta-analysis of prevalence studies from stool samples. Vet. Parasitol. 207 (3–4), 181–202.

Broglia, A., Weitzel, T., Harms, G., Cacció, S.M., Nöckler, K., 2013. Molecular typing of *Giardia duodenalis* isolates from German travellers. Parasitol. Res. 112 (10), 3449–3456.

Budu-Amoako, E., Greenwood, S.J., Dixon, B.R., Barkema, H.W., McClure, J.T., 2012. Occurrence of *Cryptosporidium* and *Giardia* on beef farms and water sources within the vicinity of the farms on Prince Edward Island, Canada. Vet. Parasitol. 184 (1), 1–9.

Cacciò, S.M., Rinaldi, L., Cringoli, G., Condoleo, R., Pozio, E., 2007. Molecular identification of *Cryptosporidium parvum* and *Giardia duodenalis* in the Italian water buffalo (*Bubalus bubalis*). Vet. Parasitol. 150, 146–149.

Cacciò, S.M., Beck, R., Lalle, M., Marinculic, A., Pozio, E., 2008. Multilocus genotyping of *Giardia duodenalis* reveals striking differences between assemblages A and B. Int. J. Parasitol. 38, 1523–1531.

Cacciò, S.M., Lalle, M., Svärd, S.G., 2018. Host specificity in the *Giardia duodenalis* species complex. Infect. Genet. Evol. 66, 335–345.

Cano, L., de Lucio, A., Bailo, B., Cardona, G.A., Muadica, A.S., Lobo, L., Carmena, D., 2016. Identification and genotyping of *Giardia* spp. and *Cryptosporidium* spp. isolates in aquatic birds in the Salburua wetlands, Álava, Northern Spain. Vet. Parasitol. 221, 144–148.

Cardona, G.A., de Lucio, A., Bailo, B., Cano, L., de Fuentes, I., Carmena, D., 2015. Unexpected finding of feline-specific *Giardia duodenalis* assemblage F and *Cryptosporidium felis* in asymptomatic adult cattle in Northern Spain. Vet. Parasitol. 209 (3–4), 258–263.

Castro-Hermida, J.A., Delafosse, A., Pors, I., Ares-Mazás, E., Chartier, C., 2005. *Giardia duodenalis* and *Cryptosporidium parvum* infections in adult goats and their implications for neonatal kids. Vet. Rec. 157 (20), 623–627.

Cheng, H.S., Shieh, Y.H., 2000. Investigation on subclinical aspects related to intestinal parasitic infections among Thai laborers in Taipei. J. Travel Med. 7, 319–324.

Chilvers, B.L., Cowan, P.E., Waddington, D.C., Kelly, P.J., Brown, T.J., 2010. The prevalence of infection of Giardia spp. and Cryptosporidium spp. in wild animals on farmland, southeastern North Island, New Zealand. Int. J. Environ. Health Res. 8 (1), 1998.

Clarke, E.L., Sundararaman, S.A., Seifert, S.N., Bushman, F.D., Hahn, B.H., Brisson, D., 2017. SWGA: a primer design toolkit for selective whole genome amplification. Bioinformatics 33 (14), 2071–2077.

Colli, C.M., Bezagio, R.C., Nishi, L., Bignotto, T.S., Ferreira, E.C., Falavigna-Guilherme, A.L., Gomes, M.L., 2015. Identical assemblage of *Giardia duodenalis* in humans, animals and vegetables in an urban area in southern Brazil indicates a relationship among them. PLoS One 10, e0118065.

Cotton, J.A., Amat, C.B., Buret, A.G., 2015. Disruptions of host immunity and inflammation by *Giardia duodenalis*: potential consequences for co-infections in the gastro-intestinal tract. Pathogens 4 (4), 764–792.

Cui, Z., Wang, L., Cao, L., Sun, M., Liang, N., Wang, H., Chang, Y., Lin, X., Yu, L., Wang, R., Zhang, S., Ning, C., Zhang, L., 2018. Genetic characteristics and geographic segregation of *Giardia duodenalis* in dairy cattle from Guangdong Province, southern China. Infect. Genet. Evol. 66, 95–100.

da Cunha, M.J.R., Cury, M.C., Santín, M., 2017. Molecular identification of *Enterocytozoon bieneusi, Cryptosporidium*, and *Giardia* in Brazilian captive birds. Parasitol. Res. 116 (2), 487–493.

De Liberato, C., Berrilli, F., Marangi, M., Santoro, M., Trogu, T., Putignani, L., Lanfranchi, P., Ferretti, F., D'Amelio, S., Giangaspero, A., 2015. *Giardia duodenalis* in alpine (*Rupicapra rupicapra rupicapra*) and apennine (*Rupicapra pyrenaica ornata*) chamois. Parasit. Vectors 8, 650.

de Lucio, A., Bailo, B., Aguilera, M., Cardona, G.A., Fernández-Crespo, J.C., Carmena, D., 2017. No molecular epidemiological evidence supporting household transmission of zoonotic *Giardia duodenalis* and *Cryptosporidium* spp. from pet dogs and cats in the province of Álava, Northern Spain. Acta Trop. 170, 48–56.

Debenham, J.J., Tysnes, K., Khunger, S., Robertson, L.J., 2017. Occurrence of *Giardia, Cryptosporidium*, and *Entamoeba* in wild rhesus macaques (*Macaca mulatta*) living in urban and semi-rural North-West India. Int. J. Parasitol. Parasites Wildl. 6, 29–34.

Deng, L., Luo, R., Liu, H., Zhou, Z., Li, L., Chai, Y., Yang, L., Wang, W., Fu, H., Zhong, Z., Cao, S., Peng, G., 2018. First identification and multilocus genotyping of *Giardia duodenalis* in pet chipmunks (*Eutamias asiaticus*) in Sichuan Province, southwestern China. Parasit. Vectors 11, 199.

Di Cristanziano, V., Santoro, M., Parisi, F., Albonico, M., Shaali, M.A., Di Cave, D., Berrilli, F., 2014. Genetic characterization of *Giardia duodenalis* by sequence analysis in humans and animals in Pemba Island, Tanzania. Parasitol. Int. 63 (2), 438–441.

Di Piazza, F., Di Benedetto, M.A., Maida, C.M., Glorioso, S., Adamo, G., Mazzola, T., Firenze, A., 2013. A study on occupational exposure of Sicilian farmers to *Giardia* and *Cryptosporidium*. J. Prev. Med. Hyg. 54 (4), 212–217.

Dixon, B.R., Parrington, L.J., Parenteau, M., Leclair, D., Santín, M., Fayer, R., 2008. *Giardia duodenalis* and *Cryptosporidium* spp. in the intestinal contents of ringed seals (*Phoca hispida*) and bearded seals (*Erignathus barbatus*) in Nunavik, Quebec, Canada. J. Parasitol. 94 (5), 1161–1163.

Du, S.Z., Zhao, G.H., Shao, J.F., Fang, Y.Q., Tian, G.R., Zhang, L.X., Wang, R.J., Wang, H.Y., Qi, M., Yu, S.K., 2015. *Cryptosporidium* spp., *Giardia intestinalis*, and *Enterocytozoon bieneusi* in captive non-human primates in qinling mountains. Korean J. Parasitol. 53, 395–402.

Ehsan, A.M., Geurden, T., Casaert, S., Parvin, S.M., Islam, T.M., Ahmed, U.M., Levecke, B., Vercruysse, J., Claerebout, E., 2015. Assessment of zoonotic transmission of *Giardia* and *Cryptosporidium* between cattle and humans in rural villages in Bangladesh. PLoS One 10 (2), e0118239.

Einarsson, E., Ma'ayeh, S., Svärd, S.G., 2016. An up-date on *Giardia* and giardiasis. Curr. Opin. Microbiol. 34, 47–52.

Erlandsen, S.L., Bemrick, W.J., 1987. SEM evidence for a new species, *Giardia psittaci*. J. Parasitol. 73, 623–629.

Erlandsen, S.L., Weisbrod, A.R., Knudson, L.W., Olereich, R., Dodge, W.E., Jakubowski, W., Bemrick, W.J., 1991. Giardiasis in wild and captive bird populations: high prevalence in herons and budgerigars. Int. J. Environ. Health Res. 1, 132–143.

Esch, K.J., Petersen, C.A., 2013. Transmission and epidemiology of zoonotic protozoal diseases of companion animals. Clin. Microbiol. Rev. 26 (1), 58–85.

Ey, P.L., Mansouri, M., Kulda, J., Nohýnková, E., Monis, P.T., Andrews, R.H., Mayrhofer, G., 1997. Genetic analysis of *Giardia* from hoofed farm animals reveals artiodactyl-specific and potentially zoonotic genotypes. J. Eukaryot. Microbiol. 44, 626–635.

Fan, Y., Wang, T., Koehler, A.V., Hu, M., Gasser, R.B., 2017. Molecular investigation of *Cryptosporidium* and *Giardia* in pre- and post-weaned calves in Hubei Province, China. Parasit. Vectors 10 (1), 519.

Fantinatti, M., Bello, A.R., Fernandes, O., Da-Cruz, A.M., 2016. Identification of giardia lamblia assemblage E in humans points to a new anthropozoonotic cycle. J. Infect. Dis. 214 (8), 1256–1259.

Fantinatti, M., Caseca, A.C., Bello, A.R., Fernandes, O., Da-Cruz, A.M., 2018. The presence of *Giardia lamblia* assemblage A in dogs suggests an anthropozoonotic cycle of the parasite in Rio de Janeiro, Brazil. Infect. Genet. Evol. 65, 265–269.

Fava, N.M., Soares, R.M., Scalia, L.A., Kalapothakis, E., Pena, I.F., Vieira, C.U., Faria, E.S., Cunha, M.J., Couto, T.R., Cury, M.C., 2013. Performance of glutamate dehydrogenase and triose phosphate isomerase genes in the analysis of genotypic variability of isolates of *Giardia duodenalis* from livestocks. Biomed. Res. Int. 2013, 875048.

Fava, N.M., Soares, R.M., Scalia, L.A., Cunha, M.J., Faria, E.S., Cury, M.C., 2016. Molecular typing of canine *Giardia duodenalis* isolates from Minas Gerais, Brazil. Exp. Parasitol. 161, 1–5.

Fayer, R., Santin, M., Trout, J.M., de Stefano, S., Koenen, K., Kaur, T., 2006. Prevalence of *Microsporidia*, *Cryptosporidium* spp., and *Giardia* spp. in beavers (*Castor canadensis*) in Massachusetts. J. Zoo Wildl. Med. 37, 492–497.

Feng, Y., Xiao, L., 2011. Zoonotic potential and molecular epidemiology of *Giardia* species and giardiasis. Clin. Microbiol. Rev. 24 (1), 110–140.

Feng, Y., Gong, X., Zhu, K., Li, N., Yu, Z., Guo, Y., Weng, Y., Kváč, M., Feng, Y., Xiao, L., 2019. Prevalence and genotypic identification of *Cryptosporidium* spp., *Giardia duodenalis* and *Enterocytozoon bieneusi* in pre-weaned dairy calves in Guangdong, China. Parasit. Vectors 12 (1), 41.

Fernandez-Alvarez, A., Martin-Alonso, A., Abreu-Acosta, N., Feliu, C., Hugot, J.P., Valladares, B., Foronda, P., 2014. Identification of a novel assemblage G subgenotype and a zoonotic assemblage B in rodent isolates of *Giardia duodenalis* in the Canary Islands, Spain. Parasitology 141, 206–215.

Filice, F.P., 1952. Studies on the cytology and life history of a *Giardia* from the laboratory rat. Univ. Calif. Publ. Zool. 57, 53–146.

Filippich, L.J., McDonnell, P.A., Munoz, E., Upcroft, J.A., 1998. *Giardia* infection in budgerigars. Aust. Vet. J. 76 (4), 246–249.

Foronda, P., Bargues, M.D., Abreu-Acosta, N., Periago, M.V., Valero, M.A., Valladares, B., Mas-Coma, S., 2008. Identification of genotypes of *Giardia intestinalis* of human isolates in Egypt. Parasitol. Res. 103, 1177–1181.

Franzén, O., Jerlström-Hultqvist, J., Castro, E., Sherwood, E., Ankarklev, J., Reiner, D.S., Palm, D., Andersson, J.O., Andersson, B., Svärd, S.G., 2009. Draft genome sequencing of giardia intestinalis assemblage B isolate GS: is human giardiasis caused by two different species? PLoS Pathog. 5 (8), e1000560.

García-Cervantes, P.C., Báez-Flores, M.E., Delgado-Vargas, F., Ponce-Macotela, M., Nawa, Y., De-la-Cruz-Otero, M.D., Martínez-Gordillo, M.N., Díaz-Camacho, S.P., 2017. *Giardia duodenalis* genotypes among schoolchildren and their families and pets in urban and rural areas of Sinaloa, Mexico. J. Infect. Dev. Ctries. 11 (2), 180–187.

Gaydos, J.K., Miller, W.A., Johnson, C., Zornetzer, H., Melli, A., Packham, A., Jeffries, S.J., Lance, M.M., Conrad, P.A., 2008. Novel and canine genotypes of *Giardia duodenalis* in harbor seals (*Phoca vitulina richardsi*). J. Parasitol. 94 (6), 1264–1268.

Gelanew, T., Lalle, M., Hailu, A., Pozio, E., Cacciò, S.M., 2007. Molecular characterization of human isolates of *Giardia duodenalis* from Ethiopia. Acta Trop. 102, 92–99.

Geurden, T., Claerebout, E., Dursin, L., Deflandre, A., Bernay, F., Kaltsatos, V., Vercruysse, J., 2006. The efficacy of an oral treatment with paromomycin against an experimental infection with **Giardia** in calves. Vet. Parasitol. 135 (3–4), 241–247.

Geurden, T., Thomas, P., Casaert, S., Vercruysse, J., Claerebout, E., 2008. Prevalence and molecular characterisation of *Cryptosporidium* and *Giardia* in lambs and goat kids in Belgium. Vet. Parasitol. 155, 142–145.

Geurden, T., Vercruysse, J., Claerebout, E., 2010a. Is *Giardia* a significant pathogen in production animals? Exp. Parasitol. 124, 98–106.

Geurden, T., Vandenhoute, E., Pohle, H., Casaert, S., De Wilde, N., Vercruysse, J., Claerebout, E., 2010b. The effect of a fenbendazole treatment on cyst excretion and weight gain in calves experimentally infected with *Giardia duodenalis*. Vet. Parasitol. 169, 18–23.

Geurden, T., Olson, M.E., O'Handley, R.M., Schetters, T., Bowman, D., Vercruysse, J., 2014. World association for the advancement of veterinary parasitology (WAAVP): guideline for the evaluation of drug efficacy against non-coccidial gastrointestinal protozoa in livestock and companion animals. Vet. Parasitol. 204 (3–4), 81–86.

Gherman, C.M., Kalmár, Z., Györke, A., Mircean, V., 2018. Occurrence of *Giardia duodenalis* assemblages in farmed long-tailed chinchillas *Chinchilla lanigera* (Rodentia) from Romania. Parasit. Vectors 11, 86.

Ghoneim, N.H., Abdel-Moein, K.A., Saeed, H., 2012. Fish as a possible reservoir for zoonotic *Giardia duodenalis* assemblages. Parasitol. Res. 110 (6), 2193–2196.

Gil, H., Cano, L., de Lucio, A., Bailo, B., de Mingo, M.H., Cardona, G.A., Fernández-Basterra, J.A., Aramburu-Aguirre, J., López-Molina, N., Carmena, D., 2017. Detection and molecular diversity of Giardia duodenalis and Cryptosporidium spp. in sheltered dogs and cats in Northern Spain. Infect. Genet. Evol. 50, 62–69.

Gillhuber, J., Pallant, L., Ash, A., Thompson, R.C., Pfister, K., Scheuerle, M.C., 2013. Molecular identification of zoonotic and livestock-specific *Giardia*-species in faecal samples of calves in Southern *Germany*. Parasit. Vectors 6 (1), 346.

Gómez-Muñoz, M.T., Cámara-Badenes, C., Martínez-Herrero Mdel, C., Dea-Ayuela, M.A., Pérez-Gracia, M.T., Fernández-Barredo, S., Santín, M., Fayer, R., 2012. Multilocus genotyping of *Giardia duodenalis* in lambs from Spain reveals a high heterogeneity. Res. Vet. Sci. 93 (2), 836–842.

Graczyk, T.K., Fayer, R., Trout, J.M., Lewis, E.J., Farley, C.A., Sulaiman, I., Lal, A.A., 1998. *Giardia* sp. cysts and infectious *Cryptosporidium parvum* oocysts in the feces of migratory Canada geese (*Branta canadensis*). Appl. Environ. Microbiol. 64 (7), 2736–2738.

Graczyk, T.K., Bosco-Nizeyi, J., Ssebide, B., Thompson, R.C.A., Read, C., Cranfield, M.R., 2002. Anthropozoonotic genotype (Assemblage) A infections in habitats of free-ranging human-habituated gorillas, Uganda. J. Parasitol. 88, 905–909.

Gultekin, M., Ural, K., Aysul, N., Ayan, A., Balikci, C., Akyildiz, G., 2017. Prevalence and molecular characterization of *Giardia duodenalis* in dogs in Aydin, Turkey. Int. J. Environ. Health Res. 27 (3), 161–168.

Hamnes, I.S., Gjerde, B.K., Forberg, T., Robertson, L.J., 2007. Occurrence of *Giardia* and *Cryptosporidium* in Norwegian red foxes (*Vulpes vulpes*). Vet. Parasitol. 143, 347–353.

Hanevik, K., Bakken, R., Brattbakk, H.R., Saghaug, C.S., Langeland, N., 2014. Whole genome sequencing of clinical isolates of *Giardia lamblia*. Clin. Microbiol. Infect. 21 (2), 192. e1-3.

Helmy, Y., Klotz, C., Wilking, H., Krücken, J., Nöckler, K., Samson-Himmelstjerna, G., Zessin, K., Aebischer, T., 2014. Epidemiology of *Giardia duodenalis* infection in ruminant livestock and children in the Ismailia province of Egypt: insights by genetic characterization. Parasit. Vectors 7, 321.

Helmy, Y.A., Spierling, N.G., Schmidt, S., Rosenfeld, U.M., Reil, D., Imholt, C., Jacob, J., Ulrich, R.G., Aebischer, T., Klotz, C., 2018. Occurrence and distribution of *Giardia* species in wild rodents in Germany. Parasit. Vectors 11, 213.

Hermosilla, C., Kleinertz, S., Silva, L.M., Hirzmann, J., Huber, D., Kusak, J., Taubert, A., 2017. Protozoan and helminth parasite fauna of free-living Croatian wild wolves (*Canis lupus*) analyzed by scat collection. Vet. Parasitol. 233, 14–19.

Hillman, A., Ash, A., Elliot, A., Lymbery, A., Perez, C., Thompson, R., 2016. Confirmation of a unique species of *Giardia*, parasitic in the quenda (*Isoodon obesulus*). Int. J. Parasitol. Parasites wildlife 5, 110–115.

Hogan, J.N., Miller, W.A., Cranfield, M.R., Ramer, J., Hassell, J., Noheri, J.B., Conrad, P.A., Gilardi, K.V., 2014. *Giardia* in mountain gorillas (*Gorilla beringei beringei*), forest buffalo (*Syncerus caffer*), and domestic cattle in Volcanoes National Park, Rwanda. J. Wildl. Dis. 50, 21–30.

Hopkins, R.M., Meloni, B.P., Groth, D.M., Wetherall, J.D., Reynoldson, J.D., Thompson, R.C.A., 1997. Ribosomal RNA sequencing reveals differences between the genotypes of *Giardia* isolates recovered from humans and dogs living in the same locality. J. Parasitol. 83, 44–51.

Hu, S., Liu, Z., Yan, F., Zhang, Z., Zhang, G., Zhang, L., Jian, F., Zhang, S., Ning, C., Wang, R., 2017. Zoonotic and host-adapted genotypes of *Cryptosporidium* spp., *Giardia duodenalis* and *Enterocytozoon bieneusi* in dairy cattle in Hebei and Tianjin, China. Vet. Parasitol. 248, 68–73.

Huang, J., Yue, D., Qi, M., Wang, R., Zhao, J., Li, J., Shi, K., Wang, M., Zhang, L., 2014. Prevalence and molecular characterization of *Cryptosporidium* spp. and *Giardia duodenalis* in dairy cattle in Ningxia, northwestern China. BMC Vet. Res. 10, 292.

Huang, J., Zhang, Z., Zhang, Y., Yang, Y., Zhao, J., Wang, R., Jian, F., Ning, C., Zhang, W., Zhang, L., 2018. Prevalence and molecular characterization of *Cryptosporidium* spp. and *Giardia duodenalis* in deer in Henan and Jilin, China. Parasit. Vectors 11, 239.

Ichikawa, R.S., Santana, B.N., Ferrari, E.D., do Nascimento, I.G., Nakamura, A.A., Nardi, A.R.M., Meireles, M.V., 2019. Detection and molecular characterization of *Giardia* spp. in captive Psittaciformes in Brazil. Prev. Vet. Med. 164, 10–12.

Inpankaew, T., Traub, R., Thompson, R.C., Sukthana, Y., 2007. Canine parasitic zoonoses in Bangkok temples. Southeast Asian J. Trop. Med. Public Health 38 (2), 247–255.

Inpankaew, T., Schär, F., Odermatt, P., Dalsgaard, A., Chimnoi, W., Khieu, V., Muth, S., Traub, R.J., 2014. Low risk for transmission of zoonotic *Giardia duodenalis* from dogs to humans in rural Cambodia. Parasit. Vectors 7, 412.

Inpankaew, T., Jiyipong, T., Thadtapong, N., Kengradomkij, C., Pinyopanuwat, N., Chimnoi, W., Jittapalapong, S., 2015. Prevalence and genotype of *Giardia duodenalis* in dairy cattle from northern and northeastern part of Thailand. Acta Parasitol. 60, 459–461.

Itagaki, T., Kinoshita, S., Aoki, M., Itoh, N., Saeki, H., Sato, N., Uetsuki, J., Izumiyama, S., Yagita, K., Endo, T., 2005. Genotyping of *Giardia intestinalis* from domestic and wild animals in Japan using glutamate dehydrogenase gene sequencing. Vet. Parasitol. 133, 283–287.

Ito, Y., Iijima, Y., Itoh, N., Kimura, Y., 2017. Multilocus genotyping of Giardia duodenalis isolates from breeding cattery cats in Japan. J. Feline Med. Surg. 3 (2), 2055116917745237.

Jacobson, C., Williams, A., Yang, R., Ryan, U., Carmichael, I., Campbell, A.J., Gardner, G.E., 2016. Greater intensity and frequency of *Cryptosporidium* and *Giardia* oocyst shedding beyond the neonatal period is associated with reductions in growth, carcase weight and dressing efficiency in sheep. Vet. Parasitol. 228, 42–51.

Jafari, H., Jalali, M.H.R., Shapouri, M.S.A., Hajikolaii, M.R.H., 2014. Determination of *Giardia duodenalis* genotypes in sheep and goat from Iran. J. Parasit. Dis. 38, 81–84.

Janeczko, S., Griffin, B., 2010. *Giardia* infection in cats. Compend. Contin. Educ. Pract. Vet. 32 (8), E4.

Jerlström-Hultqvist, J., Franzén, O., Ankarklev, J., Xu, F., Nohýnková, E., Andersson, J.O., Svärd, S.G., Andersson, B., 2010. Genome analysis and comparative genomics of a *Giardia intestinalis* assemblage E isolate. BMC Genomics 11, 543.

Jian, Y., Zhang, X., Li, X., Karanis, G., Ma, L., Karanis, P., 2018. Prevalence and molecular characterization of *Giardia duodenalis* in cattle and sheep from the Qinghai-Tibetan Plateau Area (QTPA), northwestern China. Vet. Parasitol. 250, 40–44.

Jiang, J., Ma, J.G., Zhang, N.Z., Xu, P., Hou, G., Zhao, Q., Zhang, X.X., 2018. Prevalence and risk factors of *Giardia duodenalis* in domestic rabbits (*Oryctolagus cuniculus*) in Jilin and Liaoning province, northeastern China. J. Infect. Public Health 11, 723–726.

Jin, Y., Fei, J., Cai, J., Wang, X., Li, N., Guo, Y., Feng, Y., Xiao, L., 2017. Multilocus genotyping of *Giardia duodenalis* in Tibetan sheep and yaks in Qinghai, China. Vet. Parasitol. 247, 70–76.

Johnson, D., Harms, N.J., Larter, N.C., Elkin, B.T., Tabel, H., Wei, G., 2010. Serum biochemistry, serology, and parasitology of boreal caribou (*Rangifer tarandus caribou*) in the Northwest Territories, Canada. J. Wildl. Dis. 46, 1096–1107.

Johnston, A.R., Gillespie, T.R., Rwego, I.B., McLachlan, T.L.T., Kent, A.D., Goldberg, T.L., 2010. Molecular epidemiology of cross-species *Giardia duodenalis* transmission in western Uganda. PLoS Negl. Trop. Dis. 4, e683.

Karanis, P., Kourenti, C., Smith, H., 2007. Waterborne transmission of protozoan parasites: a worldwide review of outbreaks and lessons learnt. J. Water Health 5 (1), 1–38.

Karim, M.R., Zhang, S., Jian, F., Li, J., Zhou, C., Zhang, L., Sun, M., Yang, G., Zou, F., Dong, H., Li, J., Rume, F.I., Qi, M., Wang, R., Ning, C., Xiao, L., 2014. Multilocus typing of *Cryptosporidium* spp. and *Giardia duodenalis* from non-human primates in China. Int. J. Parasitol. 44, 1039–1047.

Karim, M.R., Wang, R., Yu, F., Li, T., Dong, H., Li, D., Zhang, L., Li, J., Jian, F., Zhang, S., Rume, F.I., Ning, C., Xiao, L., 2015. Multi-locus analysis of *Giardia duodenalis* from nonhuman primates kept in zoos in China: geographical segregation and host-adaptation of assemblage B isolates. Infect. Genet. Evol. 30, 82–88.

Khan, S.M., Debnath, C., Pramanik, A.K., Xiao, L., Nozaki, T., Ganguly, S., 2011. Molecular evidence for zoonotic transmission of *Giardia duodenalis* among dairy farm workers in West Bengal, India. Vet. Parasitol. 178, 342–345.

Kilonzo, C., Li, X., Vodoz, T., Xiao, C., Chase, J.A., Jay-Russell, M.T., Vivas, E.J., Atwill, E.R., 2017. Quantitative shedding of multiple genotypes of *Cryptosporidium* and *Giardia* by Deer Mice (*Peromyscus maniculatus*) in a major agricultural region on the california central coast. J. Food Prot. 7, 819–828.

Koehler, A.V., Haydon, S.R., Jex, A.R., Gasser, R.B., 2016. *Cryptosporidium* and *Giardia* taxa in faecal samples from animals in catchments supplying the city of Melbourne with drinking water (2011 to 2015). Parasit. Vectors 9, 315.

Kostopoulou, D., Claerebout, E., Arvanitis, D., Ligda, P., Voutzourakis, N., Casaert, S., Sotiraki, S., 2017. Abundance, zoonotic potential and risk factors of intestinal parasitism amongst dog and cat populations: the scenario of Crete, Greece. Parasit. Vectors 10 (1), 43.

Kunstler, J., 1882. Sur cinq protozoaires parasites nouveaux. Comptes rendus des séances de la Société de biologie et de ses filiales, Paris 95, 347–349.

Kutz, S.J., Thompson, R.A., Polley, L., Kandola, K., Nagy, J., Wielinga, C.M., Elkin, B.T., 2008. *Giardia* assemblage A: human genotype in muskoxen in the Canadian Arctic. J. Parasitol. Vector Biol 1, 32.

Lalle, M., Pozio, E., Capelli, G., Bruschi, F., Crotti, D., Cacciò, S.M., 2005. Genetic heterogeneity at the beta-giardin locus among human and animal isolates of *Giardia duodenalis* and identification of new potentially zoonotic, genotypes. Int. J. Parasitol. 35, 207–213.

Lalle, M., Frangipane di Regalbono, A., Poppi, L., Nobili, G., Tonanzi, D., Pozio, E., Cacciò, S.M., 2007. A novel *Giardia duodenalis* assemblage A subtype in fallow deer. J. Parasitol. 93, 426–428.

Langkjaer, R.B., Vigre, H., Enemark, H.L., Maddox-Hyttel, C., 2007. Molecular and phylogenetic characterization of *Cryptosporidium* and *Giardia* from pigs and cattle in Denmark. Parasitology 134, 339–350.

Lasek-Nesselquist, E., Welch, D.M., Sogin, M.L., 2010. The identification of a new *Giardia duodenalis* assemblage in marine vertebrates and a preliminary analysis of *G. duodenalis* population biology in marine systems. Int. J. Parasitol. 40, 1063–1074.

Lebbad, M., Mattsson, J.G., Christensson, B., Ljungstrom, B., Backhans, A., Andersson, J.O., Svard, S.G., 2010. From mouse to moose: multilocus genotyping of *Giardia* isolates from various animal species. Vet. Parasitol. 168, 231–239.

Lee, S.H., VanBik, D., Kim, H.Y., Cho, A., Kim, J.W., Byun, J.W., Oem, J.K., Oh, S.I., Kwak, D., 2016. Prevalence and molecular characterisation of *Giardia duodenalis* in calves with diarrhoea. Vet. Rec. 178 (25), 633.

Lee, M.F., Cadogan, P., Eytle, S., Copeland, S., Walochnik, J., Lindo, J.F., 2017. Molecular epidemiology and multilocus sequence analysis of potentially zoonotic *Giardia* spp. from humans and dogs in Jamaica. Parasitol. Res. 116 (1), 409–414.

Lee, Y.J., Han, D.G., Ryu, J.H., Chae, J.B., Chae, J.S., Yu, D.H., Park, J., Park, B.K., Kim, H.C., Choi, K.S., 2018. Identification of zoonotic *Giardia duodenalis* in Korean native calves with normal feces. Parasitol. Res. 117 (6), 1969–1973.

Levecke, B., Dorny, P., Geurden, T., Vercammen, F., Vercruysse, J., 2007. Gastrointestinal protozoa in non-human primates of four zoological gardens in Belgium. Vet. Parasitol. 148, 236–246.

Levecke, B., Geldhof, P., Claerebout, E., Dorny, P., Vercammen, F., Cacciò, S.M., Vercruysse, J., Geurden, T., 2009. Molecular characterisation of *Giardia duodenalis* in captive non-human primates reveals mixed assemblage A and B infections and novel polymorphisms. Int. J. Parasitol. 39, 1595–1601.

Levecke, B., Meulemans, L., Dalemans, T., Casaert, S., Claerebout, E., Geurden, T., 2011. Mixed *Giardia duodenalis* assemblage A, B, C and E infections in pet chinchillas (*Chinchilla lanigera*) in Flanders (Belgium). Vet. Parasitol. 177, 166–170.

Li, W., Kiulia, N.M., Mwenda, J.M., Nyachieo, A., Taylor, M.B., Zhang, X., Xiao, L., 2011. *Cyclospora papionis*, *Cryptosporidium hominis*, and human-pathogenic *Enterocytozoon bieneusi* in captive baboons in Kenya. J. Clin. Microbiol. 49, 4326–4329.

Li, W., Liu, C., Yu, Y., Li, J., Gong, P., Song, M., Xiao, l., and Zhnag, X., 2013. Molecular characterization of *Giardia duodenalis* isolates from police and farm dogs in China. Exp. Parasitol. 135, 223–226.

Li, W., Li, Y., Song, M., Lu, Y., Yang, J., Tao, W., Jiang, Y., Wan, Q., Zhang, S., Xiao, L., 2015a. Prevalence and genetic characteristics of *Cryptosporidium, Enterocytozoon bieneusi* and *Giardia duodenalis* in cats and dogs in Heilongjiang province, China. Vet. Parasitol. 208 (3-4), 125–134.

Li, J., Qi, M., Chang, Y., Wang, R., Li, T., Dong, H., Zhang, L., 2015b. Molecular characterization of *Cryptosporidium* spp., *Giardia duodenalis*, and *Enterocytozoon bieneusi* in captive wildlife at Zhengzhou zoo, China. J. Eukaryot. Microbiol. 62, 833–839.

Li, F., Wang, H., Zhang, Z., Li, J., Wang, C., Zhao, J., Hu, S., Wang, R., Zhang, L., Wang, M., 2016a. Prevalence and molecular characterization of *Cryptosporidium* spp. and *Giardia duodenalis* in dairy cattle in Beijing, China. Vet. Parasitol. 219, 61–65.

Li, W., Yu, M., Zhong, Z., Wang, Q., Liu, X., Yu, J., Li, Q., Deng, J., Deng, L., Niu, L., Xie, N., Chen, H., Gong, C., Yang, J., Liao, L., Tan, H., Peng, G., 2016b. Isolation and identification of *Giardia* and *Cryptosporidium* genotypes from captive wild boars and Xiang pigs in Sichuan province. Chinese J. Vet. Sci. 9, 1166–1169.

Li, W., Deng, L., Wu, K., Huang, X., Song, Y., Su, H., Hu, Y., Fu, H., Zhong, Z., Peng, G., 2017a. Presence of zoonotic *Cryptosporidium scrofarum*, *Giardia duodenalis* assemblage A and *Enterocytozoon bieneusi* genotypes in captive Eurasian wild boars (*Sus scrofa*) in China: potential for zoonotic transmission. Parasit. Vectors 10, 10.

Li, J., Wang, H., Wang, R., Zhang, L., 2017b. *Giardia duodenalis* Infections in humans and other animals in China. Front. Microbiol. 8, 2004.

Liberato, C., Berrilli, F., Odorizi, L., Scarcella, R., Barni, M., Amoruso, C., Scarito, A., Filippo, M.M.D., Carvelli, A., Iacoponi, F., Scaramozzino, P., 2018. Parasites in stray dogs from Italy: prevalence, risk factors and management concerns. Acta Parasitol. 63 (1), 27–32.

Lim, Y.A.L., Mahdy, M.A.K., Tan, T.K., Xiang, T.G., Jex, A.R., Nolan, M.J., Sharma, R.S., Gasser, R.B., 2013. First molecular characterization of *Giardia duodenalis* from goats in Malaysia. Mol. Cell. Probes 27, 28–31.

Liu, A., Yang, F., Shen, Y., Zhang, W., Wang, R., Zhao, W., Zhang, L., Ling, H., amd Cao, J., 2014. Genetic analysis of the *gdh* and *bg* genes of animal-derived *Giardia duodenalis* isolates in Northeastern China and evaluation of zoonotic transmission potential. PLoS One 9 (4), e95291.

Liu, G., Su, Y., Zhou, M., Zhao, J., Zhang, T., Ahmad, W., Lu, H., Jiang, N., Chen, Q., Xiang, M., Yin, J., 2015. Prevalence and molecular characterization of *Giardia duodenalis* isolates from dairy cattle in northeast China. Exp. Parasitol. 154, 20–24.

Lucio-Forster, A., Griffiths, J.K., Cama, V.A., Xiao, L., Bowman, D.D., 2010. Minimal zoonotic risk of cryptosporidiosis from pet dogs and cats. Trends Parasitol. 26 (4), 174–179.

Lyu, Z., Shao, J., Xue, M., Ye, Q., Chen, B., Qin, Y., Wen, J., 2018. A new species of *Giardia* Künstler, 1882 (*Sarcomastigophora: Hexamitidae*) in hamsters. Parasit. Vectors 11, 202.

Ma, X., Wang, Y., Zhang, H.J., Wu, H.X., Zhao, G.H., 2018. First report of *Giardia duodenalis* infection in bamboo rats. Parasit. Vectors 11, 520.

Mahato, M.K., Singh, D.K., Rana, H.B., Acharya, K.P., 2018. Prevalence and risk factors associated with *Giardia duodenalis* infection in dairy cattle of Chitwan, Nepal. J. Parasit. Dis. 42 (1), 122–126.

Majewska, A.C., Graczyk, T.K., Słodkowicz-Kowalska, A., Tamang, L., Jedrzejewski, S., Zduniak, P., Solarczyk, P., Nowosad, A., Nowosad, P., 2009. The role of free-ranging, captive, and domestic birds of Western Poland in environmental contamination with *Cryptosporidium parvum* oocysts and *Giardia lamblia* cysts. Parasitol. Res. 104 (5), 1093–1099.

Majewska, A.C., Solarczyk, P., Moskwa, B., Cabaj, W., Jankowska, W., Nowosad, P., 2012. *Giardia* prevalence in wild cervids in Poland. Ann Parasitol 58, 207–209.

Malekifard, F., Ahmadpour, M., 2018. Molecular detection and identification of *Giardia duodenalis* in cattle of Urmia, northwest of Iran. Vet. Res. Forum 9 (1), 81–85.

Mark-Carew, M.P., Khan, Y., Wade, S.E., Schaaf, S., Mohammed, H.O., 2010. Incidence of and risks associated with Giardia infections in herds on dairy farms in the New York City Watershed. Acta Vet. Scand. 52, 44.

Mark-Carew, M.P., Wade, S.E., Chang, Y.F., Schaaf, S., Mohammed, H.O., 2012. Prevalence of *Giardia duodenalis* assemblages among dairy herds in the New York City Watershed. Vet. Parasitol. 185 (2–4), 151–157.

Martínez-Díaz, R.A., Sansano-Maestre, J., Martínez-Herrero Mdel, C., Ponce-Gordo, F., Gómez-Muñoz, M.T., 2011. Occurrence and genetic characterization of *Giardia duodenalis* from captive nonhuman primates by multi-locus sequence analysis. Parasitol. Res. 109, 539–544.

Mateo, M., de Mingo, M.H., de Lucio, A., Morales, L., Balseiro, A., Espí, A., Barral, M., Lima Barbero, J.F., Habela, M.Á., Fernández-García, J.L., Bernal, R.C., Köster, P.C., Cardona, G.A., Carmena, D., 2017. Occurrence and molecular genotyping of *Giardia duodenalis* and *Cryptosporidium* spp. in wild mesocarnivores in Spain. Vet. Parasitol. 235, 86–93.

McCarthy, S., Ng, J., Gordon, C., Miller, R., Wyber, A., Ryan, U.M., 2008. Prevalence of *Cryptosporidium* and *Giardia* species in animals in irrigation catchments in the southwest of Australia. Exp. Parasitol. 118, 596–959.

McRoberts, K.M., Meloni, B.P., Morgan, U.M., Marano, R., Binz, N., Eriandsen, S.L., Halse, S.A., Thompson, R.C., 1996. Morphological and molecular characterization of *Giardia* isolated from the straw-necked ibis (*Threskiornis spinicollis*) in Western Australia. J. Parasitol. 82 (5), 711–718.

Meerburg, B.G., Singleton, G.R., Kijlstra, A., 2009. Rodent-borne diseases and their risks for public health. Crit. Rev. Microbiol. 35, 221–270.

Minetti, C., Taweenan, W., Hogg, R., Featherstone, C., Randle, N., Latham, S.M., Wastling, J.M., 2014. Occurrence and diversity of *Giardia duodenalis* assemblages in livestock in the UK. Transbound. Emerg. Dis. 61, e60–e67.

Minvielle, M.C., Molina, N.B., Polverino, D., Basualdo, J.A., 2008. First genotyping of *Giardia lamblia* from human and animal feces in Argentina, South America. Mem. Inst. Oswaldo Cruz 103 (1), 98–103.

Monis, P.T., Andrews, R.H., Mayrhofer, G., Kulda, J., Isaac-Renton, J.L., Ey, P.L., 1998. Novel lineages of *Giardia intestinalis* identified by genetic analysis of organisms isolated from dogs in Australia. Parasitology 116, 7–19.

Monis, P.T., Andrews, R.H., Mayrhofer, G., Ey, P.L., 1999. Molecular systematics of the parasitic protozoan *Giardia intestinalis*. Mol. Biol. Evol. 16, 1114–1135.

Monis, P.T., Caccio, S.M., Thompson, R.C., 2009. Variation in Giardia: towards a taxonomic revision of the genus. Trends Parasitol 25 (2), 93–100.

Moron-Soto, M., Gutierrez, L., Sumano, H., Tapia, G., Alcala-Canto, Y., 2017. Efficacy of nitazoxanide to treat natural *Giardia* infections in dogs. Parasit. Vectors 10 (1), 52.

Muhid, A., Robertson, I., Ng, J., Yang, R., Ryan, U., 2012. Prevalence of *Giardia* spp. infection in pre-weaned and weaned calves in relation to management factors. Vet. J. 191 (1), 135–137.

Munoz, J., Mayer, D.C., 2016. *Toxoplasma gondii* and *Giardia duodenalis* infections in domestic dogs in New York City public parks. Vet. J. 211, 97–99.

Mynářová, A., Foitová, I., Kváč, M., Květoňová, D., Rost, M., Morrogh-Bernard, H., Nurcahyo, W., Nguyen, C., Supriyadi, S., Sak, B., 2017. Prevalence of *Cryptosporidium* spp., *Enterocytozoon bieneusi*, *Encephalitozoon* spp. and *Giardia intestinalis* in wild, semi-wild and captive orangutans (*Pongo abelii* and *Pongo pygmaeus*) on Sumatra and Borneo, Indonesia. PLoS One 11, e0152771.

Naguib, D., El-Gohary, A.H., Mohamed, A.A., Roellig, D.M., Arafat, N., Xiao, L., 2018. Age patterns of *Cryptosporidium* species and *Giardia duodenalis* in dairy calves in Egypt. Parasitol. Int. 67 (6), 736–741.

Nematollahi, A., Jaberi, S., Helan, J.A., Sheikhzadeh, N., 2016. Histopathological study on parasites in freshwater ornamental fishes in Iran. J. Parasit. Dis. 40 (3), 756–759.

Ng, J., Yang, R., Whiffin, V., Cox, P., Ryan, U., 2011. Identification of zoonotic *Cryptosporidium* and *Giardia* genotypes infecting animals in Sydney's water catchments. Exp. Parasitol. 128, 138–144.

Nguyen, S.T., Fukuda, Y., Nguyen, D.T., Tada, C., Nakai, T., 2016. Prevalence and first genotyping of *Giardia duodenalis* in beef calves in Vietnam. Trop. Anim. Health Prod. 48, 837–841.

Nguyen, S.T., Fukuda, Y., Nguyen, D.T., Dao, H.T., LE, D. Q., Bui, K. L., Tada, C., and Nakai, Y., 2018. Prevalence, genotyping and risk factors of *Giardia duodenalis* from dogs in Vietnam. J. Vet. Med. Sci. 80 (1), 92–97.

Nolan, M.J., Unger, M., Yeap, Y.T., Rogers, E., Millet, I., Harman, K., Fox, M., Kalema-Zikusoka, G., Blake, D.P., 2017. Molecular characterisation of protist parasites in human-habituated mountain gorillas (*Gorilla beringei beringei*), humans and livestock, from Bwindi impenetrable National Park, Uganda. Parasit. Vectors 10 (1), 340.

O'Handley, R.M., Olson, M.E., 2006. Giardiasis and cryptosporidiosis in ruminants. Vet. Clin. North Am. Food Anim. Pract. 22, 623–643.

Oates, S.C., Miller, M.A., Hardin, D., Conrad, P.A., Melli, A., Jessup, D.A., Dominik, C., Roug, A., Tinker, M.T., Miller, W.A., 2012. Prevalence, environmental loading, and molecular characterization of *Cryptosporidium* and *Giardia* isolates from domestic and wild animals along the Central California Coast. Appl. Environ. Microbiol. 78, 8762–8772.

O'Handley, R.M., Cockwill, C., Jelinski, M., McAllister, T.A., Olson, M.E., 2000. Effects of repeat fenbendazole treatment in dairy calves with giardiasis on cyst excretion, clinical signs and production. Vet. Parasitol. 89 (3), 209–218.

O'Handley, R.M., Ceri, H., Anette, C., Olson, M.E., 2003. Passive immunity and serological immune response in dairy calves associated with natural *Giardia duodenalis* infections. Vet. Parasitol. 113 (2), 89–98.

Olson, M.E., Ceri, H., Morck, D.W., 2000. Giardia vaccination. Parasitol. Today 16 (5), 213–217.

Osterholm, M.T., Forfang, J.C., Ristinen, T.L., Dean, A.G., Washburn, J.W., Godes, J.R., Rude, R.A., McCullough, J.G., 1981. An outbreak of food borne giardiasis. N. Engl. J. Med. 304, 24–28.

Pallant, L., Barutzki, D., Schaper, R., Thompson, R.C., 2015. The epidemiology of infections with *Giardia* species and genotypes in well cared for dogs and cats in Germany. Parasit. Vectors 8, 2.

Pantchev, N., Broglia, A., Paoletti, B., Globokar Vrhovec, M., Bertram, A., Nöckler, K., Cacciò, S.M., 2014. Occurrence and molecular typing of *Giardia* isolates in pet rabbits, chinchillas, guinea pigs and ferrets collected in Europe during 2006-2012. Vet. Rec. 175, 18.

Paoletti, B., Traversa, D., Iorio, R., De Berardinis, A., Bartolini, R., Salini, R., Di Cesare, A., 2015. Zoonotic parasites in feces and fur of stray and private dogs from Italy. Parasitol. Res. 114 (6), 2135–2141.

Papini, R., Girivetto, M., Marangi, M., Mancianti, F., Giangaspero, A., 2012. Endoparasite infections in pet and zoo birds in Italy. Sci. World J. 2012, 253127.

Paz e Silva, F.M., Lopes, R.S., Bresciani, K.D., Amarante, A.F., Araujo Jr., J.P., 2014. High occurrence of *Cryptosporidium ubiquitum* and *Giardia duodenalis* genotype E in sheep from Brazil. Acta Parasitol. 59 (1), 193–196.

Paziewska, A., Bednarska, M., Newegłowski, H., Karbowiak, G., Bajer, A., 2007. Distribution of *Cryptosporidium* and *Giardia* spp. In selected species of protected and game mammals from North- Eastern Poland. Ann. Agric. Environ. Med. 14, 265–270.

Peng, X.Q., Tian, G.R., Ren, G.J., Yu, Z.Q., Lok, J.B., Zhang, L.X., Wang, X.T., Song, J.K., Zhao, G.H., 2016. Infection rate of *Giardia duodenalis, Cryptosporidium* spp. and *Enterocytozoon bieneusi* in cashmere, dairy and meat goats in China. Infect. Genet. Evol. 41, 26–31.

Perec-Matysiak, A., Bunkowska-Gawlik, K., Zalesny, G., Hildebrand, J., 2015. Small rodents as reservoirs of *Cryptosporidium* spp. and *Giardia* spp. in southwestern Poland. Ann. Agric. Environ. Med. 22, 1–5.

Petersen, H.H., Jianmin, W., Katakam, K.K., Mejer, H., Thamsborg, S.M., Dalsgaard, A., Olsen, A., Enemark, H.L., 2015. *Cryptosporidium* and *Giardia* in Danish organic pig farms: seasonal and age-related variation in prevalence, infection intensity and species/genotypes. Vet. Parasitol. 214 (1–2), 29–39.

Piekarska, J., Bajzert, J., Gorczykowski, M., Kantyka, M., Podkowik, M., 2016. Molecular identification of *Giardia duodenalis* isolates from domestic dogs and cats in Wroclaw, Poland. Ann. Agric. Environ. Med. 23 (3), 410–415.

Plutzer, J., Tomor, B., 2009. The role of aquatic birds in the environmental dissemination of human pathogenic *Giardia duodenalis* cysts and *Cryptosporidium* oocysts in Hungary. Parasitol. Int. 58 (3), 227–231.

Prystajecky, N., Tsui, C.K.M., Hsiao, W.W.L., Uyaguari-Diaz, M.I., Ho, J., Tang, P., Isaac-Renton, J., 2015. *Giardia* spp. are commonly found in mixed assemblages in surface water, as revealed by molecular and whole-genome characterization. Appl. Environ. Microbiol. 81, 4827–4834.

Qi, M., Cai, J., Wang, R., Li, J., Jian, F., Huang, J., Zhou, H., Zhang, L., 2015a. Molecular characterization of *Cryptosporidium* spp. and *Giardia duodenalis* from yaks in the central western region of China. BMC Microbiol. 15, 108.

Qi, M., Xi, J., Li, J., Wang, H., Ning, C., Zhang, L., 2015c. Prevalence of *Zoonotic Giardia duodenalis* assemblage B and first identification of assemblage E in rabbit fecal samples isolates from Central China. J. Eukaryot. Microbiol. 62, 810–814.

Qi, M., Dong, H., Wang, R., Li, J., Zhao, J., Zhang, L., Luo, J., 2016. Infection rate and genetic diversity of Giardia duodenalis in pet and stray dogs in Henan Province, China. Parasitol. Int. 65 (2), 159–162.

Quadros, R.M., Weiss, P.H., Marques, S.M., Miletti, L.C., 2016. Potential cross-contamination of similar Giardia duodenalis assemblage in children and pet dogs in southern Brazil, as determined by PCR-RFLP. Rev. Inst. Med. Trop. Sao Paulo 58, 66.

Ramírez-Ocampo, S., Cotte-Alzate, J.D., Escobedo, Á.A., Rodríguez-Morales, A.J., 2017. Prevalence of zoonotic and non-zoonotic genotypes of *Giardia intestinalis* in cats: a systematic review and meta-analysis. Infez. Med. 25 (4), 326–338.

Reboredo-Fernández, A., Ares-Mazás, E., Martínez-Cedeira, J.A., Romero-Suances, R., Cacciò, S.M., Gómez-Couso, H., 2015a. *Giardia* and *Cryptosporidium* in cetaceans on the European Atlantic coast. Parasitol. Res. 114 (2), 693–698.

Reboredo-Fernández, A., Ares-Mazás, E., Caccio, S.M., Gómez-Couso, H., 2015b. Occurrence of *Giardia* and *Cryptosporidium* in wild birds in Galicia (Northwest Spain). Parasitology 142, 917–925.

Reboredo-Fernández, A., Ares-Mazás, E., Galán, P., Cacciò, S.M., Gómez-Couso, H., 2017. Detection of zoonotic and livestock-specific assemblages of *Giardia duodenalis* in free-living wild lizards. Rev. Bras. Parasitol. Vet. 26, 395–399.

Rehbein, S., Klotz, C., Ignatius, R., Müller, E., Aebischer, A., Kohn, B., 2019. *Giardia duodenalis* in small animals and their owners in Germany: a pilot study. Zoonoses Public Health 66 (1), 117–124.

Robertson, L.J., Forberg, T., Hermansen, L., Hamnes, I.S., Gjerde, B., 2007. *Giardia duodenalis* cysts isolated from wild moose and reindeer in Norway: genetic characterization by PCR-RFLP and sequence analysis at two genes. J. Wildl. Dis. 43, 576–585.

Rodriguez-Rivera, L.D., Cummings, K.J., McNeely, I., Suchodolski, J.S., Scorza, A.V., Lappin, M.R., Mesenbrink, B.T., Leland, B.R., Bodenchuk, M.J., 2016. Prevalence and diversity of *Cryptosporidium* and *Giardia* identified among feral pigs in Texas. Vector Borne Zoonotic Dis. 16 (12), 765–768.

Ryan, U., Cacciò, S.M., 2013. Zoonotic potential of *Giardia*. Int. J. Parasitol. 43 (12–13), 943–956.

Ryan, U.M., Bath, C., Robertson, I., Read, C., Elliot, A., McInnes, L., Traub, R., Besier, B., 2005. Sheep may not be an important zoonotic reservoir for *Cryptosporidium* and *Giardia* parasites. Appl. Environ. Microbiol. 71, 4992–4997.

Sak, B., Petrzelkova, K.J., Kvetonova, D., Mynarova, A., Shutt, K.A., Pomajbikova, K., Kalousova, B., Modry, D., Benavides, J., Todd, A., Kvac, M., 2013. Long term monitoring of *Microsporidia*, *Cryptosporidium* and *Giardia* infections in western lowland gorillas (*Gorilla gorilla gorilla*) at different stages of habituation in Dzanga Sangha protected areas, central African Republic. PLoS One 8, e71840.

Saleh, M.N., Thomas, J.E., Heptinstall, J.R., Herbein, J.F., Wolf, R.F., Reichard, M.V., Zajac, A.M., 2017. Immunologic detection of *Giardia duodenalis* in a specific pathogen-free captive olive baboon (*Papio cynocephalus anubis*) colony. J. Vet. Diagn. Invest. 29, 916–919.

Santin, M., Dargatz, D., Fayer, R., 2012. Prevalence of *Giardia duodenalis* assemblages in weaned cattle on cow-calf operations in the United States. Vet. Parasitol. 183 (3-4), 231–236.

Scalia, L.A., Fava, N.M., Soares, R.M., Limongi, J.E., da Cunha, M.J., Pena, I.F., Kalapothakis, E., Cury, M.C., 2016. Multilocus genotyping of *Giardia duodenalis* in Brazilian children. Trans. R. Soc. Trop. Med. Hyg. 110, 343–349.

Schug, K., Krämer, F., Schaper, R., Hirzmann, J., Failing, K., Hermosilla, C., Taubert, A., 2018. Prevalence survey on lungworm (*Angiostrongylus vasorum, Crenosoma vulpis, Eucoleus aerophilus*) infections of wild red foxes (*Vulpes vulpes*) in central Germany. Parasit. Vectors 11, 85.

Scorza, A. V., and Lappin, M. R. (2017). Prevalence of selected zoonotic and vector-borne agents in dogs and cats on the pine ridge reservation. Vet. Sci. 4(3), 43.

Serradell, M.C., Saura, A., Rupil, L.L., Gargantini, P.R., Faya, M., Furlan, P.J., Lujan, H.D., 2016. Vaccination of domestic animals with a novel oral vaccine prevents *Giardia* infections, alleviates signs of giardiasis and reduces transmission to humans. NPJ Vaccin. 1, 16018.

Shin, J.C., Reyes, A.W., Kim, S.H., Kim, S., Park, H.J., Seo, K.W., Song, K.H., 2015. Molecular Detection of *Giardia intestinalis* from stray dogs in animal shelters of Gyeongsangbuk-do (province) and Daejeon, Korea. Korean J. Parasitol. 53 (4), 477–481.

Simonato, G., Frangipane di Regalbono, A., Cassini, R., Traversa, D., Beraldo, P., Tessarin, C., Pietrobelli, M., 2015. Copromicroscopic and molecular investigations on intestinal parasites in kenneled dogs. Parasitol. Res. 114 (5), 1963–1970.

Simonato, G., Frangipane di Regalbono, A., Cassini, R., Traversa, D., Tessarin, C., Di Cesare, A., Pietrobelli, M., 2017. Molecular detection of *Giardia duodenalis* and *Cryptosporidium* spp. in canine faecal samples contaminating public areas in Northern Italy. Parasitol. Res. 116 (12), 3411–3418.

Siwila, J., 2017. Giardiasis: livestock and companion animals. In: Rodriguez-Morales, A.J. (Ed.), Current Topics in Giardiasis. IntechOpen. https://doi.org/10.5772/intechopen. 70874. Available from: https://www.intechopen.com/books/current-topics-in-giardiasis/giardiasis-livestock-and-companion-animals.

Soares, R.M., de Souza, S.L.P., Silveira, L.H., Funada, M.R., Richtzenhain, L.J., Gennari, S.M., 2011. Genotyping of potentially zoonotic *Giardia duodenalis* from exotic and wild animals kept in captivity in Brazil. Vet. Parasitol. 180, 344–348.

Solarczyk, P., 2009. Occurrence of *Giardia* species and genotypes in humans and animals in Wielkopolska region, Poland. Wiad. Parazytol. 55, 459–462.

Solarczyk, P., Majewska, A.C., Moskwa, B., Cabaj, W., Dabert, M., Nowosad, P., 2012. Multilocus genotyping of *Giardia duodenalis* isolates from red deer (*Cervus elaphus*) and roe deer (*Capreolus capreolus*) from Poland. Folia Parasitol. 59 (3), 237–240.

Solarczyk, P., Majewska, A.C., Słodkowicz-Kowalska, A., 2014. Axenic in vitro culture and molecular characterization of *Giardia duodenalis* from red deer (*Cervus elaphus*) and Thomson's gazelle (*Gazella thomsonii*). Acta Parasitol. 59 (4), 763–766.

Sommer, M.F., Rupp, P., Pietsch, M., Kaspar, A., Beelitz, P., 2018. *Giardia* in a selected population of dogs and cats in Germany—diagnostics, coinfections and assemblages. Vet. Parasitol. 249, 49–56.

Song, G.Y., Qin, S.Y., Zhao, G.H., Zhu, X.Q., Zhou, D.H., Song, M.X., 2016. Molecular characterization of *Giardia duodenalis* from white yaks in China. Acta Parasitol. 61 (2), 397–400.

Song, Y., Li, W., Liu, H., Zhong, Z., Luo, Y., Wei, Y., Fu, W., Ren, Z., Zhou, Z., Deng, L., Cheng, J., Peng, G., 2018. First report of *Giardia duodenalis* and *Enterocytozoon bieneusi* in forest musk deer (*Moschus berezovskii*) in China. Parasit. Vectors 11, 204.

Souza, S.L., Gennari, S.M., Richtzenhain, L.J., Pena, H.F., Funada, M.R., Cortez, A., Gregori, F., Soares, R.M., 2007. Molecular identification of *Giardia duodenalis* isolates from humans, dogs, cats and cattle from the state of São Paulo, Brazil, by sequence analysis of fragments of glutamate dehydrogenase (*gdh*) coding gene. Vet. Parasitol. 149 (3–4), 258–264.

Sprong, H., Caccio, S.M., van der Giessen, J.W., 2009. Identification of zoonotic genotypes of *Giardia duodenalis*. PLoS Negl. Trop. Dis. 3, e558.

Squire, S.A., Yang, R., Robertson, I., Ayi, I., Ryan, U., 2017. Molecular characterization of *Cryptosporidium* and *Giardia* in farmers and their ruminant livestock from the Coastal Savannah zone of Ghana. Infect. Genet. Evol. 55, 236–243.

Sricharern, W., Inpankaew, T., Keawmongkol, S., Supanam, J., Stich, R.W., Jittapalapong, S., 2016. Molecular detection and prevalence of *Giardia duodenalis* and *Cryptosporidium* spp. among long-tailed macaques (*Macaca fascicularis*) in Thailand. Infect. Genet. Evol. 40, 310–314.

Stojecki, K., Sroka, J., Cencek, T., Dutkiewicz, J., 2015a. Epidemiological survey in Łęczyńsko Włodawskie Lake District of eastern Poland reveals new evidence of zoonotic potential of *Giardia intestinalis*. Ann. Agric. Environ. Med. 22, 594–598.

Stojecki, K., Sroka, J., Caccio, S.M., Cencek, T., Dutkiewicz, J., Kusyk, P., 2015b. Prevalence and molecular typing of *Giardia duodenalis* in wildlife from eastern Poland. Folia Parasitol. 62, 042.

Štrkolcová, G., Mad'ar, M., Hinney, B., Goldová, M., Mojžišová, J., Halánová, M., 2015. Dog's genotype of **Giardia** duodenalis in human: first evidence in Europe. Acta Parasitol 60 (4), 796–799.

Sulaiman, I.M., Fayer, R., Bern, C., Gilman, R.H., Trout, J.M., Schantz, P.M., Das, P., Lal, A.A., Xiao, L., 2003. Triosephosphate isomerase gene characterization and potential zoonotic transmission of *Giardia duodenalis*. Emerg. Infect. Dis. 9, 1444–1452.

Sweeny, J.P.A., Ryan, U.M., Robertson, I.D., Jacobson, C., 2012. *Cryptosporidium* and *Giardia* associated with reduced lamb carcase productivity. Vet. Parasitol. 182, 127–139.

Tan, T.K., Low, V.L., Ng, W.H., Ibrahim, J., Wang, D., Tan, C.H., Chellappan, S., Lim, Y.A.L., 2019. Occurrence of zoonotic *Cryptosporidium* and *Giardia duodenalis* species/genotypes in urban rodents. Parasitol. Int. 69, 110–113.

Tangtrongsup, S., Scorza, V., 2010. Update on the diagnosis and management of *Giardia* spp infections in dogs and cats. Top. Companion Anim. Med. 25 (3), 155–162.

Tangtrongsup, S., Scorza, A. V., Reif, J S., Ballweber, L. R., Lappin, M. R., and Salman, M. D. (2017). Prevalence and multilocus genotyping analysis of *Cryptosporidium* and *Giardia* isolates from dogs in Chiang Mai, Thailand. Vet. Sci. 4(2), 26.

Thompson, R.C., Monis, P., 2012. *Giardia*—from genome to proteome. Adv. Parasitol. 78, 57–95.

Thompson, R.C., Palmer, C.S., O'Handley, R., 2008. The public health and clinical significance of *Giardia* and *Cryptosporidium* in domestic animals. Vet. J. 177, 18–25.

Thompson, R.C., Kutz, S.J., Smith, A., 2009a. Parasite zoonoses and wildlife: emerging issues. Int. J. Environ. Public Health 6, 678–693.

Thompson, R.C., Colwell, D.D., Shury, T., Appelbee, A.J., Read, C., Njiru, Z., Olson, M.E., 2009b. The molecular epidemiology of *Cryptosporidium* and *Giardia* infections in coyotes from Alberta, Canada, and observations on some cohabiting parasites. Vet. Parasitol. 159, 167–170.

Thompson, R.C., Smith, A., Lymbery, A.J., Averis, S., Morris, K.D., Wayne, A.F., 2010. *Giardia* in western Australian wildlife. Vet. Parasitol. 170, 207–211.

Traub, R.J., Monis, P.T., Robertson, I., Irwin, P., Mencke, N., Thompson, R.C., 2004. Epidemiological and molecular evidence supports the zoonotic transmission of *Giardia* among humans and dogs living in the same community. Parasitology 128 (Pt. 3), 253–262.

Trout, J.M., Santin, M., Fayer, R., 2003. Identification of assemblage A *Giardia* in white tailed deer. J. Parasitol. 89, 1254–1255.

Tsui, C. K., Miller, R., Uyaguari-Diaz, M., Tang, P., Chauve, C., Hsiao, W., Isaac-Renton, J., Prystajecky, N. (2018). Beaver fever: whole-genome characterization of waterborne outbreak and sporadic isolates to study the zoonotic transmission of giardiasis. mSphere 3(2), e00090-18.

Tzanidakis, N., Sotiraki, S., Claerebout, E., Ehsan, A., Voutzourakis, N., Kostopoulou, D., Stijn, C., Vercruysse, J., Geurden, T., 2014. Occurrence and molecular characterization of *Giardia duodenalis* and *Cryptosporidium* spp. in sheep and goats reared under dairy husbandry systems in Greece. Parasite 21, 45.

Upcroft, J.A., McDonnell, P.A., Gallagher, A.N., Chen, N., Upcroft, P., 1997. Lethal *Giardia* from a wild-caught sulphur-crested cockatoo (*Cacatua galerita*) established in vitro chronically infects mice. Parasitology 114 (Pt. 5), 407–412.

Utaaker, K.S., Myhr, N., Bajwa, R.S., Joshi, H., Kumar, A., Robertson, L.J., 2017. Goats in the city: prevalence of *Giardia duodenalis* and *Cryptosporidium* spp. in extensively reared goats in northern India. Acta Vet. Scand. 59, 86.

van der Giessen, J.W., de Vries, A., Roos, M., Wielinga, P., Kortbeek, L.M., Mank, T.G., 2006. Genotyping of *Giardia* in Dutch patients and animals: a phylogenetic analysis of human and animal isolates. Int. J. Parasitol. 36 (7), 849–858.

van Keulen, H., Feely, D.E., Macechko, P.T., Jarroll, E.L., Erlandsen, S.L., 1998. The sequence of *Giardia* small subunit rRNA shows that voles and muskrats are parasitized by a unique species *Giardia microti*. J. Parasitol. 84, 294–300.

Vermeulen, E.T., Ashworth, D.L., Eldridge, M.D., Power, M.L., 2015. Investigation into potential transmission sources of *Giardia duodenalis* in a threatened marsupial (*Petrogale penicillata*). Infect. Genet. Evol. 31, 277–280.

Veronesi, F., Piergili Fioretti, D., Morganti, G., Bietta, A., Moretta, I., Moretti, A., Traversa, D., 2012. Occurrence of *Giardia duodenalis* infection in chinchillas (*Chincilla lanigera*) from Italian breeding facilities. Res. Vet. Sci. 93, 807–810.

Volotao, A.C.C., Souza Júnior, J.C., Grassini, C., Peralta, J.M., Fernandes, O., 2008. Genotyping of *Giardia duodenalis* from southern brown howler monkeys (*Alouatta clamitans*) from Brazil. Vet. Parasitol. 158, 133–137.

Wade, S.E., Mohammed, H.O., Schaaf, S.L., 2000. Epidemiologic study of *Giardia* sp. infection in dairy cattle in southeastern New York State. Vet. Parasitol. 89 (1-2), 11–21.

Wait, L.F., Fox, S., Peck, S., Power, M.L., 2017. Molecular characterization of *Cryptosporidium* and *Giardia* from the Tasmanian devil (*Sarcophilus harrisii*). PLoS One 12, e0174994.

Wang, H., Zhao, G., Chen, G., Jian, F., Zhang, S., Feng, C., Wang, R., Zhu, J., Dong, H., Hua, J., Wang, M., Zhang, L., 2014. Multilocus genotyping of *Giardia duodenalis* in dairy cattle in Henan, China. PLoS One 9 (6), e100453.

Wang, X.T., Wang, R.J., Ren, G.J., Yu, Z.Q., Zhang, L.X., Zhang, S.Y., Lu, H., Peng, X.Q., Zhao, G.H., 2016a. Multilocus genotyping of *Giardia duodenalis* and *Enterocytozoon bieneusi* in dairy and native beef (Qinchuan) calves in Shaanxi province, northwestern China. Parasitol. Res. 115 (3), 1355–1361.

Wang, H., Qi, M., Zhang, K., Li, J., Huang, J., Ning, C., Zhang, L., 2016b. Prevalence and genotyping of *Giardia duodenalis* isolated from sheep in Henan Province, central China. Infect. Genet. Evol. 39, 330–335.

Wang, X., Cai, M., Jiang, W., Wang, Y., Jin, Y., Li, N., Guo, Y., Feng, Y., Xiao, L., 2017a. High genetic diversity of *Giardia duodenalis* assemblage E in pre-weaned dairy calves in Shanghai, China, revealed by multilocus genotyping. Parasitol. Res. 116 (8), 2101–2110.

Wang, S.S., Yuan, Y.J., Yin, Y.L., Hu, R.S., Song, J.K., Zhao, G.H., 2017b. Prevalence and multilocus genotyping of *Giardia duodenalis* in pigs of Shaanxi Province, northwestern China. Parasit. Vectors 10 (1), 490.

Wang, G., Wang, G., Li, X., Zhang, X., Karanis, G., Jian, Y., Ma, L., Karanis, P., 2018. Prevalence and molecular characterization of *Cryptosporidium* spp. and *Giardia duodenalis* in 1-2-month-old highland yaks in Qinghai Province, China. Parasitol. Res. 117 (6), 1793–1800.

Wegayehu, T., Karim, M.R., Erko, B., Zhang, L., Tilahun, G., 2016. Multilocus genotyping of *Giardia duodenalis* isolates from calves in Oromia Special Zone, Central Ethiopia. Infect. Genet. Evol. 43, 281–288.

Wegayehu, T., Karim, M.R., Li, J., Adamu, H., Erko, B., Zhang, L., Tilahun, G., 2017. Prevalence and genetic characterization of *Cryptosporidium* species and *Giardia duodenalis* in lambs in Oromia Special Zone, Central Ethiopia. BMC Vet. Res. 13 (1), 22.

Wielinga, C., Thompson, R.C.A., Monis, P., Ryan, U., 2015. Identification of polymorphic genes for use in assemblage B genotyping assays through comparative genomics of multiple assemblage B *Giardia duodenalis* isolates. Mol. Biochem. Parasitol. 201 (1), 1–4.

Wu, Y., Chang, Y., Chen, Y., Zhang, X., Li, D., Zheng, S., Wang, L., Li, J., Ning, C., Zhang, L., 2018. Occurrence and molecular characterization of *Cryptosporidium* spp., *Giardia duodenalis*, and *Enterocytozoon bieneusi* from Tibetan sheep in Gansu, China. Infect. Genet. Evol. 64, 46–51.

Xiao, L., Herd, R.P., 1994. Infection pattern of *Cryptosporidium* and *Giardia* in calves. Vet. Parasitol. 55, 257–262.

Xie, S.C., Zou, Y., Chen, D., Jiang, M.M., Yuan, X.D., Li, Z., Zou, F.C., Yang, J.F., Sheng, J.L., Zhu, X.Q., 2018. Occurrence and multilocus genotyping of *Giardia duodenalis* in Yunnan black goats in China. Biomed. Res. Int. 2018, 4601737.

Yang, R., Reid, A., Lymbery, A., Ryan, U., 2010. Identification of zoonotic Giardia genotypes in fish. Int. J. Parasitol. 40 (7), 779–785.

Yang, R., Jacobson, C., Gardner, G., Carmichael, I., Campbell, A.J.D., Ryan, U., 2014. Development of a quantitative PCR (qPCR) for *Giardia* and analysis of the prevalence: cyst shedding and genotypes of Giardia present in sheep across four states in Australia. Exp. Parasitol. 137, 46–52.

Yang, R., Ying, J.L., Monis, P., Ryan, U., 2015. Molecular characterisation of *Cryptosporidium* and *Giardia* in cats (*Felis catus*) in Western Australia. Exp. Parasitol. 155, 13–18.

Ye, J., Xiao, L., Ma, J., Guo, M., Liu, L., Feng, Y., 2012. Anthroponotic enteric parasites in monkeys in public park, China. Emerg. Infect. Dis. 18, 1640–1643.

Ye, J., Xiao, L., Li, J., Huang, W., Amer, S.E., Guo, Y., Roelling, D., Feng, Y., 2014. Occurrence of human-pathogenic *Enterocytozoon bieneusi*, *Giardia duodenalis* and *Cryptosporidium* genotypes in laboratory macaques in Guangxi, China. Parasitol. Int. 63, 132–137.

Ye, J., Xiao, L., Wang, Y., Guo, Y., Roellig, D.M., Feng, Y., 2015. Dominance of *Giardia duodenalis* assemblage A and *Enterocytozoon bieneusi* genotype BEB6 in sheep in inner Mongolia, China. Vet. Parasitol. 210 (3–4), 235–239.

Yin, Y.L., Zhang, H.J., Yuan, J., Tang, H., Chen, D., Jing, S., Wu, H.X., Wang, S.S., Zhao, G.H., 2018. Prevalence and multi-locus genotyping of *Giardia duodenalis* from goats in Shaanxi province, northwestern China. Acta Trop. 182, 202–206.

Yu, Z., Ruan, Y., Zhou, M., Chen, S., Zhang, Y., Wang, L., Zhu, G., Yu, Y., 2018. Prevalence of intestinal parasites in companion dogs with diarrhea in Beijing, China, and genetic characteristics of *Giardia* and *Cryptosporidium* species. Parasitol. Res. 117 (1), 35–43.

Zahedi, A., Paparini, A., Jian, F., Robertson, I., Ryan, U., 2016. Public health significance of zoonotic *Cryptosporidium* species in wildlife: critical insights into better drinking water management. Int. J. Parasitol. Parasites Wildl. 5 (1), 88–109.

Zahedi, A., Field, D., Ryan, U., 2017. Molecular typing of *Giardia duodenalis* in humans in Queensland—first report of assemblage E. Parasitology 144 (9), 1154–1161.

Zhang, W., Zhang, X., Wang, R., Liu, A., Shen, Y., Ling, H., Cao, J., Yang, F., Zhang, X., Zhang, L., 2012a. Genetic characterization of *Giardia duodenalis* in sheep and goats in Heilongjiang Province, China and possibility of zoonotic transmission. PLoS Negl. Trop. Dis. 6, e1826.

Zhang, W., Shen, Y., Wang, R., Liu, A., Ling, H., Li, Y., Cao, J., Zhang, X., Shu, J., Zhang, L., 2012b. *Cryptosporidium* cuniculus and *Giardia duodenalis* in rabbits: genetic diversity and possible zoonotic transmission. PLoS One 7, e31262.

Zhang, X.X., Tan, Q.D., Zhao, G.H., Ma, J.G., Zheng, W.B., Ni, X.T., Zhao, Q., Zhou, D.H., Zhu, X.Q., 2016a. Prevalence, risk factors and multilocus genotyping of *Giardia intestinalis* in Dairy Cattle, Northwest China. J. Eukaryot. Microbiol. 63 (4), 498–504.

Zhang, X.X., Zheng, W.B., Ma, J.G., Yao, Q.X., Zou, Y., Bubu, C.J., Zhao, Q., Zhu, X.Q., 2016b. Occurrence and multilocus genotyping of *Giardia intestinalis* assemblage C and D in farmed raccoon dogs, *Nyctereutes procyonoides,* in China. Parasit. Vectors 9, 471.

Zhang, Y., Zhong, Z., Deng, L., Wang, M., Li, W., Gong, C., Fu, H., Cao, S., Shi, X., Wu, K., Peng, G., 2017. Detection and multilocus genotyping of *Giardia duodenalis* in dogs in Sichuan province, China. Parasite 24, 31.

Zhao, J., Qi, M., Wang, H., Feng, C., Zhang, L., 2011. Prevalence of intestinal parasites in captive macaques (*Macaca mulatt*). J. Henan Agric. Sci. 40, 135–138.

Zhao, Z., Dong, H., Wang, R., Zhao, W., Chen, G., Li, S., Qi, M., Zhang, S., Jian, F., Zhao, J., Zhang, L., Wang, H., Liu, A., 2014. Genotyping and subtyping *Cryptosporidium parvum* and *Giardia duodenalis* carried by flies on dairy farms in Henan, China. Parasit. Vectors 7, 190.

Zhao, Z., Wang, R., Zhao, W., Qi, M., Zhao, J., Zhang, L., Li, J., Liu, A., 2015. Genotyping and subtyping of *Giardia* and *Cryptosporidium* isolates from commensal rodents in China. Parasitology 142, 800–806.

Zheng, G., Hu, W., Liu, Y., Luo, Q., Tan, L., Li, G., 2015. Occurrence and molecular identification of *Giardia duodenalis* from stray cats in Guangzhou, southern China. Korean J. Parasitol. 53 (1), 119–124.

Zhong, Z., Tian, Y., Li, W., Huang, X., Deng, L., Cao, S., Geng, Y., Fu, H., Shen, L., Liu, H., Peng, G., 2017. Multilocus genotyping of *Giardia duodenalis* in captive non-human primates in Sichuan and Guizhou provinces, Southwestern China. PLoS One 12, e0184913.

Zhong, Z., Tu, R., Ou, H., Yan, G., Dan, J., Xiao, Q., Wang, Y., Cao, S., Shen, L., Deng, J., Zuo, Z., Ma, X., Zhou, Z., Liu, H., Yu, S., Ren, Z., Hu, Y., Peng, G., 2018. Occurrence and genetic characterization of *Giardia duodenalis* and *Cryptosporidium* spp. from adult goats in Sichuan Province, China. PLoS One 13 (6), e0199325.

Further reading

Gu, Y.F., Wang, L.K., Li, Y., Li, L., Chu, X.H., Xin, D.W., Ma, C.X., Xu, W.H., Wu, S.B., Wang, H.Y., Li, W.C., 2014. Prevalence and molecular characterization of *Giardia lamblia* isolates from goats in Anhui Province. Chinese J. Parasitol. Parasit. Dis. 32, 401–403.

Qi, M., Yu, F., Li, S., Wang, H., Luo, N., Huang, J., Zhang, L., 2015b. Multilocus genotyping of potentially zoonotic *Giardia duodenalis* in pet chinchillas (*Chinchilla lanigera*) in China. Vet. Parasitol. 208, 113–117.

Ruiz, A., Foronda, P., González, J.F., Guedes, A., Abreu-Acosta, N., Molina, J.M., Valladares, B., 2008. Occurrence and genotype characterization of *Giardia duodenalis* in goat kids from the Canary Islands, Spain. Vet. Parasitol. 154, 137–141.

Solarczyk, P., Majewska, A.C., Jędrzejewski, S., Górecki, M.T., Nowicki, S., Przysiecki, P., 2016. First record of *Giardia* assemblage D infection in farmed raccoon dogs (*Nyctereutes procyonoides*). Ann. Agric. Environ. Med. 23 (4), 696–698.

Van Keulen, H., Macechko, P.T., Wade, S., Schaaf, S., Wallis, P.M., Erlandsen, S.L., 2002. Presence of human Giardia in domestic, farm and wild animals: and environmental samples suggests a zoonotic potential for giardiasis. Vet. Parasitol. 108, 97–107.

Kolibri 360 GmbH
Ferdinand-Jühlke-Straße 7
99095 Erfurt, Deutschland
produktsicherheit@kolibri360.de